**Second Edition**

# Physical Agent Modalities

Theory and Application for the
Occupational Therapist

**Second Edition**

# Physical Agent Modalities

Theory and Application for the
Occupational Therapist

Alfred G. Bracciano, EdD, OTR/L, FAOTA

*Associate Professor*
*School of Pharmacy and Health Professions*
*Creighton University*
*Department of Occupational Therapy*
*Omaha, Nebraska*

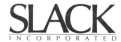

*Delivering the best in health care information*
*and education worldwide*

ISBN: 978-1-55642-649-0

Contact SLACK Incorporated for more information about other books in this field or about the availability of our books from distributors outside the United States.

Published by:    SLACK Incorporated
                 6900 Grove Road
                 Thorofare, NJ 08086 USA
                 Telephone: 856-848-1000
                 Fax: 856-853-5991
                 www.slackbooks.com

Library of Congress Cataloging-in-Publication Data

Bracciano, Alfred G., 1956-
    Physical agent modalities : theory and application for the occupational therapist / Alfred G. Bracciano. -- 2nd ed.
        p. ; cm.
    Includes bibliographical references and index.
    ISBN 978-1-55642-649-0 (soft cover : alk. paper)  1.  Medicine, Physical. 2.  Physical therapy. 3. Occupational therapists. I. Title.
    [DNLM: 1. Occupational Therapy--methods. 2. Cryotherapy. 3. Electric Stimulation Therapy. 4. Heat--therapeutic use. 5. Ultrasonic Therapy.  WB 555 B796p 2008]

RM700.B68 2008
615.8'2--dc22
                              2007048787

Printed in the United States of America.

Last digit is print number: 10 9 8 7 6 5 4

# Dedication

This book is dedicated to my father, Alfred F. Bracciano, the first "author" in our family, who led by example, and whose quiet strength, persistence, vision, support, and love has influenced and impacted my life, my career, and my writing.

# Contents

# Acknowledgments

I would like to thank Dr. Joy Voltz, OTR/L for her thorough review of this text and her assistance. My thanks to Dr. Kirk Peck for his able review and assistance with the chapter on electrotherapy, and to my colleagues at Creighton University who have set the bar for me in their research, writing, and scholarly activities. I would also like to thank the team at SLACK Incorporated, particularly Amy McShane for her persistence and support. My deepest appreciation to my patients and their families through all of these years for allowing me to learn from their conditions, be a part of their lives, and for supporting my professional growth and that of my students. I am always amazed at their generosity and patience.

I would also like to thank my wife Tamara and my children—Chris, Elizabeth, Alfred, and Matthew—for their patience and support and for putting up with my hours, days, and weeks behind the computer screen working on this project.

# About the Author

*Alfred G. Bracciano, EdD, OTR/L, FAOTA* received his undergraduate degree in occupational therapy from Wayne State University in Detroit, Michigan; his Master of Science in Hospital and Health Administration from Central Michigan University, Mt. Pleasant, Michigan; and his Doctorate in Education from Western Michigan University. Dr. Bracciano holds an academic appointment as an Associate Professor at Creighton University, Omaha, Nebraska; Clinical Associate Professor, Stony Brook University, New York; and Visiting Professor at Jinan University, in Guangzhou, China. Dr. Bracciano was the Founding Chair and Professor of the Occupational Therapy Program at Saginaw Valley State University in Michigan.

Dr. Bracciano has always had an active private practice specializing in orthopedics and upper extremity injuries in addition to his academic appointments. He was inducted into the Roster of Fellows in the AOTA for his work in education and international occupational therapy. He has published and lectured extensively on physical agent modalities and orthopedic conditions throughout the United States and in China and Asia. Dr. Bracciano serves on a number of editorial boards including *American Journal of Occupational Therapy* and the *Chinese Journal of Clinical Rehabilitative Tissue Engineering Research*. Dr. Bracciano also serves on a variety of medical advisory boards. Dr Bracciano has served as a content expert for the Department of Defense, and developed a series of training modules on physical agents for the US Army, Navy and Air Force occupational therapists. He coauthored the AOTA's *Position Statement on Physical Agent Modalities* and has consulted for a number of state licensing and regulatory boards relative to physical agent licensing laws.

# Contributing Author

*Kirk Peck PT, PhD, CSCS* holds a Baccalaureate degree in Exercise Science, a Masters degree in Physical Therapy, and a PhD in Higher Education. He is also credentialed as a strength and conditioning specialist through the National Strength and Conditioning Association. Dr. Peck has practiced physical therapy in a variety of clinical settings with a primary focus in outpatient orthopedics and sports medicine. He has lectured extensively in the academy, and has presented several post-graduate continuing education courses on the use of electrical stimulation for practitioners in the professions of physical and occupational therapy. Dr. Peck is currently an Assistant Professor in the Department of Physical Therapy at Creighton University.

# Preface to the Second Edition

Often, the profession of occupational therapy appears to be at a crossroads with the numerous challenges facing it and dire predictions of what the future may hold. There have been multiple threats and opportunities to the profession over the course of its existence ranging from changes in reimbursement, managed care, accreditation issues, personnel shortages, practice arenas, infringement by other disciplines into our traditional practice areas, debate over "traditional" versus nontraditional practice, community-based practice, value of the medical model, the apparent dichotomy between education and practice, as well as the dramatic societal and cultural changes that have occurred over the past century and into the new millenium. Initially, physical agents were viewed with skepticism and apprehension by many in the profession. As with any culture shift, the acceptance of physical agent modality (PAM) use as an adjunct to clinical practice occurred from the grass roots. The clinicians were responsible for branching out into hospitals, programs, regulatory boards, and eventually into academia and education. Clinicians have always been at the forefront of the profession by expanding the base of knowledge and practice, and pushing the envelope for better, more effective interventions and strategies. It is these people, through their perseverance and diligence, who have brought about a change in the profession leading to acceptance of physical agents as another "tool" that can be used by clinicians to facilitate occupational performance and outcomes.

There have been many changes since the publication of the first edition, with increasing numbers of state regulatory bodies requiring occupational therapists to obtain additional training and/or credentialing in physical agent modalities. Manufacturers have responded to the exigencies and casualties of war through advances in technology and research. The American Occupational Therapy Association's (AOTA) Accreditation Council for Occupational Therapy Education (ACOTE) has finally, though watered down somewhat, revised the educational standards to include PAMs, and the National Board for the Certification of Occupational Therapists (NBCOT) has included PAMs in their "snapshot" of clinical practice. However, there is still a long way to go. The incorporation of physical agents as part of clinical practice is often viewed as a technical skill and many therapists use physical agents without using the clinical reasoning skills necessary to effect positive change in their patients. Issues regarding competency in the use of physical agents has always been one of the leading arguments limiting greater use and acceptance of physical agents.

Therapists must possess the foundational knowledge of the scientific basis and physiological effects of physical agents in order to apply them correctly. Concurrent with this is the ability to be able to differentially diagnose the condition and underlying components of the injury or illness to determine which physical agent would be most appropriate to use and to determine what physiological response we are attempting to impact. The use of physical agents is an inexact science with often apparently conflicting research. It is the responsibility of the therapist to determine the appropriate selection, parameters, and application of the physical agent based on their knowledge of the disease process and influence of the physical agent on the tissue. There are often no right or wrong answers, and clinicians often want a "cookbook" with which they can select various interventions or treatment parameters. There is no true "cookbook" approach to the use and application of physical agents, as there is diversity in the patients and conditions with which we will use them. There are general parameters and guidelines, and this text will provide the reader with a framework with which to begin to safely and effectively use physical agents with their patients. This book will provide the framework which will require a paradigm shift for many occupational therapists—one from a perspective of accommodation and adaptation to a perspective of healing and repair. This will require high levels of clinical skills in diagnosis, evaluation, and treatment. Selecting and applying the correct physical agent to the appropriate tissue, at the appropriate time, and using the appropriate parameters is vital to ensure improvement in our patients and outcomes. Occupational therapists cannot continue to apply physical agents in a technical, linear fashion without understanding the principles underlying the science, and art, of physical agents and the conditions therapists treat.

Feedback from readers of the first edition commented how user-friendly it was and how easy it was to understand often complex concepts. I have continued to keep the text functional and understandable. I have always worn two "hats"—one as an academician and researcher, but another as a clinician. Though I teach, I continue to treat patients clinically, and I have used all of these interventions with my patients. Like you, I need to use the equipment, to adjust the parameters, and to see what the outcomes are going to be. Use of physical agents as a part of treatment is often an inexact science that requires creativity and flexibility to shift your clinical reasoning and applications based on the tissue's response or the patient's response.

This text will also address the new ACOTE standards for education and training for occupational therapists and occupational therapy assistants. This text provides the latest research on each physical agent, and the physiological basis for use; the clinical applications, precautions, and contraindications; and specific application techniques and parameters. Each modality also has a case study and questions that are posed to facilitate the reader's clinical reasoning process. My sincerest appreciation, also, to my patients who allowed me to use their conditions as a teaching tool.

I have included a new chapter providing a framework and theoretical basis for the use of physical agent modalities within occupational therapy. I will never forget colleagues arguing that physical agent modalities are "not occupational" in nature and should not be considered a "part" of occupational therapy; and the addendum to "write" a theoretical perspective before they would consider using or teaching physical agents. Chapter 1 is my response to that request. I am certain that I will continue to revise and modify it as the science and technology progresses. However, it does provide a starting point.

I have also added a chapter on laser therapy and expanded all of the existing chapters in response to advances in technology, research, and clinical practice. Each chapter discusses the various concepts, principles, and theories that under-gird physical agent modalities and are supported by research, clinical evidence, and experience. The text will be useful for clinicians who are looking for specific parameters for physical agents, as well as for the student who is developing his or her clinical reasoning skills. Competency in the use of physical agents requires thorough and accurate diagnosis and frequent thoughtful and clinically sound application with a variety of patients. It is through the skillful and reflective use of these agents that occupational therapists will expand their scope of practice and facilitate occupational outcomes and performance.

# Chapter 1

# PHYSICAL AGENT MODALITIES
## A THEORETICAL FRAMEWORK

## Learning Objectives

1. Discuss the philosophical trends related to physical agent modalities (PAMs) within occupational therapy.
2. Discuss the relationship between PAMs and the American Occupational Therapy Association (AOTA) *Occupational Therapy Practice Framework.*
3. Articulate a theoretical and philosophical connection between client factors and physical agent modalities.
4. Outline the historical trends in PAM use and occupational therapy.
5. Define biophysiological client factors and their impact on occupational performance.

## Terminology

| | |
|---|---|
| Biophysiological factors | Performance skills |
| Client factors | Reductionism |
| Pathogenesis | |

## Background

The profession of occupational therapy continues to evolve and mature due to a variety of internal and external forces that affect clinical practice, theory development, and education. The United States health care system continues to be faced with multiple challenges related to an aging population, an influx of aging "baby boomers" reaching retirement age, escalating health care costs, economic competition from overseas outsourcing, advances in technology and medicine, growing emphasis on evidence-based practice, quality of life issues, cost containment by the health care industry, and growing federal and state budget deficits (Unruh & Fottler, 2005; *Shortage of specialists worsens, ACEP says*, 2006). These dynamic changes to the health care system are directly impacting clinical practice for occupational therapists and all health professions. All health professionals, including occupational therapists, are seeing shifts in professional responsibilities and practice patterns with greater emphasis on physician extenders. Where it was once thought that there would be an oversupply of health professionals, such as physicians, nurses, and allied health professionals, there is now fear of a growing shortage. There are also concerns that the global economy is contributing to a world health care shortage as well as inequities in the distribution of health care workers (Sheldon, 2006). Other health professions continue to aggressively expand their reach and scope of practice through revised lexicon and training, an entrepreneurial focus to practice, or directly through challenges and modification to regulatory language and reimbursement. Occupational therapy has also seen changes in educational standards, a renewed emphasis on "occupation," debate between community-based practice versus reliance on traditional hospital-based health care venues, and attempts at increased collaborative and collegial relationships between agencies such as NBCOT and AOTA, which represent and influence practice.

# Definitions

An often-debated topic in occupational therapy, physical medicine, and rehabilitation in general has been the efficacy and use of PAMs in the treatment process and the occupational therapist's role in their use. There have been proponents as well as critics for the use of physical agents within the practice of occupational therapy, though the dialogue between the competing positions has been less vociferous in recent years. Within clinicians and students, an apparent critical mass has been reached leading to a general consensus that occupational therapists can use physical agents, though there appears to be some apprehension from academic circles and theorists that worry that physical agents aren't "occupational" in nature. The primary issue, from a regulatory or licensing standpoint is determining the appropriate training and credentialing necessary to demonstrate competency in physical agent application during occupational therapy treatments. This issue has been approached from a variety of diverse viewpoints and regulations, though there are some consistent patterns. The generalized acceptance of physical agents as an area of practice within occupational therapy has not always been the case.

Before a further discussion related to PAMs can occur, it is important to define what PAMs are and what they encompass. *PAMs* are those procedures and interventions that are systematically applied to modify specific client factors that may be limiting occupational performance; which use various forms of energy in order to modulate pain, modify tissue healing, increase tissue extensibility, modify skin and scar tissue, decrease edema, inflammation, or decreased occupational performance secondary to musculoskeletal or skin conditions; and which are used as an adjunctive method preparatory to engagement in occupation. There are specific categories of physical agents, including superficial thermal and electrotherapeutic agents as an example. As there is often controversy and confusion as to what constitutes an electrotherapeutic modality, it is important that we define this category of physical agent as well. *Electrotherapeutic agents* are those procedures or interventions that are systematically applied to modify specific client factors which may be limiting occupational performance; that use electricity and the electromagnetic spectrum to facilitate tissue healing, improve muscle strength and endurance, decrease edema, modulate pain, decrease the inflammatory process and modify the healing process; and that are used as an adjunctive method prior to engagement in occupation.

There is a wide discrepancy among educational programs and occupational therapists in training and education in PAMs. Physical agents are frequently used in the treatment of musculoskeletal injuries, or by "hand" therapists, but are often overlooked by many clinicians. This is limiting to both the profession and the patient.

The basic, underlying physiological principles related to normal healing and the influence of physical agents on that process, are consistent whether the tissue is located in the hand, shoulder, knee, or back. To isolate physical agent use to only "the hand" is a flawed paradigm. An appreciation of the impact physical agents can have on physiological and systemic processes will facilitate clinical reasoning and generalization of the interventions to other conditions and injuries. Occupational therapists possess the unique perspective of occupation and performance to the use and application of these agents as part of the treatment process. With dramatic advances in technology, equipment, and research related to physical agents, it is both limiting to the profession and a disservice to the patient to neglect their use as a part of treatment or overlook their potential impact to facilitate healing and performance.

## History of Physical Agent Modalities in Occupational Therapy

The AOTA developed a Physical Agent Modality Task Force in 1990 to explore the issues related to physical agents and the philosophical positions of the involved constituents. One aspect of the Task Force was to undertake an AOTA member data survey to determine specific use of physical agents. Results showed that therapists in private practice used modalities with greater frequency than those therapists in nonmental health practice. Hot packs (44%), cold packs (42%), and paraffin (39%) were the modalities most frequently used by nonmental health practitioners, followed by contrast baths (34%), electrical stimulation (28%), and fluidotherapy (22%). Therapists in private practice cited the use of electrical stimulation (45%), contrast baths (42%), ultrasound (32%), and whirlpool (32%) as more frequently used modalities (AOTA, 1991b). The AOTA official policy statement at the time concluded that PAMs could be used as an adjunct to purposeful activity to enhance occupational performance, but that the practice was not considered "entry-level" (AOTA, 1991a).

Many leaders of the profession, however, were opposed to the use of physical agents, believing them inconsistent with the profession's theory and philosophy of occupation. Taylor and Humphry found that 80% of the 650 respondents in physical disability practice believed that the use of physical agents reflected a natural evolution of the profession toward new technologies, and a full 58% thought that the use of physical agents was consistent with the philosophical base of occupational therapy (Taylor & Humphry, 1991). Interestingly, the respondents who identified themselves as educators were less ardent than clinicians that physical agents should be taught as part of academic curricula. Other educators surveyed also disagreed with the inclusion of physical agents in clinical practice (Vogel, 1991). Cornish-Painter, Peterson, and Lindstrom-Hazel (1997) surveyed occupational therapists from the physical disabilities special interest section regarding their use of, education in, competency testing for, and opinion on eight physical agents. They found that the most common method of education in use of physical agents was through on-the-job training, and the least common was higher-level accredited education.

At that time, AOTA's *A Guide for the Preparation of Occupational Therapy Practitioners for the Use of Physical Agent Modalities* described the basis for information and knowledge necessary to use physical agents, the skill and experience required, and the preparation spanning the therapists' career (AOTA, 1994). AOTA's recommendation for appropriate mechanisms to obtain the requisite knowledge was through formal academic course work or continuing education. Cornish-Painter and colleagues survey found that the AOTA's recommendations were inconsistent with the most commonly reported methods used: informal on-the-job training, self-taught, or observations of physical therapists (Cornish-Painter et al., 1997). A study by Glauner, Ekes, James, & Holm (1997) on the theoretical and technical competence and education of physical agents in occupational therapy practice found that the level and type of education needed to obtain competence in physical agent use varied widely and was dependent on the type of agent. Glauner et al. also recommended that occupational therapy educational programs be provided with a mechanism to ensure that content in physical agents would be developed. Funk also reported that respondents in their study believed that entry-level occupational therapy programs should educate students in the use of PAMs (Funk, 1994). This apparent inconsistency between the desire of clinicians to obtain basic information regarding physical agents at an academic level and the reality of on-the-job training, contributed to many states adopting regulatory language to outline the necessary training and skills needed by occupational therapists to use physical agents. There continued to be an apparent divide, however, between education and clinical practice and the arguments for and against use of physical agents continues at a somewhat less vociferous level.

# Philosophical Perspectives

PAMs are defined as the interventions or technologies that produce a response in soft tissue through the use of light, water, temperature, sound, or electricity. PAMs include, but are not limited to, paraffin baths, cold packs, hot packs, fluidotherapy, contrast baths, ultrasound, whirlpool, electrical stimulation, neuromuscular stimulation (NMES), and transcutaneous electrical nerve stimulation (TENS) (McPhee, Bracciano, Rose, Brayman, & Commission on Practice, 2003). The AOTA has long advocated the use of physical agents as an adjunctive method used in preparation for or in conjunction with patient involvement in purposeful activity or occupation. These "adjunctive methods" support occupational performance components that allow the patient to participate in activities of daily living (ADLs) and facilitate occupational performance. The AOTA states that these methods may be used as a precursor to activity or occupational engagement. Administering PAMs as a treatment method without application to functional outcome or occupational performance is not considered occupational therapy, or sound practice.

Arguments against the use of physical agents in occupational therapy revolve around the contention that physical agents are not consistent with the basic philosophy of occupation, the hallmark being the use of purposeful activity (or occupation) to influence health and healing. One school of thought contends that the use of PAMs is inconsistent with the basic philosophy of occupational therapy: that of purposeful activity, or occupation, to influence health and healing (McGuire, 1991; Ahlscwede, 1992; West & Weimer, 1991; West, 1984). The use of occupation and purposeful activity is paramount to the profession and, as such, should not be abandoned. To this faction, physical agents alone do not address the basic human needs of independence in daily activities. Incorporating physical agents into our repertoire of treatment will open the profession to criticism, public confusion, political issues, and confrontation with physical therapy. This viewpoint, however, fails to address the issue that was articulated by Meyer who proposed in 1922 that occupation facilitates an individual's search for actuality, reality, a balance of time, and, ultimately, health and well being (Meyer,

1922). Physical agents can facilitate occupation by increasing the ability to function during activity through their influence on occupational performance components—on those individual, unique client factors (e.g., through pain reduction or tissue repair).

Others have contended that occupational therapists have an ethical responsibility to use new technologies and interventions with patients. These proponents have argued that the concept of occupational therapy to "diminish or correct pathology" places the onus of responsibility on the occupational therapist to utilize all mechanisms of intervention to facilitate occupational performance (Ahlscwede, 1992). Failure to do so, in effect, would violate the *Code of Ethics*. The revised AOTA PAM position statement clarifies and explicitly states that occupational therapists have an ethical responsibility to apply physical agents in a safe and competent manner and therapists should keep current with emerging knowledge relevant to their practice (McPhee et al., 2003). The issue and use of physical agents within the scope of practice for occupational therapy is, in fact, being driven in part by changes in health care and societal trends. With the growth of managed care and its impetus to contain costs and limit health care expenditures, third party intermediaries and the federal government are less concerned with who provides what type of service, as long as it is safely, effectively, and appropriately provided. Additionally, the service must be consistent with appropriate standards of practice and service delivery, as well as being efficacious. The federal government, managed care organizations, and third party intermediaries are demanding that therapeutic interventions facilitate and be related to functional outcomes in our patients. Additionally, occupational therapists can be reimbursed by health care insurance intermediaries including Medicare and Medicaid for use of physical agents and are not deemed exclusive to any single discipline.

The challenge in today's dynamic health care environment is to treat patients and clients with the most effective, yet low-cost, technologies and interventions available, with the ultimate goal being improved occupational performance. By improving occupational performance, occupational therapists facilitate the patient's ability to interact with his or her environment, perform occupations and roles of choice, and improve and enhance the individual's quality of life. Though other health professions that use physical agents espouse "function" and pay cursory attention to functional outcomes, the occupational therapist's unique perspective encompasses occupational performance issues at the level of the person-environment interaction, which is invaluable in selecting and utilizing physical agents in the treatment process.

# Dynamics Between Education and Practice

The profession of occupational therapy has a long and colorful history grounded in occupation, but receptive to inquiry and inclusion of new concepts and approaches. Just as the founding fathers of occupational therapy implemented a unique approach to treatment based on "doing," clinicians have always pushed the envelope of practice, expanding into underserved and emerging areas and incorporating new technology, interventions, and techniques. Occupational therapy has always been a dynamic, nonlinear profession, recreating and adjusting itself to meet societal changes and patient needs. This independence and activism has often contributed to the underlying tension between academics and clinicians over the issue of "who" or "what" drives practice—education and academia or clinical practice and clinicians. There often appears to be a dichotomy over what is being "taught" in academic programs and what is being practiced in the clinic. Students often complain that what they have been taught—

frames of reference, theoretical issues, a lexicon of occupation, and an approach to practice—are not being observed or used in the clinic. Clinicians and students often comment about the discrepancy between what they "learn" academically and the exigencies and realities of clinical practice. Students and clinicians often lament about bridging academia and practice.

Because of the dynamism and variability within the profession, occupational therapy often appears to be at a crossroads with a dynamic tension guiding and influencing the direction, scope, vision of the profession, and, ultimately, practice. Clinicians are often at the forefront of learning, refining, and implementing new techniques and technologies which expand the scope and effectiveness of practice. This underlying tension—the apparent discrepancy or dichotomy between education/academics, and clinicians—also presents the profession with the opportunity to grow and expand the scope of practice and base of knowledge.

Occupational therapy has evolved through both internal and external influences impacting the profession. Change within the profession frequently occurs gradually, due in part to the diversity of competing theories, frames of reference, and language that we use as occupational therapists. In addition, accreditation, educational requirements, local and state licensing, and regulatory issues also influence practice and education. There are a variety of issues and motivations that propel the field of occupational therapy to reflect and evolve in response to dialogue and assimilation of theoretical and practical knowledge. These issues may initially be divisive, but as discussion and integration occur, unifying themes and realities emerge.

PAMs have been an initially divisive issue, and some would contend that it still remains a discordant issue. As occupational therapists began specializing in hand and upper extremity injuries, physicians and other health care professionals recognized the important contributions occupational therapists could make with these clinical conditions. Therapists began to advocate for acknowledgement by AOTA of the "right" to use physical agents and expand their practice and repertoire of interventions. As challenges to the use of physical agents as part of occupational therapy practice became increasingly vocalized by other health professionals, regulatory bodies, and within the field of occupational therapy itself, the AOTA reviewed the issue and drafted the initial statement on PAM use. In the initial 1991 position statement, PAM use was not considered "entry level," but postprofessional, requiring education and training beyond the initial entry-level degree (AOTA, 1991a).

As occupational therapy education evolved and adapted to postbaccalaureate levels, so did the AOTA's position on physical agents. The revised AOTA position statement contends that, "occupational therapists and occupational therapy assistants must have demonstrated verifiable competence in order to use PAMs in occupational therapy practice" (AOTA, 2003). Additionally, preparation for using physical agents include the "foundational knowledge necessary for proper use of these modalities requires appropriate documented professional education, such as continuing education, in-service training, or accredited higher education programs" (AOTA, 2003). Conspicuously missing in the revised statement was the caveat that physical agents are "not" considered entry-level practice. In part, the recognition that physical agents be considered another "tool" in the vast toolbox of occupational therapy interventions was motivated by the greater acceptance in the use of physical agents. An additional factor leading to this recognition was in part due to increasing state regulatory oversight on physical agent use by occupational therapists that has occurred. Changes in education and training of occupational therapists, with the move to postbaccalaureate education at the masters or entry-level doctorate and with increased emphasis on evidence-based practice, fostered the recognition that these physical agents could be taught at the academic level and could be integrated into clinical practice and theory.

In the new revisions to occupational therapy education, the Accreditation Council for Occupational Therapy Education (ACOTE) included PAMs as a component of occupational therapy academic programs. The ACOTE standards (AOTA, 2006) for the occupational therapist include PAMs under:

➤ **B.5.13.** Explain the use of superficial thermal and mechanical modalities as a pre-paratory measure to improve occupational performance, including foundational knowledge, underlying principles, indications, contraindications, and precautions. Demonstrate safe and effective application of superficial thermal and mechanical modalities.

➤ **B.5.14.** Explain the use of deep thermal and electrotherapeutic modalities as a preparatory measure to improve occupational performance, including indications, contraindications, and precautions.

The ACOTE standards for the occupational therapy assistant (OTA) in PAMs include:

➤ **B.5.13.** Recognize the use of superficial thermal and mechanical modalities as a preparatory measure to improve occupational performance. Based on the intervention plan, demonstrate safe and effective administration of superficial thermal and mechanical modalities to achieve established goals while adhering to contra-indications and precautions.

Though this is a start, the new ACOTE standards do not include the need for occupational therapy graduates to "demonstrate safe and effective application" of electro-therapeutic or deep thermal modalities—areas that are seeing rapid increases in the research and application of these agents to facilitate healing and performance. This lack of consistency regarding educational standards in PAMs will continue to cause variability among graduates in meeting specific state regulatory and licensing requirements and further impede those graduates wishing to use physical agents as a component of clinical practice.

## Theoretical Issues Related to Physical Agent Modalities

Occupational therapy has never been a "static" field with a clearly-defined, singular, or uniform base of knowledge, theory, language, and approach. The profession is dynamic and evolving, while steeped in the uniqueness of occupation. Occupational therapists have readily incorporated and expanded their repertoire of techniques and ideas by gleaning and modifying theory, concepts, and approaches from other health and human service professions, disciplines, and theoreticians. This theoretical interdependence has been one of the more controversial aspects when discussing the profession's base of knowledge, particularly as it relates to the lexicon or language of occupational therapy. The argument that there is no "unique" body of knowledge or base, aside from "occupation," that is clearly identified with occupational therapy has often been an apparent point of contention and argument within and outside the profession.

Detractors often argue that occupational therapists use "bits and pieces" of other disciplines theories and approaches and that as occupational therapists, we should focus and emphasize occupation. This would seem to exclude occupational therapists from using interventions or approaches which may have been aligned with other professions, such as physical agents. In academia, there is frequently-encountered resistance or hesitancy to using or teaching PAMs as they may be aligned closely with other health professions besides occupational therapy. The argument often made is that physical agents are not intrinsic or unique to our profession and base of knowledge and are not "occupational" in nature in-and-of themselves; therefore, they should not be taught or used.

Other health professions, however, appear to be less confined by historical and emotional dogma and readily adapt to changes in service provision or external opportunities in an attempt to expand their practice domain. Many health professions expand and adapt in language, theory base, and clinical interventions based on perceived changes in social and environmental factors. When the American Physical Therapy Association (APTA) released their *Guide to Physical Therapy Practice* (APTA, 2001), there were concerns voiced by occupational therapists and other professions over the apparent encroachment into areas historically considered unique to a specific discipline such as occupational therapy. The APTA, however, continued to refine their position and expansion into areas of evaluation, education, and treatment that had been traditionally considered "occupational" in nature and in service delivery. These contentious areas are now considered by physical therapy educators to be "entry-level," and are required curricular content. Challenges to occupational therapy's standing as the profession of "occupational" or "functional" tasks and abilities, continue as various state associations attempt to reopen and modify regulatory language that defines physical therapy and other health professionals' practices. In part, this is driven by third party intermediaries who are stressing more "functional" based goals and outcomes that require a more universal language or lexicon. Occupation is defined as "the uniquely human task behavior that is characterized by the qualities of personal meaning and purpose used in the context of occupational therapy. Occupation is the means through which a patient/client (consumer) achieves therapeutic goals for maximum independence and life satisfaction. Successful engagement in occupation is the desired end product for intervention" (ACOTE, 2001). Though we have progressed and adapted to serve a variety of different patients, populations, and communities, it has long been argued that occupational therapy's knowledge must be further developed and its societal value better communicated (West, 1984).

Though occupational therapists and others profess to be unique in their respective therapeutic approach and body of expertise and knowledge, much of allied health's foundation, knowledge, and practice are based on theory and applications derived from the social sciences, medicine, psychology, and the arts. Allied health professions readily adopt and adapt information, theory, technology, and interventions that facilitate and strengthen their outcomes and efficacy. The profession of occupational therapy espouses that practice is based on a framework of occupation and daily life activities (AOTA, 2002), which is what makes the profession "unique" in the health and social sciences. Conversely, other professions have surreptitiously integrated core concepts of *occupation* or *function* into their knowledge base and approach. Though terminology has been modified or revised, there is little doubt that most health professionals espouse the primary importance and significance of improving function or functional abilities as the underpinning of their clinical outcomes. This revisionist thinking is based on a variety of factors, one of which is the motivating influence of reimbursement and the interplay with quality of life issues. This renewed focus on a function/dysfunction continuum of health and wellness, rather than on reductionism and pathology, has motivated many individuals to refocus on occupational therapy's historical roots. This often creates an underlying tension and dissonance related to incorporation of nontraditional technology and interventions into this historical framework. Because other disciplines and health professions are so quick to adapt new languages and lexicons, it is somewhat ironic that as occupational therapists, we continue to disagree on whether physical agents are "occupational in nature," when in fact, they are merely another tool that can be used to impact specific client factors and represent advancements in technology and treatment.

This conceptual retrenchment can strengthen the profession and clarify the inherent uniqueness of the profession, but can also leave occupational therapy vulnerable to encroachment by other disciplines more astute at utilizing a socially understandable lexicon and one more adept at maneuvering through the regulatory and reimbursement systems. This in part is why evidenced-based practice has been strengthened and articulated as a vital component to demonstrate occupational therapy's efficacy and its therapeutic approaches. Occupational therapy must continue to be open to new ideas and concepts, to recognize trends and needs, and to integrate change into the practice and profession. This process of professional growth and maturation is dynamic and transformational, and is vital to ensure the continued growth and success of occupational therapy.

## Holism or Reductionism: A Clinical Balancing Act

Occupational therapists should always use physical agents as an adjunctive method to the overall plan of treatment. Physical agents are not a means to an end in and of themselves. The goal of treatment may vary, but the impetus and outcome should always be successful and rewarding engagement in occupations. Occupational therapists are trained and adept at modifying an individual's performance based on our knowledge of disease, disability, and evidence-based practice. Engagement in meaningful, contextual activity is universal. The World Health Organization (WHO) recognized the significance of the effect of disease and disability on health and the ability or inability to carry out activities or participate in life situations (WHO, 2001). Occupational therapists "fit" into this perspective through a focus on engaging the individual in "occupations," in home, school, workplace, and community. Occupational therapists are skillful at seeing the "big picture" with patients, but may, because of training, fail to look at or consider the smaller, underlying subcomponents that make up part of the problem.

Occupational therapists are adept at assessing the performance skills and patterns; the contextual issues; and the physical, cognitive, and psychosocial factors that influence performance and occupation. We appreciate the use of occupation as a means to an end. We have developed and continue to develop a language, framework, and mechanism for approaching a "clinical problem" and identifying and implementing occupation-based interventions to ameliorate or address the deficit or impact on the individual. The question and argument that has often been made by proponents of physical agent use is a rhetorical question: "tell me how physical agents fit into the framework and language of occupational therapy."

The *Occupational Therapy Practice Framework* (AOTA, 2002) was developed to provide a common language describing the profession's focus on occupation, daily activity and the intervention process to strengthen and facilitate occupational function and engagement. The *Framework* describes the domain that grounds the profession's focus and outlines the process of evaluation and intervention, emphasizing the significance and use of occupation. The *Framework* also articulates to internal and external readers the factors that influence performance and the profession's focus on facilitating function and performance in daily life activities. The *Framework* gives us a mechanism with which to describe issues related to an individual's performance, but does not directly specify therapeutic interventions such as physical agents. The *Framework*, while providing a common language and perspective to the profession, does not directly address the underlying, fundamental, and cellular components of performance.

# Performance Skills and Activity Demands

According to Mosey (1992), the "domain...consists of those areas of human experience in which practitioners of the profession offer assistance to others" (p. 852). As occupational therapists, our focus is facilitating engagement in daily life activities that have meaning and purpose to the individual. As articulated in the *Framework* (AOTA, 2002), the term used to describe "everyday life activity" is occupation, which encompasses "[A]ctivities...of everyday life, named, organized, and given value and meaning by individuals and a culture" (Law, Polatajko, Baptistse, & Townsend, 1997, p. 32). Activity is considered a goal-directed action undertaken by an individual, but may not hold primary significance or importance to the individual.

To undertake these activities and engage in meaningful occupations that have specific and unique activity demands, an individual must possess a level of performance skills (motor, process, and communication/interaction), which allows successful completion of the activity or occupation. A "skill" is an incremental unit or component of performance such as moving, looking, or selecting which is part of an activity. These components, when organized and carried out in a sequential fashion, allow for successful completion of an activity. The most obvious performance skill is the motor component, and allows the individual to maneuver and manipulate through their environment. Motor skills consist of posture, mobility, coordination, strength, effort, and energy that will vary across the lifespan.

## Activity Demands

The unique components and characteristics of the activity that is being engaged will determine the "demand" of the activity and will have an impact on the "skill" and/or potential success or completion of the performance. In the past, occupational therapists and occupational therapy education emphasized and utilized the process of "task analysis" to determine the basic components and demands of an activity. The activity demands are closely linked to the specific client factors, those components which "reside" within or are the unique biophysiological factors of the individual. These "client factors" affect the individual's ability to engage in occupations.

In the AOTA *Framework*, client factors are described as the components that include body functions and body structures, initially articulated in the *International Classification of Functioning, Disability and Health* by the WHO (2001). Body functions consist of the "physiological function of body systems (including psychological functions), while body structures consist of the "anatomical parts of the body such as organs, limbs, and their components [that support body function]" (2001, p. 10).

Under the general heading of Client Factors, the subcategory of body function includes the components of mental or thought functions, both global and specific, such as attention, memory, perception, thought, and consciousness, as well as the sensory functions such as taste, smell, touch, pain, and vision. Neuromusculoskeletal and movement-related functions refer to those components and factors that allow an individual to physically move and engage in or manipulate their environment. These factors or components include mobility, reflexes, and voluntary and involuntary movements and are concerned with the stability or instability of many of these components. Cardiovascular, hematological, immunological, and respiratory system functions are given rudimentary acknowledgement within the *Framework* with the caveat that therapists have "knowledge" of these functions and "understand broadly the interaction that occurs between these functions and engagement in occupation to support participation" (AOTA, 2002, p. 625). Because of their impact on the biophysiological functions of tissue, physical agents influence the cardiovascular, hematological, and immunological systems. Within the conceptual organization of the *Framework*, physical agents impact client factors and physiological systems and can be used preparatory to treating a variety of neuromusculoskeletal, movement related, and sensory functions.

## Biophysiological Client Factors

When using physical agents, we are impacting the individual's performance at the cellular or tissue level. We are influencing the biophysiological client factors of the cardiovascular, hematological, and immunological systems. Through appropriate selection and application of physical agents, we can modify cellular and histochemical activity within the body. When using PAMs as part of clinical treatment, we need to look at the disease and disability in a more focused and reductionistic manner and appreciate the pathogenesis of the conditions. Reductionism can be characterized as attempting to explain complex facts or phenomena by reducing them into a smaller, simpler set. This reductionistic concept and process has been used by occupational therapists in the form of activity analysis. This is a characteristic of the activity analysis where we break down an activity into subcomponents to better understand the basic make up and components of an activity or occupation. As occupational therapists, we need to understand the pathogenesis of the conditions that we are treating, including both cellular and clinical presentations. We need to review and appreciate the impact of disease or disability on the basic biophysiological components of the neurological, cardiovascular, pulmonary and integumentary, and musculoskeletal systems.

The WHO defines body functions as "the physiological functions of body systems (including psychological functions)" (2001, p. 10). The *Framework* (AOTA, 2002) defines client factors as those factors residing "within" the client, and those which may affect performance in areas of occupation. As part of our assessment, we need to determine not only what is being impacted from a larger, functional, or occupational standpoint, but decide what client factors and performance skill are being affected and why? We need to be able to critically evaluate, clinically reason, and as part of our clinical reasoning, differentially diagnose and identify the biophysiological components—those unique client factors that are affecting the individual's performance within the greater context.

Occupational therapists have become astute at modifying an individual's worksite, or providing adaptive equipment or modifications and training necessary to treat, for example, an individual with repetitive motion disorders such as epicondylitis or carpal tunnel. However, if we can appreciate exactly "what" is occurring at a tissue or cellular level and how we can manipulate the tissue and influence the healing process, we can intervene more effectively at a different level and improve our outcomes. Through our selection and application of appropriate physical agents as part of the treatment process, we can, in effect, prevent further tissue damage, costly modifications, and potentially expensive or unnecessary surgery. Using our example of a referral for epicondylitis: if all we do as occupational therapists is determine what performance skills, patterns, and activities have been affected, we have failed to fully explore all therapeutic options for the individual. We have not treated and corrected the underlying causal pathology.

As occupational therapists, we need to move beyond a mere "knowledge" of these specific client functions (or body systems) to impact occupational performance. We need to advance beyond a "broad" understanding of the interaction that these systems have on occupational performance to determine what is occurring at the underlying, specific biophysiological client factors. We need to be able to modify these biophysiological client factors—those body functions and structures that have been impacted by disease, disuse, or illness—before we can expect change as a result of engaging in an occupation or activity. We can use physical agents to prepare the tissue and area rather than just facilitating adaptation to the condition before an individual engages in meaningful occupations and activity and facilitates the healing process.

Occupational therapists have an ethical responsibility to provide a thorough, accurate and complete assessment of an individual's complete function and abilities to determine appropriate therapeutic interventions. As occupational therapists, we need to understand the biophysiological client factors, including not only the sensory, neuromusculoskeletal, and movement-related functions, but those cardiovascular, hematological, immunological, and respiratory system functions (i.e., the biophysiological client factors) that make up the essential components and foundations that allow for full participation in occupation and activity.

By using physical agents in a judicious and efficacious manner, we can positively impact the structure or functions that have been impacted by disease or disability. Through appropriate selection and intervention of PAMs as an adjunctive method to our treatment, we can facilitate engagement and active participation in life situations and occupational tasks and activities. PAMs are never an end; they are an additional tool in the occupational therapist's greater toolbox that can facilitate occupational performance and engagement in meaningful and satisfying ways.

# References

Ahlscwede, K. (1992). The issue is—views on physical agent modalities and specialization within occupational therapy: A rebuttal. *American Journal of Occupational Therapy, 46*, 650-652.

American Occupational Therapy Association. (1991a). Official: AOTA statement on physical agent modalities. *American Journal of Occupational Therapy, 45*, 1075.

American Occupational Therapy Association. (1991b). *Physical agent modality task force report.* Bethesda, MD: Author.

American Occupational Therapy Association. (1994). *A guide for the preparation of occupational therapy practitioners for the use of physical agent modalities.* Bethesda, MD: Author.

American Occupational Therapy Association. (2002). Occupational therapy practice framework: Domain and process. *American Journal of Occupational Therapy, 56*, 609-639.

American Occupational Therapy Association. (2003).

American Occupational Therapy Association. (2006). *Accreditation council for occupational therapy education (ACOTE®) standards and interpretive guidelines.* Bethesda, MD: Author.

American Physical Therapy Association. (2001). Guide to physical therapist practice, Second edition. *Physical Therapy, 81*, 9-746.

Cornish-Painter, C., Peterson, C. Q., & Lindstrom-Hazel, D. K. (1997). Skill acquisition and competency testing for physical agent modality use. *American Journal of Occupational Therapy, 51*, 681-685.

Funk,  D. R. (1994). Occupational therapists' attitudes toward and use of physical agent modalities. *Journal of Occupational Therapy Students*, *8*, 35-47.

Glauner, J. H., Ekes, A. M., James, A. E., & Holm, M. B. (1997). A pilot study of the theoretical and technical competence and appropriate education for the use of nine physical agent modalities in occupational therapy practice. *American Journal of Occupational Therapy, 51*, 767-774.

McGuire, M. J. (1991). AOTA releases draft position paper: Physical agent modalities. *OT Week, 6*, 7.

McPhee, S. D., Bracciano, A. G., Rose, B. W., Brayman, S. J., & Commission on Practice. (2003). Physical agent modalities: A position paper (2003). *American Journal of Occupational Therapy, 57*, 650-651.

Meyer A. (1922). The philosophy of occupation therapy. *Archives of Occupational Therapy, 1*, 1-10.

Mosey, A. C. (1992). Partition of occupational science and occupational therapy. *American Journal of Occupational Therapy, 46,* 851-853.

Sheldon, G. F. (2006). Globalization and the health workforce shortage. *Surgery, 140*, 354-358.

Shortage of specialists worsens, ACEP says (2006). *ED Management: The Monthly Update on Emergency Department Management, 18*, 91-93.

Taylor, E., & Humphry, R. (1991). Survey of physical agent modality use. *American Journal of Occupational Therapy, 45*, 924-931.

Unruh, L. Y., & Fottler, M. D. (2005). Projections and trends in RN supply: What do they tell us about the nursing shortage? *Policy, Politics & Nursing Practice, 6*, 171-182.

Vogel, K. (1991). Perceptions of practitioners, educators, and students concerning the role of the occupational therapy practitioner. *American Journal of Occupational Therapy, 45*, 130-136.

West, W., & Weimer, R. (1991). The issue is—should the representative assembly have voted as it did, when it did, on occupational therapists' use of physical agent modalities? *American Journal of Occupational Therapy, 45*, 1143-1147.

West, W. L. (1984). A reaffirmed philosphy and practice of occupational therapy for the 1980's. *American Journal of Occupational Therapy, 38*, 15-23.

World Health Organization. (2001).

# REGULATORY GUIDELINES FOR THE USE OF PHYSICAL AGENTS

## Learning Objectives

1. Discuss the professional issues related to physical agent modality (PAM) use in occupational therapy.
2. Identify the challenges and changes in the health care system impacting the profession and practice.
3. Discuss the ethical responsibilities in using physical agents.
4. Discuss the AOTA position on physical agent use and educational preparation.
5. Identify state regulatory agencies which govern the use of physical agents by occupational therapists.

## Terminology

| | | |
|---|---|---|
| Competency | License | Regulatory standards |
| Ethics | PAMs | |

## Background

Occupational therapy is a diverse and unique profession whose members practice in a variety of clinical and nonclinical settings. Occupational therapists practice in "traditional" settings such as outpatient and inpatient hospital settings, community mental health, and school districts, as well as in emerging areas of practice such as assisted living, industrial rehabilitation, community-based care, and private practice arenas. Because of the diversity of practice areas and interventions that we use as occupational therapists, regulatory language and requirements vary from state to state and it is imperative that therapists know and understand the specific requirements of their respective states. In addition to conventional licensing and regulation of occupational therapists, many states have implemented new regulations and guidelines related to PAMs that define specific training, requirements, or credentialing. These guidelines may require an additional license or certification to be able to use PAMs in clinical practice. Therapists have an ethical and legal responsibility to be aware of any additional licensing or training requirements before beginning to incorporate and implement physical agents into their toolbox of interventions. Failure to comply with the additional physical agent requirements can make the practitioner susceptible to legal and disciplinary action.

# Regulatory Oversight

Regulatory oversight of occupational therapists can take many forms and occurs at the local, state, or national level. Depending on the area of practice, departmental and institutional rules and regulations may exist that occupational therapists must follow. Broader requirements of regulatory bodies such as accrediting agencies, state and national licensing boards, and organizations, such as NBCOT, also apply. Internal, departmental, and institutional regulation depends upon the clinical site and the area of practice. For example, an occupational therapist practicing in an outpatient hospital setting may need to abide by not only the department and hospital rules and regulations, but may also have to comply with the specifics of external regulatory bodies such as the Joint Commission on Accreditation of Healthcare Organizations (JCAHO) or other regulatory bodies such as Medicare, third-party intermediaries, and state health care agencies. In addition, the therapist will also have to comply with the respective state licensing or regulatory board requirements. Occupational therapists must have an understanding of the laws that govern the practice of occupational therapy in their respective practice setting and state, and stay abreast of any changes to the statutes or regulations that may define or limit their practice. "Ignorance of the law" is not considered an "excuse" for any legal action that may occur should the therapist perform an activity outside of the legal definition of their respective state guidelines or laws.

Occupational therapists have a legal and ethical responsibility to understand and abide by all laws, rules, and the AOTA *Code of Ethics* (AOTA, 2005). Principle 5 of the AOTA Code of Ethics states that occupational therapists must "comply with laws and Association policies guiding the profession of occupational therapy." Occupational therapists have a legal, moral, and ethical responsibility to abide by all rules and regulations governing occupational therapy practice and to know and understand those specific to the scope or area of practice and the state and institution.

In the United States, each state has the responsibility to regulate health care professionals' practice. This regulatory oversight may take many forms including licensing, registration, or certification. Within each state, health professional practice acts are statutory laws that establish licensing or regulatory agencies or boards. These boards then develop rules that regulate both medical practice and health care professionals. The intent of most licensing regulation is to protect uninformed consumers from ill-prepared or unqualified health professionals, thereby improving the quality and safety of the services being provided (Willmarth & Smith, 2003). Regulatory guidelines also restrict entry into a profession by setting the minimum level of education, experience, or training required to practice. Many states have also adopted special regulatory guidelines to regulate advanced practice skills, such as PAMs, that are considered beyond the realm of entry-level practice. Depending on the form of regulation adopted by a state, regulatory oversight may also define or specify the legally permissible boundaries of practice for the health care profession. Regulatory language can also help to define the legally-allowed scope of practice and, thereby, specify the allowed business practices of health care professionals.

There are essentially five types of regulatory oversight for occupational therapy. These include *licensure/practice acts, mandatory certification, mandatory registration, voluntary certification or registration*, and *title control (or trademark acts)* with decreasing levels of rigor, respectively. The primary intention of regulation or oversight of occupational therapy is to ensure protection of the public by unscrupulous or incompetent therapists.

Licensure or practice acts provide the highest level of public protection and are often the most proscriptive. Licensure prohibits unlicensed individuals from practicing occupational therapy or referring to themselves as occupational therapists or assistants. Licensure laws identify a specific scope of practice for those who are issued a license and mandate what level of entry level competence is required. State health departments often oversee these forms of regulation and delegate authority to an occupational therapy board or advisory board to promulgate rules and guidelines and the regulatory functions. To assist state regulatory agencies with oversight responsibilities, the AOTA has drafted a definition of occupational therapy practice, the AOTA Model Practice Act (2006a), which serves as a starting point and guide for delineating occupational therapy practice for promulgating state specific regulatory laws, definitions, and guidelines for the profession. The Practice Act defines occupational therapy and outlines the practice of occupational therapy including methods or strategies to direct the intervention process, the evaluation of factors affecting activities of daily living including the performance skills and client factors, and also defines the interventions and procedures used as part of occupational therapy treatment.

Physical agents are identified within the context of item C:13: "Interventions and procedures to promote or enhance safety and performance in activities of daily living (ADLs), instrumental activities of daily living (IADLs), education, work, play, leisure, and social participation. Item number 13 specifically identifies application of PAMs, and use of a range of specific therapeutic procedures (such as wound care management; techniques to enhance sensory, perceptual, and cognitive processing; manual therapy techniques) to enhance performance skills" (AOTA, 2006a, p. 4). This section provides the starting point and validation that occupational therapists base their use of physical agents upon. This language also serves as the basis for the development of more restrictive laws and regulations related to PAM use within a state.

# Professional Trends

PAMs have gained greater support and use as clinical practice and specialty areas have expanded. There appears to be a "critical mass" that has been reached regarding use of physical agents by occupational therapists, but until recently, had not been clearly addressed by either occupational therapy education in the form of ACOTE or by the National Board for Certification in Occupational Therapy (NBCOT), the agency responsible for occupational therapy credentialing. To the apparent consternation of some academic programs, occupational therapy students have reported seeing physical agents used within clinical practice during their fieldwork rotations or have been asked to apply them. In response to greater use and acceptance of physical agents, increasing numbers of state regulatory agencies have drafted licensing guidelines to ensure competency and safe use of these interventions. In a significant change, ACOTE and NBCOT have also identified PAM use as an area deserving further review and recognition as a part of clinical practice and education. Both of these agencies have reviewed the scope of occupational therapy practice and education and have responded to the greater use of physical agents by occupational therapists by surveying practice and delineating academic needs.

The NBCOT serves the public interest by developing, administering, and reviewing a certification process that reflects current standards of competent practice in occupational therapy. The NBCOT also works with state regulatory authorities, providing information on credentials, disciplinary actions, and regulatory and certification renewal issues. As part of its responsibility to ensure psychometrically sound and defensible certification examinations, NBCOT regularly examines the practice of occupational therapy in 6-year cycles. This review of current entry-level practice identifies the domains, tasks, knowledge areas, and interventions that occupational therapists are using in everyday practice. The survey of occupational therapy practice assists the NBCOT in preparing and ensuring the content and basis of the tasks and knowledge of the certification examination (Bent, Crist, Florey, & Strickland, 2005).

# National Board for Certification in Occupational Therapy Practice Analysis

In the most recent practice analysis study (2002 to 2003) of occupational therapists that have been practicing for 3 years or less, what many therapists believed was long overdue, the NBCOT questioned therapists and assistants on their use of physical agents as therapeutic interventions. The NBCOT reported that 75% or more registered occupational therapist respondents did not use the nine interventions listed on the survey to a great extent. These physical agents listed included electrical stimulation, fluidotherapy, hydroptherapy, iontophoresis, and ultrasound. It should be noted, though, that the same group of therapists also reported not using other nontraditional interventions such as work hardening/work conditioning, or work transition (Bent et al., 2005). Conversely, their findings would also mean that in its most recent practice analysis of "new" therapists, approximately 25% of those surveyed were using some form of physical agents as part of their clinical practice. This is an interesting result of the practice survey as those surveyed were considered by the NBCOT as being "recent" graduates. This becomes somewhat problematic, since at the time of the survey, the AOTA considered physical agent use a postprofessional skill and intervention requiring postprofessional education and training.

What this may indicate is that recent graduates, contrary to the 1997 AOTA *PAM Position Paper* (AOTA, 1997), were using physical agents at an earlier stage in their careers than expected, with greater frequency and potentially less academic preparation or training. Physical agent use occurs with greater frequency by those occupational therapists practicing in acute care, outpatient, settings where many of the cases may be orthopedic in nature (Glauner, Ekes, James, & Holm, 1997). Further research and clarification is needed to more adequately determine PAM use by experienced clinicians in order to clarify frequency of use and clinical setting. A review of academic preparation of therapists in physical agents and the format of training and preparation "new" graduates are receiving prior to use would also benefit the profession and assist in clarifying educational and licensing requirements. With the changes occurring in clinical practice related to PAMs and the recognition by ACOTE that physical agents are a component of occupational therapy practice and education, inclusion of questions related to the topic will likely be a part of the certification examination in the near future.

# Academic Requirements

The apparent dichotomy and tension between practice and academics has frequently been a point of concern when students begin preparation for the registration examination upon graduation from an accredited program in occupational therapy. Students are aware that the NBCOT examination is based, in part, on a survey of clinical practice, while their academic training may have been more theoretically and institutionally developed. Philosophical differences and approaches in educational programs exist as academic content is based, in part, on the unique philosophy and background of the academic staff and institution within the overarching structure provided by the ACOTE standards.

Academic education is based on the ACOTE's *Standards for an Accredited Educational Program for the Occupational Therapist/Occupational Therapy Assistant* (AOTA, 2006b), which has been in a process of review and revision. These standards establish the critical competencies necessary to prepare individuals to become entry-level occupational therapists or occupational therapy assistants. The *Standards* are formatively and summatively reviewed to ensure that they remain current and effective. Academic programs have some leeway in designing their curriculum and coursework which is unique to their program and institutional mission, philosophy, service area, and background and interests of their faculty. In ACOTE's newest revision of the *Standards*, the area of PAMs was added (AOTA, 2006b). ACOTE identified the need for graduates of occupational therapy programs to be able to understand the principles and applications of physical agents. The standard [OT B5.13] states: "Explain the use of superficial thermal and mechanical modalities as a preparatory measure to improve occupational performance, including foundational knowledge, underlying principles, indications, contraindications, and precautions. Demonstrate safe and effective application of superficial thermal and mechanical modalities." B5.14 states: "Explain the use of deep thermal and electrotherapeutic modalities as a preparatory measure to improve occupational performance, including indications, contraindications, and precautions."

For the occupational therapy assistant, standard B5.13 states: "Recognize the use of superficial thermal and mechanical modalities as a preparatory measure to improve occupational performance. Based on the intervention plan, demonstrate safe and effective administration of superficial thermal and mechanical modalities to achieve established goals while adhering to contraindications and precautions" (AOTA, 2006b).

This addition will support the use of physical agents by occupational therapists as allowed by regulatory bodies and will facilitate the use of therapeutic techniques as an additional mechanism to enhance performance skills. Both the NBCOT and ACOTE are proactively responding to concerns from regulatory agencies, institutional administrations, clinicians, and educators to identify and articulate consistent educational and practice requirements related to the safe use of physical agents. In addition, there has been a greater emphasis by both organizations to effectively collaborate and use consistent language across the scope of occupational therapy practice and within occupational therapy's documents. This heightened sense of collaboration between ACOTE and NBCOT will assist in alleviating the perceived discrepancies between entry-level practice and education. This renewed focus and interest will further strengthen the profession while ameliorating some of the concerns regulatory boards often cite with regard to inconsistencies related to PAM training. The ACOTE acknowledgment that PAMs can be a part of the intervention plan for occupational therapists will also facilitate the movement for greater academic preparation in physical agents by educational programs, though it still falls short of specifying application and training of all physi-cal agents. By incorporating academic standards on physical agents, there will be less incongruence with regulatory bodies overseeing PAM use by occupational therapists and will lead to greater expansion of physical agent use as a viable treatment option.

## Competency Issues

Aside from the philosophical issues inherent in PAM use within the profession, the other primary argument against the widespread acceptance of physical agents relates to the issue of competency. In addition to inconsistencies with academic and professional preparation, competency is an issue that has led to a plethora of states adding regulatory oversight and specialized credentialing and education in PAMs. This regulatory drive is often led by occupational therapists and other health profes-sionals with the intent of ensuring or clarifying appropriate training and education of physical agents by occupational therapists who choose to use physical agents in treatment. Occupational therapists' strong background in performance and psycho-social issues, activity analysis, and appreciation of occupation provide the therapist with a unique and valuable perspective on the use and application of physical agents. Research into many of the applications common for physical agents has demonstrated a relationship between outcomes and functional activity and improvement. Combining physical agents with occupation can improve the efficacy of many of the interventions and promote better outcomes (Aoyagi & Tsubahara, 2004; Bhakta, 2000; Blyth, March, Nicholas, & Cousins, 2005; Chae, 2003; Chae, Fang, Walker, & Pourmehdi, 2001). Many individuals continue to hold the position that occupational therapists are not trained in physical agents and that they are not occupational in nature.

Many of the arguments against the use of physical agents by occupational therapists revolve around the misperception that these interventions are used singularly and without regard to active engagement of the patient in the treatment process. These individuals argue that physical agents are passive in nature and decry the fact that the patient is sitting there passively during treatment. These same critics, however, often use tools and techniques that appear passive in nature, yet allow the client to develop the ability to perform occupational tasks, or prevent dysfunction, such as splinting and adaptive equipment. Conversely, adherents of physical agent use by occupational therapists, argue that the patients are engaged in active range of motion (ROM) exer-cises during scar management, ultrasound, or whirlpool treatments, and if not, the interlude can be spent discussing occupational performance issues, collaborative goal setting, or patient education (Ahlscwede, 1992). Rarely is the occupational therapist at a loss during this narrative phase of clinical reasoning or therapist-patient interaction. The occupational therapist's ability to merge function and physical agents as part of the therapeutic intervention to ameliorate or compensate for deficits in occupational performance components is unique and valuable.

Competency of occupational therapists is an issue that has been controversial within the profession and has often led to disagreements and ill-will between profes-sional organizations representing occupational therapists and practice. Occupational therapists have an ethical responsibility to provide occupational therapy services that are "appropriate and beneficial" and "do no harm" (AOTA, 2005). In addition, Principle 6A of the *OT Code of Ethics* (Veracity) outlines the concept that "Occupational therapy personnel shall represent their credentials, qualifications, education, experience, training, and competence accurately" (AOTA, 2005). Inconsistent preparation and training in the area of PAMs of occupational therapists has influenced the proliferation of regulatory oversight in PAM use.

Inconsistent definitions of competency as it relates to physical agents have also prevented occupational therapists from incorporating these agents and technologies into clinical practice. Proscriptive licensing laws and regulations have often limited the ability of occupational therapists to use physical agents, and may vary by state. Differences in licensing requirements and regulatory guidelines may also impact an occupational therapists ability to relocate without carefully reviewing the licensing requirements of the specific state. Therapists enter clinical practice with a variety of backgrounds and clinical and academic training in physical agents. There is no stated education standard that defines or requires PAMs be taught within the academic setting. This inconsistency and variability in training and preparation was apparent to the Department of Defense, United States Army Medical Department (AMMEDD) which approached the author to develop a mechanism for standardizing the training and education of the occupational therapists in the "tri-services": Army, Navy, and Air Force. AMMEDD had noted a wide variation in academic and clinical training of therapists and set out to standardize the competency and educational requirements within their system to ensure appropriate, safe, and efficacious application of physical agents by occupational therapists.

The inconsistency and variability in the training and preparation of occupational therapists in PAMs (i.e., the competency issue) also impacts licensing and regulatory issues between states. There is no set standard or general consensus on reciprocity between states with competing regulatory guidelines related to physical agents at this time. Occupational therapists and assistants are cautioned to always review specific state requirements for physical agents prior to using them in clinical practice or before relocating. Additionally, some states will require a specific number of continuing education units or some other mechanism to maintain licensure and prove continuing competency. The NBCOT maintains a Professional Development Provider Registry to assist therapists certified as Occupational Therapist Registered (OTR), or Certified Occupational Therapy Assistant (COTA) in meeting their required 36 professional development units to maintain their registration.

## American Occupational Therapy Association
### *Position Paper*

Until recently, the AOTA had identified standards requiring occupational therapy practitioners to receive specialized training for the proper use of physical agents. The AOTA contended that selection, application, and adjustment of physical agents was not considered entry-level practice, and required continued training as the therapist's professional career evolved. Skill and training in physical agents could be achieved through fieldwork experience, on-the-job training, or postprofessional education, such as continuing education, in-service training, or graduate education (AOTA, 1997). The AOTA also holds that practitioners have an ethical responsibility to possess basic information and the knowledge base, skills, or experience to safely and competently use physical agents.

Until the new *Standards* were approved in 2006, the AOTA contended that the theoretical background needed to use physical agents should include course work in anatomy and physiology; principles of chemistry and physics related to the properties of light, water, temperature, sound, and electricity; the physiological, neurophysiological, and electrophysiological changes that occur with the use of physical agents; and the response of normal and abnormal tissue to the agents. Course content should include information on pain control theories, wound healing principles, biophysical principles of thermal agents, and neurophysiologic mechanisms related to electrical stimulation (AOTA, 1994). In 2003, The AOTA's Representative Assembly in Washington D.C. adopted the revised Commission on Practice document, *PAMs: A Position Paper* (AOTA, 2003). This document clarified the appropriate context for use of PAMs in occupational therapy. This important document clarified and outlined the AOTA's position on PAMs. The *Position Paper* has been used by state regulatory boards as a resource in determining appropriate requirements for the use of PAMs in states (Glauner et al., 1997).

Unfortunately, the vast majority of occupational therapists who use physical agents learn on the job with little training occurring during higher education. In addition, a lack of competency testing exists, as well as any particular guidelines with regard to testing or frequency of continuing education. There is little controversy among therapists about the necessity for training or education to acquire theoretical and technical competence with physical agents. Continuing education courses are currently considered the best method for gaining the skills necessary for use of deep thermal agents and those agents using the electromagnetic spectrum, such as neuromuscular electrical stimulation (AOTA, 1997). Though there has been recognition that PAMs may be addressed to varying degrees by academic programs, many therapists believe that physical agents should be considered part of entry-level occupational therapy programs and taught in the academic environment (Ahlscwede, 1992; Taylor & Humphry, 1991). Though controversial, it would appear that the profession and educators are moving from their comfort area to ensure that future therapists have the knowledge base and expertise to employ physical agents as part of occupational therapy treatments. The challenge to the practitioner is not the acquisition of the technical skill in using physical agents, but in obtaining and developing the knowledge and clinical reasoning required to use physical agents as an adjunctive method with or in preparation for patient involvement in purposeful activity or occupation.

## Specific State Regulatory Guidelines

Due to all of the changes inherent within the profession and the increasing demands for competency and evidence-based practice, licensing and regulatory oversight of occupational therapists using PAMs as a part of clinical practice is growing rapidly. Many states have adopted specific licensing laws and regulations outlining the specific requirements for competency, continuing education, and preparation for physical agent use. It is important to remember, that in those states regulated by such laws, it is illegal to apply PAMs without the requisite license for the respective state. Many of the states with existing laws or language related to physical agents have strengthened or expanded their licensing regulations. Most recently, California, New Hampshire, Nebraska, Montana, South Dakota, and Kentucky have added regulatory guidelines or language specific to PAMs to their licensing laws (Willmarth, 2005).

Many of the new state regulations specify a certain number of hours of continuing education or training that is required, as well as requiring a specified number of clinical applications in order to meet the licensing requirements for PAMs. States such as Florida, Georgia, Minnesota, and others specify training and competency standards for the use of physical agents by occupational therapists. In what may be a growing trend, the Nebraska Licensing Board also identified competency testing through both formative and summative evaluation as part of their requirements of their licensing guidelines. This added requirement was due in response to the concerns regarding competency and preparation of occupational therapists. Local, state, or institutional regulations and guidelines supersede the AOTA position statement on physical agents and therapists should be aware of the regulations specific to their state and clinical practice. A primary difficulty with many of the regulatory laws is that they vary in scope and clinical application and may lack reciprocity. South Dakota, for example, requires that "supervised mentorship to include five case studies on each class of modality to be incorporated into patient care" (SB 179, 2005).

By contrast, California,  in a highly controversial addition to their licensing law, mandated that occupational therapists that are going to use physical agents complete a minimum of 240 hours of additional training. Competency and educational requirements are additional factors that state regulatory boards have struggled to clarify and strengthen. Many of the laws specify that providers of education or training in PAMs must be approved by the licensing board or by national bodies such as the AOTA. The board may specify specific content or other requirements that must be met by the agency or individual providing the continuing education.

# Summary of States Requiring Competency in Physical Agents

## Alabama

> Defines occupational therapy intervention to include "modalities."

> No competency requirements.

> No restrictions on modalities.

Specific occupational therapy treatment techniques include activities of daily living (ADLs); the design, fabrication, and application of selected splints or orthotics, or both; sensorimotor activities and exercise; the use of specifically designed goal-oriented arts and crafts; design, fabrication, selection, and use of adaptive equipment; therapeutic activities, modalities, and exercises to enhance functional performance; and work readiness evaluation and training (The Code of Alabama 1975, Section 34-39-3).

## Delaware

Defines application of "thermal agent modalities." These services may require assessment of the need for use of interventions such as the design, development, adaptation, application or training in the use of assistive technology devices; the design, fabrication, or application of rehabilitative technology such as selected orthotic devices; training in the use of assistive technology, orthotic, or prosthetic devices; the application of thermal agent modalities, including, but not limited to, paraffin, hot and cold packs, and fluidotherapy, as an adjunct to or in preparation for purposeful activity; the use of ergonomic principles; the adaptation of environments and processes to enhance functional performance; or the promotion of health and wellness (TITLE 24 Professions and Occupations, Chapter 20. Occupational Therapy, Subchapter I. Board of Occupational Therapy Practice). Delaware's law does not define electrotherapeutic interventions.

## Florida

➤ Requires a minimal competency level and training for the use of "electrical stimulation devices" and "ultrasound."

These services may require assessment of the need for use of interventions such as the design, development, adaptation, application, or training in the use of assistive technology devices; the design, fabrication, or application of rehabilitative technology such as selected orthotic devices; training in the use of assistive technology; orthotic or prosthetic devices; the application of PAMs as an adjunct to or in preparation for purposeful activity; the use of ergonomic principles; the adaptation of environments and processes to enhance functional performance; or the promotion of health and wellness (2005 Florida Statutes, Title XXXII, Part 3, Chapter 468).

## California

### 4152. PAMs

(m) "PAMs" means techniques that produce a response in soft tissue through the use of light, water, temperature, sound, or electricity. These techniques are used as adjunctive methods in conjunction with, or in immediate preparation for, occupational therapy services.

(d) An occupational therapist may provide advanced practices if the therapist has the knowledge, skill, and ability to do so and has demonstrated to the satisfaction of the board that he or she has met educational training and competency requirements. These advanced practices include the following:

1. Hand therapy.
2. The use of PAMs.
3. Swallowing assessment, evaluation, or intervention.

(f) An occupational therapist using PAMs shall demonstrate to the satisfaction of the board that he or she has completed postprofessional education and training in all of the following areas:

1. Anatomy and physiology of muscle, sensory, vascular, and connective tissue in response to the application of physical agent modalities.
2. Principles of chemistry and physics related to the selected modality.
3. Physiological, neurophysiological, and electrophysiological changes that occur as a result of the application of a modality.
4. Guidelines for the preparation of the patient, including education about the process and possible outcomes of treatment.
5. Safety rules and precautions related to the selected modality.
6. Methods for documenting immediate and long-term effects of treatment.
7. Characteristics of the equipment, including safe operation, adjustment, indications of malfunction, and care.

(g) An occupational therapist in the process of achieving the education, training, and competency requirements established by the board for providing hand therapy or using PAMs may practice these techniques under the supervision of an occupational therapist who has already met the requirements established by the board, a physical therapist, or a physician and surgeon.

(a) PAMs may be used only when an occupational therapist has demonstrated to the board that he or she has met the postprofessional education and training requirements established by this section as follows:

    1. Education: Completion of 30 contact hours in the subjects listed in Code section 2570.3(f).

    2. Training: Completion of 240 hours of supervised on-the-job training, clinical internship or affiliation, which may be paid or voluntary, pertaining to PAMs.

(b) An occupational therapist may use only those PAMs he or she is competent to use.

Note: Authority Cited: Sections 2570.3 and 2570.20, Business and Professions Code. Reference: Sections 2570.2 and 2570.3, Business and Professions Code.

## Minnesota

Minnesota revised their licensing law for PAMs. It specifies education, training and clinical requirements for "superficial physical agents," "electrotherapy," and "ultrasound." An occupational therapy assistant may also use PAMs if they meet specific requirements and demonstrates "service competency" and works under the direct supervision of an occupational therapist. The Minnesota regulations specify:

### 148.6440 PAMs.

#### Subdivision 1. General Considerations.

(a) Occupational therapists who use superficial PAMs must comply with the requirements in subdivision 3. Occupational therapists who use electrotherapy must comply with the requirements in subdivision 4. Occupational therapists who use ultrasound devices must comply with the requirements in subdivision 5. Occupational therapy assistants who use PAMs must comply with subdivision 6.

(b) Use of superficial PAMs, electrical stimulation devices, and ultrasound devices must be on the order of a physician.

(c) The commissioner shall maintain a roster of persons licensed under sections 148.6401 to 148.6450 who use PAMs. Prior to using a PAM, licensees must inform the commissioner of the PAM they will use. Persons who use PAMs must indicate on their initial and renewal applications the PAMs that they use.

## Oregon

The Occupational Therapy Licensing Board has the responsibility to generally supervise the practice of occupational therapy in this state under ORS 675.320 (10). The Occupational Therapy Licensing Board, therefore, has established a position statement to further interpret the Practice Act as follows:

> *"PAMs may be used by occupational therapy practitioners when used as an adjunct to/or in preparation for purposeful activity to enhance the occupational therapy performance and when applied by a practitioner who has documented evidence of possessing the theoretical background and technical skills for safe and competent integration of the modality into an occupational therapy intervention plan."*

Failing to obtain a physician's referral in situations where an OT is using a modality not specifically defined in ORS 675.210(3) Specifies education, training and documentation for using "sound or electrical PAMs," must be "board approved," and requires:

## 24.165.513 Approval to Use Sound and Electrical Physical Agent Modalities

(a)  20 hours of instruction or training in sound PAM devices;

(b)  20 hours of instruction or training in electrical PAM devices; and

(c)  either: (i) certification by the hand certification commission, inc.; or (ii) the successful completion of 10 proctored treatments consisting of:

(A)  Five proctored treatments under the direct supervision of a licensed medical practitioner in sound PAM devices; and

(B)  Five proctored treatments under the direct supervision of a licensed medical practitioner in electrical PAM devices. (History: 37-24-201, 37-24-202, MCA; IMP, 37-24-106, MCA; NEW, 2005 MAR p. 447,Eff. 4/1/05.)

An occupational therapist must also have additional training and education in the use of topical medications and iontophoresis. The guidelines specify:

## 24.165.514 Qualifications to Apply Topical Medications—Clinician Defined

(1)  Prior to the administration or use of topical medications, an occupational therapist desiring to administer or use topical medications on a patient shall, in addition to the instruction or training provided for in 37-24-106, MCA and ARM 4.165.513, successfully complete five hours of instruction or training approved by the board in:

(a)  principles of topical drug interaction;

(b)  adverse reactions and factors modifying response;

(c)  actions of topical drugs by therapeutic classes; and

(d)  techniques by which topical drugs are administered.

(2)  In addition to the 5 hours of instruction required by (1), a licensee shall, pursuant to 37-24-107, MCA, prior to administering topical edication, perform one proctored treatment in direct application of topical medications under the direct supervision of a licensed medical practitioner, as described in ARM 24.156.510 (2), and either:

(a)  two proctored treatments in phonophoresis under the direct supervision of a licensed medical practitioner; or

(b)  three proctored treatments of iontophoresis under the direct supervision of a licensed medical practitioner.

(3)  For the purposes of the rules related to application of topical medications by occupational therapists, the term "clinician" means an occupational therapy licensee who has been approved by the board to administer topical medications. (History: 37-24-201, 37-24-202, MCA; IMP, 37-24-106, 37-24-107,MCA; NEW, 2005 MAR p. 447, Eff. 4/1/05.) Rule 24.165.515 reserved 24.165.516 US.

## Ohio

The Ohio Licensing Board has determined that occupational therapists may use ultrasound and electrical stimulation in their treatments.

A.  Pursuant to (A) (3) of 4755.01, it is the position of the Occupational Therapy Section that occupational therapy practitioners may use PAMs in the provision of occupational therapy services so long as competency is documented and the clinician is practicing within the scope of practice.

## Georgia

Defines physical agents as,

*"treatment techniques which utilize heat, light, sound, cold, electricity, or mechanical devices and also means electrical therapeutic modalities which include heat, or electrical current beneath the skin, including but not limited to therapeutic ultrasound, galvanism, microwave, diathermy, and electromuscular stimulation, and also means hydrotherapy."*

Specifies topics and subjects required for the 90 hours of instruction with no less than 36 contact hours being related to specific theories. Specifies acceptable instruction to include any activity relevant to the practice of PAMs in OT and may include in-service education, conferences, workshops, seminars, and formal education. Therapists must submit documentation of training.

### 671-6-.01 Definitions

PAMs means treatment techniques as specified in Code Section 43-28-3(9). Authority O.C.G.A. Sec. 43-28-3(9). **History.** Original Rule entitled "Definitions" adopted. F. Nov. 20,1991; eff. Dec. 10, 1991. (2)

### 671-6-.02 Requirements

Any occupational therapist and occupational therapy assistant who wishes to utilize OT techniques involving PAMs must document successful completion of a minimum of 90 contact hours of instruction or training approved by the board.

## Illinois

### Professions and Occupations (225 ILCS 75/) Illinois Occupational Therapy Practice Act (Source: P.A. 83-696.)

(e) For the occupational therapists or occupational therapy assistant possessing advanced training, skill, and competency as demonstrated through examinations that shall be determined by the department, applying PAMs as an adjunct to or in preparation for engagement in occupations.

### Title 68: Professions And Occupations, Chapter VII: Department Of Professional Regulation, Part 1315 Illinois Occupational Therapy Practice Act

#### Section 1315.162 Modalities In Occupational Therapy

Occupational therapy services include the use of PAMs for occupational therapists and occupational therapy assistants who have the training, skill, and competency to apply these modalities.

a) PAMs:

1) Refer to those modalities that produce a response in soft tissue through the use of light, water, temperature, sound, or electricity;

2) Are characterized as adjunctive methods used in conjunction with or in immediate preparation for: patient involvement in purposeful activity; the use of ergonomic principles; the adaptation of environments and processes to enhance functional performance; or the promotion of health and wellness; and

3) Include but are not limited to the following:

A) Electrical stimulation;

B) Iontophoresis;

C) Superficial heating agents;

D) Cryotherapy; and

E) Deep heating agents.

b) Following is the training required for the use of PAMs used by occupational therapists and occupational therapy assistants.

1) Modalities

A) Modalities using electricity would cover: pain control, edema reduction, and muscle reeducation. Examples include, but are not limited to: biofeedback, NMES/FES, TENS, HVGS, interferential, and iontophoresis. The training shall include:

i)   a minimum of 12 hours of didactic training in a program defined in this section that includes demonstration and return demonstration and an examination; and

ii)  5 treatments in each modality supervised by a licensed health care professional trained in the use of the modality.

B) Thermal modalities would include superficial and deep heat and cyrotherapy. Examples include, but are not limited to, hot and cold packs, ice massage, fluidotherapy, warm whirlpool, cool whirlpool, ultrasound, phonophoresis, paraffin, and contrast baths.

i)   a minimum of 3 hours of didactic training in a program defined in this section that includes demonstration and return demonstration and an examination. The training session should include the mechanics and precautions of using the modality safely as well as case studies and problem solving on when to use. The ethics, economics, liability, and insurance issues related to using modalities should also be addressed in the educational process.

ii)  5 treatments in each modality supervised by a licensed health care professional trained in the use of the modality.

2) The didactic training shall be obtained through educational programs, workshops, or seminars offered by a college or university, Illinois Occupational Therapy Association, the AOTA and its affiliates, Illinois Physical Therapy Association, the APTA or its chapters, NBCOT, or the Hand Therapy Certification Commission.

3) The training shall be documented and made available to the Department or board upon request. Training shall be completed prior to the use of these modalities.

# Kansas

## 65-5402. Definitions

As used in K.S.A. 65-5401 to 65-5417, inclusive, and K.S.A. 65-5418 to 65-5420, inclusive, and amendments thereto: 5) applying PAMs as an adjunct to or in preparation for engagement in occupations.

## Kentucky

### Kentucky Revised Statutes 319A.010 Definitions for Chapter.

(6) "Occupational therapy services" include, but are not limited to:

(e) Applying superficial PAMs as an adjunct to or in preparation for engagement in occupations

(f) Applying deep PAMs as an adjunct to or in preparation for engagement in occupations, in accordance with KRS 319A.080

(8) "Deep PAMs" means any device that uses sound waves or agents which supply or induce an electric current through the body, which make the body a part of the circuit, including iontophoresis units with a physician's prescription, ultrasound, transcutaneous electrical nerve stimulation units and functional electrical stimulation, or microcurrent devices; and

(9) "Superficial PAMs" means hot packs, cold packs, ice, fluidotherapy, paraffin, water, and other commercially available superficial heating and cooling devices.

**Effective**: July 15, 2002

**History**: Amended 2002 Ky. Acts ch. 14, sec. 1, effective July 15, 2002.—Amended 1994 Ky. Acts ch. 405, sec. 84, effective July 15, 1994.—Amended 1988 Ky. Acts ch. 311, sec. 1, effective July 15, 1988.—Created 1986 Ky. Acts ch. 78, sec. 1, effective July 15, 1986.

(2) The supervised treatment sessions shall include one (1) session for each of the following areas:

(a) Iontophoresis;

(b) Ultrasound; and

(c) Electrical stimulation.

(3) The remaining two (2) sessions may cover any deep physical agent identified in KRS 319A.010(8).

1. The person is an occupational therapist licensed under this chapter who has successfully completed a minimum of thirty-six (36) hours of training or instruction that meets the requirements specified in administrative regulations promulgated by the board, as well as five (5) treatments under supervision;

2. The person is an occupational therapist licensed under this chapter who has successfully completed the certified hand therapist examination approved by the Hand Therapy Certification Commission, and who has successfully completed a minimum of twelve (12) hours of training or instruction that meets the requirements specified in administrative regulations promulgated by the board, as well as five (5) treatments under supervision; or

3. The person is an occupational therapy assistant licensed under this chapter who has successfully completed a minimum of seventy-two (72) hours of training or instruction that meets the requirements specified in administrative regulations promulgated by the board, as well as five (5) treatments under supervision.

# Maryland

(3) Electrical PAMs.

    (a) "Electrical PAMs" means therapeutic modalities which induce heat or electrical current beneath the skin.

    (b) "Electrical PAMs" includes, but is not limited to:

        (i) Therapeutic ultrasound;

        (ii) Iontophoresis;

        (iii) Phonophoresis; and

        (iv) Electromuscular stimulation.

## Competence Requirements

(1) Before applying PAMs under this chapter, a licensee shall:

    (a) Complete 15 contact hours of continuing education for each specific modality; and

    (b) Apply a minimum of five patient treatments per modality under direct supervision.

## .06 Superficial PAMs

A licensee may apply superficial PAMs including, but not limited to, hot packs, cold packs, paraffin, fluidotherapy, and icing.

(2) Proof of education;

(3) Proof of 15 contact hours of continuing education for each specific modality;

(4) Certificate of completion;

(5) An official grade report, or official transcript to verify academic education;

(6) Written verification from the supervisor of five treatments performed applying each specific modality.

## Administrative History

Effective date:

Regulations .01 through .06 adopted as an emergency provision effective June 1, 2001 (28:12 Md. R. 1102); adopted permanently effective September 17, 2001 (28:18 Md. R. 1621) Board of Occupational Therapy Practice 10.46.06.06 55.

# Massachusetts

**Treatment**. A treatment program shall be consistent with the statutory scope of practice and shall:

    (a) Include the therapeutic use of goal-directed activities, exercises, and techniques and the use of group process to enhance occupational performance. Treatment also includes the use of therapeutic agents or techniques in preparation for, or as an adjunct to, purposeful activity to enhance occupational performance.

    (c) Include, where appropriate for such purposes and under appropriate conditions, therapeutic agents and techniques based on approaches taught in an occupational therapy curriculum, included in a program of professional education in occupational therapy, specific certification programs, continuing education, or in-service education. Such continuing education or in-service education must include documented educational goals and objective testing (written examination, practical examination, and/or written simulation or case study) to ascertain a level of competence. Therapeutic procedures provided must be consistent with the individual's level of competence.

## Regulatory Authority

259 CMR 3.00: M.G.L. c. 112, § 23A.

# Minnesota

Practitioners are prohibited from using PAMs independently until granted approval as provided in Minn. Stat. §148.6440, Subd. 7, of the licensing regulations. State regulations require written documentation verifying *educational* (theoretical) and *clinical application* requirements prior to use of PAMs. There are three modality areas: superficial physical agents, ultrasound and electrotherapy. The occupational therapist may apply for use of one, two, or all three areas.

## Physical Agent Modalities

The Commissioner is required by Minnesota Statutes §148.6440, Subdivision 1, (c) to maintain a roster of licensees using PAMs. Please follow *Written Documentation Required* section below when you meet the requirements and are ready to submit documents to be reviewed for approval to use any PAM (superficial, electrical stimulation, ultrasound). Prior to use of PAMs, you must submit to the Commissioner documentation verifying that you have met the educational requirements described in Minnesota Statutes §148.6440, Subds. 3 to 5 *and* have been granted approval as provided in subdivison 7. Minnesota Statutes §148.6440, Subdivision 1 (b), requires that PAMs be provided only under a physician's order. Please review the following information before completing the statement below.

*Superficial PAMs* are therapeutic media which produce a temperature change in skin and underlying subcutaneous tissues within a depth of 0-3 centimeters for the purposes of rehabilitation of neuromusculoskeletal dysfunction.

Superficial PAMs may include, but are not limited to: paraffin baths, hot packs, cold packs, fluidotherapy, contrast baths, and whirlpool baths. Superficial PAMs do not include the use of electrical stimulation devices, ultrasound, or quick icing.

*Electrotherapy* means the use of electrical stimulation devices for a therapeutic purpose.

*Ultrasound* means a device intended to generate and emit high frequency acoustic vibrational energy for the purposes of rehabilitation of neuromusculoskeletal dysfunction.

## Written Documentation Required

Prior to use of PAMs, an occupational therapist must provide to the commissioner documentation verifying that the occupational therapist has met the educational and clinical requirements described in subdivisions 3 to 5, depending on the modality or modalities used. Both theoretical training and clinical application objectives must be met for each modality used. Documentation must include the name and address of the individual or organization sponsoring the activity; the name and address of the facility at which the activity was presented; and a copy of the course, workshop, or seminar description, including learning objectives and standards for meeting the objectives.

In the case of clinical application objectives, teaching methods must be documented, including actual supervised practice. Documentation must include a transcript or certificate showing successful completion of the course work. Practitioners are prohibited from using PAMs independently until granted approval as provided in Minnesota Statutes §148.6440, Subdivision 7.

## Occupational Therapy Assistant

Occupational therapy assistants using any PAM must work under the direct supervision of an approved occupation therapist and are limited to set up and implementation of treatment. Prior to using PAMs as an occupational therapy assistant you must meet the requirements described in Minnesota Statutes §148.6440, Subd. 6.

*PLEASE NOTE: You are responsible for submitting required documentation separate from your application and gaining approval from the Commissioner prior to independent practice of each type of PAM.*

## Minnesota Statutes 2002, Chapter 148

➤ 148.6404 Scope of practice. The practice of occupational therapy by an occupational therapist or occupational therapy assistant includes, but is not limited to, intervention directed toward: (12) employing PAMs, in preparation for or as an adjunct to purposeful activity, within the same treatment session or to meet established functional occupational therapy goals, consistent with the requirements of section 148.6440; and (13) promoting health and wellness. HIST: 2000 c 361 s 42.

➤ Subd. 10. Direct supervision. "Direct supervision" of an occupational therapy assistant using PAMs means that the occupational therapist has evaluated the patient and determined a need for use of a particular PAM in the occupational therapy treatment plan, has determined the appropriate PAM application procedure, and is available for in-person intervention while treatment is provided.

➤ Subd. 11. Electrical stimulation device. "Electrical stimulation device" means any device which generates pulsed, direct, or alternating electrical current for the purposes of rehabilitation of neuromusculoskeletal dysfunction.

➤ Subd. 12. Electrotherapy. "Electrotherapy" means the use of electrical stimulation devices for a therapeutic purpose.

➤ Subd. 17. PAMs. "PAMs" mean modalities that use the properties of light, water, temperature, sound, or electricity to produce a response in soft tissue. The PAMs referred to in sections 148.6404 and 148.6440 are superficial PAMs, electrical stimulation devices, and ultrasound.

➤ Subd. 24. Superficial PAM. "Superficial PAM" means a therapeutic medium which produces temperature changes in skin and underlying subcutaneous tissues within a depth of zero to three centimeters for the purposes of rehabilitation of neuromusculoskeletal dysfunction. Superficial PAMs may include, but are not limited to: paraffin baths, hot packs, cold packs, fluidotherapy, contrast baths, and whirlpool baths. Superficial PAMs do not include the use of electrical stimulation devices, ultrasound, or quick icing.

➤ Subd. 26. Ultrasound device. "Ultrasound device" means a device intended to generate and emit high frequency acoustic vibrational energy for the purposes of rehabilitation of neuromusculoskeletal dysfunction. HIST: 2000 c 361 s 2; 2001 c 7 s 35,36=148.6440.

➤    148.6440 PAMs.

(b) Use of superficial PAMs, electrical stimulation devices, and ultrasound devices must be on the order of a physician. Before use of PAMs, an occupational therapist must provide to the commissioner documentation verifying that the occupational therapist has met the educational and clinical requirements described in subdivisions 3 to 5, depending on the modality or modalities used. Both theoretical training and clinical application objectives must be met for each modality used. Documentation must include the name and address of the individual or organization sponsoring the activity; the name and address of the facility at which the activity was presented; and a copy of the course, workshop, or seminar description, including learning objectives and standards for meeting the objectives. In the case of clinical application objectives, teaching methods must be documented, including actual supervised practice. Documentation must include a transcript or certificate showing successful completion of the coursework. Practitioners are prohibited from using PAMs independently until granted approval as provided in subdivision 7.

➤ Subd. 3. Educational and clinical requirements for use of superficial PAMs. (a) An occupational therapist may use superficial PAMs if the occupational therapist has received theoretical training and clinical application training in the use of superficial PAMs. (b) Theoretical training in the use of superficial PAMs must: (1) explain the rationale and clinical indications for use of superficial PAMs; (2) explain the physical properties and principles of the superficial PAMs; (3) describe the types of heat and cold transference; (4) explain the factors affecting tissue response to superficial heat and cold; (5) describe the biophysical effects of superficial PAMs in normal and abnormal tissue; (6) describe the thermal conductivity of tissue, matter, and air.

➤ Subd. 6. Occupational therapy assistant use of PAMs. An occupational therapy assistant may set up and implement treatment using PAMs if the assistant meets the requirements of this section, has demonstrated service competency for the particular modality used, and works under the direct supervision of an occupational therapist. An occupational therapy assistant who uses superficial PAMs must meet the requirements of subdivision 3. An occupational therapy assistant who uses electrotherapy must meet the requirements of subdivision 4. An occupational therapy assistant who uses ultrasound must meet the requirements of subdivision 5. An occupational therapist may not delegate evaluation, reevaluation, treatment planning, and treatment goals for PAMs to an occupational therapy assistant.

## Montana

(8) "PAMs" means those modalities that produce a response in soft tissue through the use of light, water, temperature, sound, or electricity. PAMs are characterized as adjunctive methods used in conjunction with or in immediate preparation for patient involvement in purposeful activity. Superficial PAMs include hot packs, cold packs, ice, fluidotherapy, paraffin, water, and other commercially available superficial heating and cooling devices. Use of superficial PAMs is limited to the shoulder, arm, elbow, forearm, wrist, and hand and is subject to the provisions of 37-24-105. Use of sound and electrical PAM devices is limited to the shoulder,

arm, elbow, forearm, wrist, and hand and is subject to the provisions of 37-24-106.

## 37-24-105. Use of Superficial PAMs

(1) Except as provided in subsection (2), a person may not use occupational therapy techniques involving superficial PAMs unless the person:

   (a) Is a licensed occupational therapist under this chapter;

   (b) Limits application of superficial agent modalities to the shoulder, arm, elbow, forearm, wrist, and hand; and

   (c) Has successfully completed 16 hours of instruction or training in superficial PAMs and documents competency, as approved by the board, in the following areas:

     (i) Principles of physics related to specific properties of light, water, temperature, sound, or electricity, as indicated by selected modalities;

     (ii) Physiological, neurophysiological, and electrophysiological changes that occur as a result of the application of selected modalities;

     (iii) The response of normal and abnormal tissue to the application of selected modalities;

     (iv) Indications and contraindications related to the selection and application of the modality;

     (v) Guidelines for the treatment or administration of the modality within the philosophical framework of occupational therapy;

     (vi) Guidelines for educating the patient, including information about risks and benefits of the occupational therapy techniques;

     (vii) Safety rules and precautions related to the selected modalities;

     (viii) Methods for documenting the effectiveness and immediate and long-term effects of treatment in relation to task-oriented activities; and

     (ix) Characteristics of and guidelines for the use of therapy equipment, including safe operation, adjustment, and care and maintenance of the equipment.

(2) A certified occupational therapy assistant who works under the direct supervision of a qualified occupational therapist may apply superficial PAMs to the shoulder, arm, elbow, forearm, wrist, and hand.

**History**: En. Sec. 2, Ch. 297, L. 1993.

## 37-24-106. Use of Sound and Electrical PAMs

(1) Except as provided in subsection (2), a person may not utilize occupational therapy techniques involving sound or electrical PAM devices unless the person:

   (a) Is licensed under this chapter;

   (b) Limits application of sound and electrical PAMs to the shoulder, arm, elbow, forearm, wrist, or hand to restore and enhance upper extremity function; and

   (c) (i) Provides to the board documentation of certification by the hand certification commission, inc., and has successfully completed 40 hours of instruction or training in sound and electrical PAM devices and documents competency, as approved by the board, in the areas provided in 37-24-105(1)(c); or (ii) has successfully completed 20 hours of instruction or training and five proctored treatments under the direct supervision of a licensed medical practitioner in sound PAM devices and 20 hours of instruction or training and five proctored treatments under the direct supervision of a licensed medical practitioner in electrical PAM devices and documents competency, as approved by the board, in the areas provided in 37-24-105(1)(c).

(2) A certified occupational therapy assistant who works under the direct supervision of a qualified occupational therapist may apply deep PAMs to the shoulder, arm, elbow, forearm, wrist, and hand.

**History**: En. Sec. 3, Ch. 297, L. 1993; amd. Sec. 2, Ch. 101, L. 2003.

## 37-24-108. Application and Administration of Topical Medications—Prescription, Purchasing, and Recordkeeping Requirements

(1) A licensed occupational therapist who meets the requirements of 37-24-106 may apply or administer topical medications by:

(a) Circect application;

(b) Iontophoresis, a process in which topical medications are applied through the use of electricity; or

(c) Phonophoresis, a process in which topical medications are applied through the use of ultrasound.

(2) A licensed occupational therapist may apply or administer the following topical medications:

(a) Bactericidal agents;

(b) Debriding agents;

(c) Anesthetic agents;

(d) Anti-inflammatory agents;

(e) Antispasmodic agents; and

(f) Adrenocorticosteroids.

(3) (a) Topical medications applied or administered by a licensed occupational therapist must be prescribed on a specific or standing basis by a licensed medical practitioner authorized to order or prescribe topical medications and must be purchased from a pharmacy certified under 37-7-321.

(b) Topical medications dispensed under this section must comply with packaging and labeling guidelines developed by the board of pharmacy under Title 37, chapter 7.

(4) A licensed occupational therapist who applies or administers topical medications shall keep appropriate records with respect to those medications.

**History**: En. Sec. 4, Ch. 101, L. 2003.

## Nebraska

### 71-6122. PAMs; Certification Required

(1) In order to apply PAMs, an occupational therapist shall be certified pursuant to this section. The department shall issue a certificate to an occupational therapist to administer a PAM if the occupational therapist:

(a) Has successfully completed a training course approved by the board and passed an examination approved by the board on the PAM;

(b) Is certified as a hand therapist by the Hand Therapy Certification Commission or other equivalent entity recognized by the board;

(c) Has a minimum of five years of experience in the use of the PAM and has passed an examination approved by the board on the PAM; or

(d) Has completed education during a basic educational program which included demonstration of competencies for application of the PAM.

(2) The department shall issue a certificate to authorize an occupational therapy assistant to set up and implement treatment using superficial thermal agent modalities if the occupational therapy assistant has successfully completed a training course approved by the board and passed an examination approved by the board. Such set up and implementation shall only be done under the onsite supervision of an occupational therapist certified to administer superficial thermal agent modalities.

(3) An occupational therapist shall not delegate evaluation, reevaluation, treatment planning, and treatment goals for PAMs to an occupational therapy assistant.

**Source**: Laws 2004, LB 1005, § 128. Operative date July 16, 2004.

## New York

### §76.7 Definition of Occupational Therapy Practice

1. Include the therapeutic use of goal-directed activities, exercises, or techniques to maximize the client's physical and/or mental functioning in life tasks. Treatment is directed toward maximizing functional skill and task-related performance for the development of a client's vocational, avocational, daily living, or related capacities.

2. Relate to physical, perceptual, sensory, neuromuscular, sensory-integrative, cognitive, or psychosocial skills.

3. Include, where appropriate for such purposes and under appropriate conditions, modalities and techniques based on approaches taught in an occupational therapy curriculum and included in a program of professional education in occupational therapy registered by the department, and consistent with areas of individual competence. These approaches are based on:

   i. The neurological and physiological sciences as taught in a registered occupational therapy professional education program. Modalities and techniques may be based on, but not limited to, any one or more of the following:

      a. Sensory integrative approaches;

      b. Developmental approaches;

      c. Sensorimotor approaches;

      d. Neurophysiological treatment approaches;

      e. Muscle reeducation;

      f. Superficial heat and cold; or

      g. Cognitive and perceptual remediation.

# Ohio

## 4755.01 Definitions.

As used in sections 4755.01 to 4755.12 and section 4755.99 of the Revised Code:

(A) "Occupational therapy" means the evaluation of learning and performance skills and the analysis, selection, and adaptation of activities for an individual whose abilities to cope with daily living, perform tasks normally performed at the individual's stage of development, and perform vocational tasks are threatened or impaired by developmental deficiencies, the aging process, environmental deprivation, or physical, psychological, or social injury or illness, through specific techniques which include:

(1) Planning and implementing activities and programs to improve sensory and motor functioning at the level of performance normal for the individual's stage of development;

(2) Teaching skills, behaviors, and attitudes crucial to the individual's independent, productive, and satisfying social functioning;

(3) Designing, fabricating, applying, recommending, and instructing in the use of selected orthotic or prosthetic devices and other equipment which assists the individual to adapt to the individual's potential or actual impairment;

(4) Analyzing, selecting, and adapting activities to maintain the individual's optimal performance of tasks and to prevent further disability.

(5) Administration of topical drugs that have been prescribed by a licensed health professional authorized to prescribe drugs, as defined in section 4729.01 of the Revised Code.

# South Dakota

## 36-31-1. Definition of Terms

Terms used in this chapter mean:

(1) "Association," the South Dakota Occupational Therapy Association.

(2) "Board of examiners," the South Dakota State Board of Medical and Osteopathic Examiners.

(3) "Occupational therapists," any person licensed to practice occupational therapy as defined in this chapter and whose license is in good standing; "Occupational therapy," the evaluation, planning, and implementation of a program of purposeful activities to develop or maintain adaptive skills necessary to achieve the maximal physical and mental functioning of the individual in his or her daily pursuits. The practice of occupational therapy includes consultation, evaluation, and treatment of individuals whose abilities to cope with the tasks of living are threatened or impaired by developmental deficits, the aging process, learning disabilities, poverty and cultural differences, physical injury or disease, psychological and social disabilities, or anticipated dysfunction. Occupational therapy services include such treatment techniques as task-oriented activities to prevent or correct physical or emotional deficits or to minimize the disabling effect of these deficits in the life of the individual; such evaluation techniques as assessment of sensory integration and motor abilities, assessment of development of self-care and feeding, activities and capacity for independence, assessment of

the physical capacity for prevocational and work tasks, assessment of play and leisure performance, and appraisal of living areas for the handicapped; PAMs limited to the upper extremities to enhance physical functional performance, if certified in accordance with § 36-31-6; and specific occupational therapy techniques such as activities of daily living skills, designing, fabricating, or applying selected orthotic devices or selecting adaptive equipment, sensory integration and motor activities, the use of specifically designed manual and creative activities, specific exercises to enhance functional performance, and treatment techniques for physical capabilities for work activities.

(8) "PAMs," modalities that produce a biophysiological response through the use of light, water, temperature, sound, or electricity, or mechanical devices. PAMs include:

 (a) Superficial thermal agents such as hydrotherapy/whirlpool, cryotherapy (cold packs/ice), fluidotherapy, hot packs, paraffin, water, infrared, and other commercially available superficial heating and cooling technologies;

 (b) Deep thermal agents such as therapeutic ultrasound, phonophoresis, and other commercially available technologies;

 (c) Electrotherapeutic agents such as biofeedback, neuromuscular electrical stimulation, functional electrical stimulation, transcutaneous electrical nerve stimulation, electrical stimulation for tissue repair, high-voltage galvanic stimulation, and iontophoresis and other commercially available technologies;

 (d) Mechanical devices such as vasopneumatic devices and CPM (continuous passive motion).

**Source**: SL 1986, ch 323, § 1; SL 2005, ch 205, § 1.

## Tennessee

(16) Electrical Stimulation Certification—An authorization issued by the committee when a licensed occupational therapist or occupational therapy assistant has successfully completed requirements to use a device, for which a federally required prescription is necessary, that employs transcutaneous electrical current (direct, alternating, or pulsatile) for the purpose of eliciting muscle contraction, alleviating pain, reducing edema, or drug delivery.

(29) Thermal Agents Certification—An authorization issued by the committee when a licensed occupational therapist or occupational therapy assistant has successfully completed requirements to use thermal agents, for which a federally required prescription is necessary, that include superficial heating agents (e.g., hot packs, paraffin), cryotherapy, and deep heating agents (e.g., ultrasound).

(3) Certification in the use of PAMs

 (a) Electrical stimulation certification—To be eligible for certification in electrical stimulation, an applicant must:

  1. Meet all qualifications in paragraph (1) or (2) of this rule and all applicable procedures in rule 1150-2-.05; and

  2. Submit documentation of current certification from the American Society of Hand Therapists; or

  3. Successfully complete committee-approved training that shall consist of a total of twenty-five (25) contact hours of didactic and laboratory experiences which include five (5) treatments on clinical patients to be super-

vised by licensees who hold certification pursuant to subparagraph (a) or by a physical therapist currently licensed in the United States. The treatments shall be from the following categories, and at least one (1) treatment shall be from each category:

(i) Neuromuscular electrical stimulation

(ii) Electrical stimulation for pain control

(iii) Edema reduction

(iv) Iontophoresis

(b) Thermal agents certification—To be eligible for certification in the use of thermal agents, an applicant must:

  1. Meet all qualifications in paragraph (1) or (2) of this rule and all applicable procedures in rule 1150-2-.05; and

  2. Submit documentation of current certification from the American Society of Hand Therapists; or

  3. Successfully complete Committee-approved training that shall consist of a total of twenty (20) contact hours of didactic and laboratory experiences which include ten (10) treatments on clinical patients to be supervised by licensees who hold certification pursuant to subparagraph (b) or by a physical therapist currently licensed in the United States. Five (5) of the ten (10) treatments shall utilize ultrasound. The treatments shall be from the following categories, and at least one (1) treatment shall be from each category:

  (i) Superficial heating agents

  (ii) Cryotherapy

  (iii) Deep heating agents

(c) Training

  1. Approval of all training courses shall be made by the committee. The required training for electrical stimulation and thermal agents certification may be obtained through:

  (i) Colleges and universities approved for training occupational therapists and occupational therapy assistants by the AOTA, or physical therapists and physical therapy assistants by the APTA, or at clinical facilities affiliated with such accredited colleges or universities; or

  (ii) The American Society of Hand Therapists; or

  (iii) Any approved provider offering a committee-approved course.

  2. The training for the therapeutic use of electrical stimulation devices shall provide competency in the following areas:

  (i) Standards

  (I) The expected outcome or treatments with therapeutic electrical current (TEC) must be consistent with the goals of treatment.

  (II) Treatment of TEC must be safe, administered to the correct area, and be of proper dosage.

  (ii) Correct dosage and mode

  (I) Ability to determine the duration and mode of current appropriate to the patient's neurophysiological status while understanding Ohm's law of electricity, physical laws related to the passage of current through various media, as well as impedance.

    (II)  Ability to describe normal electrophysiology of nerve and muscle, understanding generation of bioelectrical signals in nerve and muscle, recruitment of motor units in normal muscle and in response to a variety of external stimuli.

    (III)  Ability to describe normal and abnormal tissue responses to external electrical stimuli while understanding the differing responses to varieties of current duration, frequency, and intensity of stimulation.

(iii)  Selection of method and equipment

    (I)  Ability to identify equipment with the capability of producing the preselected duration and mode.

    (II)  Ability to describe characteristics of electrotherapeutic equipment and understanding of the therapeutic value of different electrotherapeutic equipment.

    (III)  Ability to describe safety regulations governing the use of electrotherapeutic equipment.

    (IV)  Ability to describe principles of electrical currents.

    (V)  Ability to describe requirements/idiosyncrasies of body areas and pathological conditions with respect to electrotherapeutic treatment.

(iv)  Preparation of treatment

    (I)  Ability to prepare the patient for treatment through positioning and adequate instructions

    (II)  Ability to explain to the patient the benefits expected of the electrotherapeutic treatment.

(v)  Treatment administration

    (I) Ability to correctly operate equipment and appropriately adjust the intensity and current while understanding rate of stimulator, identification of motor points, and physiological effects desired.

    (II) Ability to adjust the intensity and rate to achieve the optimal response, based on the pertinent evaluative data.

(vi)  Documentation of treatments—Ability to document treatment including immediate and long-term effects of therapeutic electrical current.

3. The training for the therapeutic use of thermal agents shall provide competency in the following areas:

(i)  Standards

    (I)  The expected outcome or treatments with thermal agents must be consistent with the goals of treatment.

    (II)  Treatment with thermal agents must be safe, administered to the correct area, and be the proper dosage.

    (III)  Treatment with thermal agents be adequately documented.

(ii)  Instrumentation

    (I)  Ability to describe the physiological effects of thermal agents as well as differentiate tissue responses to the various modes of application.

    (II)  Ability to select the appropriate thermal agent considering the area and conditions being treated.

(III) Ability to describe equipment characteristics, indications, and contraindications for treatment, including identifying source and mechanisms of generation of thermal energy and its transmission through air and physical matter.

(iii) Preparation for treatment

(I) Ability to prepare the patient for treatment through positioning and adequate instruction.

(II) Ability to explain to the patient the benefits expected of the thermal treatment.

(iv) Determination of dosage—Ability to determine dosage through determination of target tissue depth, stage of the condition (acute vs. chronic), and application of power/dosage calculation rules as appropriate.

(v) Treatment administration—Ability to administer treatment through identification of controls, sequence of operation, correct application techniques, and application of all safety rules and precautions.

(vi) Documentation of treatments—Ability to document treatment including immediate and long-term effects of thermal agents.

(4) In determining the qualifications of applicants for certification as an occupational therapist or as an occupational therapy assistant, only a majority vote of the committee of occupational therapy shall be required. Authority: T.C.A. §§ 4-5-202, 4-5-204, 63-13-102, 63-13-103, 63-13-108, 63-13-202, 63-13-203, 63-13-206, and 63-13-213. Administrative History: Original rule filed March 15, 1996; effective May 29, 1996. Amendment filed July 31, 2000; effective October 14, 2000. Amendments filed March 10, 2005; effective May 24, 2005.

## 1150-2-.05 Procedures For Certification

To become certified as a occupational therapist or occupational therapy assistant in Tennessee, a person must comply with the following procedures and requirements.

(1) Occupational therapist and occupational therapy assistant by examination.

(a) An application packet shall be requested from the Committee's administrative office.

(b) An applicant shall respond truthfully and completely to every question or request for information contained in the application form and submit it along with all documentation and fees required by the form and these rules to the committee's administrative office. It is the intent of these rules that all steps necessary to accomplish the filing of the required documentation be completed prior to filing an application and that all documentation be filed simultaneously.

(c) Applications will be accepted throughout the year and completed files will ordinarily be processed at the next committee meeting scheduled for the purpose of reviewing files.

(d) An applicant shall pay the nonrefundable application fee and state regulatory fee as provided in rule 1150-2-.06 when submitting the application.

(e) An applicant shall submit with his application a "passport"-style photograph taken within the preceding 12 months.

(f) It is the applicant's responsibility to request that a graduate transcript from his degree granting institution, pursuant to T.C.A. §63-13-202, be submitted directly from the school to the committee's administrative office. The institution granting the degree must be accredited by the AOTA at the time the degree was granted. The transcript must show that the degree has been conferred and carry the official seal of the institution and reference the name under which the applicant has applied for certification.

(g) An applicant shall submit an original letter of recommendation attesting to the applicant's good moral character. The letter cannot be from a relative.

(h) Examination verification:

1. It is the responsibility of the applicant to request a copy of his certification examination results from the National Board for Certification in Occupational Therapy Examination be sent directly to the Committee's administrative office.

2. For examinations taken prior to January, 1985, the applicant shall request the NBCOT send a verification of certification examination results to the Committee of Occupational Therapy. For an examination taken in January, 1985, or later, the applicant shall request that Professional Exam Service send verification of certification examination results to the Committee of Occupational Therapy.

   (i) PAM certification:

   (I) If an applicant is seeking certification in the use of PAMs, as provided in paragraph (3) of rule 1150-2-.04, the applicant shall cause to have proof of successful training completion be submitted directly from the training provider to the committee's administrative office.

   (II) Current licensees who are presently using PAMs may continue to do so for eighteen (18) months from the effective date of these rule amendments. After that date certification shall be required.

(j) When necessary, all required documents shall be translated into English. Both translation and original document, certified as to authenticity by the issuing source must be submitted.

(k) Personal resumes are not acceptable and will not be reviewed.

   (l) Application review and licensure decisions shall be governed by Rule 1150

# References

Ahlscwede, K. (1992). The issue is—views on PAMs and specialization within occupational therapy: A rebuttal. *American Journal of Occupational Therapy, 46,* 650-652.

American Occupational Therapy Association. (2006a). *Model occupational therapy act.* Bethesda, MD: AOTA.

American Occupational Therapy Association. (2006b). *Accreditation Council for Occupational Therapy Education (ACOTE®) standards and interpretative guidelines* (2006 ed.). Bethesda, MD: AOTA.

American Occupational Therapy Association. (2005). *Code of ethics.* Bethesda, MD: AOTA.

American Occupational Therapy Association. (1997). Physical agent modalities position paper. *American Journal of Occupational Therapy, 51,* 10.

American Occupational Therapy Association. (1994). *A guide for the preparation of occupational therapy practitioners for the use of physical agent modalities.* Bethesda, MD: AOTA.

Aoyagi, Y., & Tsubahara, A. (2004). Therapeutic orthosis and electrical stimulation for upper extremity hemiplegia after stroke: A review of effectiveness based on evidence. *Top Stroke Rehabilitation, 11,* 9-15.

Bent, M., Crist, P., Florey, L., & Strickland, L. R. (2005). A practice analysis of occupational therapy and impact on certification examination. *OTJR: Occupation, Participation and Health, 25*, 105-118.

Bhakta, B. B. (2000). Management of spasticity in stroke. *British Medical Bulletin, 56,* 476-485.

Blyth, F. M., March, L. M., Nicholas, M. K., & Cousins, M. J. (2005). Self-management of chronic pain: A population-based study. *Pain, 113,* 285-292.

Chae, J. (2003). Neuromuscular electrical stimulation for motor relearning in hemiparesis. *Physical Medicine and Rehabilitation Clinics of North America, 14,* S93-109.

Chae, J., Fang, Z. P., Walker, M., & Pourmehdi, S. (2001). Intramuscular electromyographically controlled neuromuscular electrical stimulation for upper limb recovery in chronic hemiplegia. *American Journal of Physical Medicine & Rehabilitation, 80*, 935-941.

Glauner, J. H., Ekes, A. M., James, A. E., & Holm, M. B. (1997). A pilot study of the theoretical and technical competence and appropriate education for the use of nine PAMs in occupational therapy practice. *American Journal of Occupational Therapy, 51*, 767-774.

SB 179. (2005). Chapter 205; SB179 (Senate Bill ed.) South Dakota.

Taylor, E., & Humphry, R. (1991). Survey of PAM use. *American Journal of Occupational Therapy, 45,* 924-931.

Willmarth, C. & Smith. (2003). *AOTA state issues update.* Bethesda, MD: AOTA.

Willmarth, C. (2005). *AOTA state issues update.* Bethesda, MD: AOTA.

# Chapter 3

# WOUND HEALING

## Learning Objectives

1. Identify the phases of wound healing and the physiological changes that occur.
2. Describe the anatomy of the skin.
3. List the classification systems describing pressure ulcers and wounds.
4. Identify the factors which influence or impair the healing process.
5. Discuss the clinical decision-making in assessing wounds and wound healing.

## Terminology

| | | |
|---|---|---|
| Approximation | Granulation tissue | Proliferation |
| Dermis | Hypertrophic scar | Purulent |
| Epidermis | Inflammation | Remodeling |
| Epithelialization | Keloid | Serosanguanous |
| Fibroblasts | Partial-thickness | Serous |
| Full-thickness | Picture frame | Wound classification |

An important component and goal of any occupational therapy intervention is to decrease pain following an injury, illness, or disease. Though the patient's pain is one of the outward expressions of the condition, it is important to remember that pain is a symptom and that the underlying dysfunction or problem lies in the basic "client factors" that impact the patient's occupational performance. Unless we determine the primary cause and treat the underlying problem, we are merely compensating for a loss of function or masking the symptoms. Often, many of the conditions that we treat as occupational therapists have pain as a component or involve the musculoskeletal system and involve injury or damage to soft tissue. It is crucial that occupational therapists have an understanding of the underlying dysfunction and client factors involved in the clinical condition being treated as this will assist in determining appropriate interventions and timing of those interventions. The determination of which therapeutic modality to use is based on a number of considerations including the goals for treatment, the stage of healing for the specific injury or condition, determining which tissues are involved and at what depth, the patients' tolerance and preference, and the ease and convenience of application. A thorough understanding of the process of tissue healing is crucial to assist in the clinical reasoning and application of PAMs. Using PAMs will impact the healing process, and by doing so, manipulate these unique client factors that further impact occupational performance.

Injury to a highly vascularized part of the body leads to a series of interconnected events known as inflammation and repair. The sequence of events that occur after an injury are the body's attempt to control the negative effects of the injury and attempt to return the affected tissue to a "normal" state. An understanding of the wound healing process and an appreciation of the sequence of events that occurs following injury are necessary to be able to determine appropriate interventions and technologies which may facilitate healing and positively influence the process. Wound healing is a complex process involving myriad events and is influenced by both physical and psychological components. Initial insult or injury to the body causes a series of physiologic responses which are overlapping and sequenced, ultimately resulting in normal healing.

The healing process has been arbitrarily divided into three phases, which are not distinct but overlap considerably with one another and include inflammation, repair and regeneration, and maturation. Though there is great variability within each patient and case, the three phases provide a starting point for determining the healing process. We ultimately hope to have viable tissue and a healed wound, but not all tissue can regenerate into normal tissue. When this occurs, the process of scar formation occurs with scar tissue taking the place of the tissue and providing tensile strength to the injured area. Scar tissue, however, is devoid of physiological function and will result in a repair which may become tight, disfiguring, and negatively affect movement or organ function. Influencing wound healing is dependent upon the therapist understanding the process of repair and the factors that affect the repair process, and then clinically reasoning through the interventions and technologies that may impact the outcome.

# Skin Anatomy

Skin is the most frequently injured tissue of the body. Skin thickness and appearance will vary according to the anatomical site. We often experience scratches, bruising, and mild burns to the skin that are healed by the process of epidermal regeneration. In normal skin, there is a balance between the rate of cell division and growth and differentiation. Following an injury, the normal homeostasis is disrupted and the body attempts to heal the affected area (Chang, Andrews, Carter, & Dagnino, 2006; Read & Watt, 1988). As part of the process, special cells respond to the injury by producing a *collagenous glue*, which is called granulation scar tissue. Maintaining the homeostasis of our skin depends on our body's ability to sense a disruption to the skin or underlying structure, alert the appropriate cells to action, and oversee the sequence of repair without complications. Our bodies are composed of 14 different types of collagen. Mature scar tissue is formed from type-I collagen; however, the greatest contribution to the healing process is its ability to imitate the structure of other collagen types. The scar formed in dense tissue "senses" the need for strength and attempts to mimic the surrounding tissue structure. Likewise, a scar filling a defect in loose, flexible tissue will change in its last phase of healing to reproduce, as much as possible, those physical characteristics. Thus, in response to certain internal and external influences, scar tissue does differentiate to become quasispecific to the surrounding tissue (Steenvoorde, Calame, & Oskam, 2006).

The skin is composed of two primary layers, the *epidermis* and the *dermis*. The skin is the largest organ of the body and functions as a barrier between the body and the external environment. The epidermis is approximately 0.04 mm thick, and the dermis is approximately 0.5 mm thick. The epidermis is the outer epithelial layer that provides a protective barrier to injury, contamination, and light. The epidermis is avascular and also functions to prevent dehydration of the underlying tissues. The dermis is vascularized and composed of collagen and elastin fibrous connective tissues which give the skin its strength and resilience. The vascular supply of the dermis also nourishes the epidermis and is responsible, in part, for regulating body temperature. Hair follicles, sebaceous glands, and sweat glands are located in the dermis and help to provide the secretions which lubricate and keep the skin soft and flexible. Nerve endings are also located in the dermis, along with the receptors for pain, touch, heat, and cold. Subcutaneous layers consisting of fat tissues and connective tissues are located below the dermis. These subcutaneous layers protect the underlying tissue and provide insulation, support, and cushioning to withstand pressure and stress.

# Wound Classification

There are a number of wound classification systems used to describe the etiology and severity of a wound. The most common classifications used by therapists are from the National Pressure Ulcer Advisory Panel (NPUAP), which is based on the tissue layers and depth of tissue destruction (Van Rijswijk, 1995), and Marion Laboratories red/yellow/ black color system, which is based on wound color (NPUAP, 1989; Wagner, 1981). Some clinical conditions, such as spinal cord injuries, have a higher incidence of pressure ulcer occurrence and require the occupational therapist and health care team to appreciate the unique circumstances and context of the patient for prevention and treatment (Clark et al., 2006; Reddy, Gill, & Rochon, 2006).

## Pressure Ulcers: Four-Stage System

The NPUAP pressure ulcer staging system is most frequently used to classify ulcers. This system of classification is recommended for use with wounds caused by pressure or tissue perfusion such as diabetic neuropathic ulcers (Bergstrom, 1994). The NPUAP classification uses a four-stage system that describes pressure ulcers by anatomic depth and the soft tissue layers which are involved. Pressure ulcers are often referred to as bedsores, decubitus ulcers, or pressure sores. Pressure ulcers are caused by localized areas of tissue necrosis, which are often associated with compression between a bony prominence and an external surface for an extended period of time (Figure 3-1). The four-stage system is commonly used to describe wound severity and to establish treatment protocols and interventions (Shea, 1975; Eager, 1997). A primary difficulty inherent in the stage system of wound classification is that identification of the wound cannot be done if the area is covered by eschar or necrotic tissue until it is removed. Staging of the wound should be used only as a diagnostic tool to describe the severity of the wound, not the healing of the wound (Ankrom et al., 2005; Krasner & Weir D., 1997)

## Depth of Tissue Involvement

Wounds can also be classified according to the depth of the tissue involved and the thickness of the skin loss—partial- or full-thickness. This classification system is most often used for skin tears, donor sites, surgical wounds, and burns. Partial-thickness wounds involve the epidermal layer and may include the superficial layer of the dermis.

**Figure 3-1.** Stages of healing: Decubitus ulcer. Note periosteum of bone visible in the initial image at the base of the wound. (Stage 4 ulcer) Over the course of several months, the wound slowly healed (Content and photograph by Charlie Goldberg, M.D., UCSD School of Medicine and VA Medical Center, San Diego, California, 92093-0611).

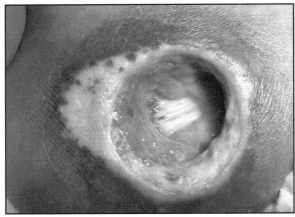

Partial-thickness wounds do not extend through the dermis, the second layer of the skin. Partial-thickness wounds heal by regeneration, known as epithelialization, and may be characterized by a crust or covering consisting of blood and debris particles.

Because of their superficial nature, partial-thickness wounds heal faster than full-thickness wounds. Partial-thickness wounds are shallow, moist, and may be painful due to the loss of the epidermal coverings with exposure of the nerve endings. The wound base often appears as bright pink-red. By contrast, full-thickness wounds involve the epidermis, dermis, and subcutaneous tissues. Subcutaneous tissue wounds may extend into muscles, fascia, tendons, and bone, depending on the depth of injury. Full-thickness wounds may involve necrotic tissue or infection. Full-thickness wound healing is a complex process often referred to as secondary intention healing. This process consists of three phases: *inflammatory, proliferative*, and *remodeling*. These phases of the healing process are not singular events and may overlap. Full-thickness wounds heal by secondary intention, which involves fibroplasia or the formation of granulation tissue with contraction of the wound (Benbow, 2006; Bielecki, Skowronski, & Skowronski, 2006).

## Red/Yellow/Black Wound Classification

Wounds that are classified according to their surface color are described using the three-color concept of red, yellow, or black. This system is frequently used in the clinic due to its simplicity. Red wounds are clean, healing, and granulating appropriately without complications. The goal is to provide a moist wound environment and minimize any damage to the newly formed tissue. Yellow wounds may indicate the possibility of infection and the need for debridement and cleaning of the area. Yellow may also indicate the presence of necrotic tissue. The yellow tissue contains devitalized slough, or fibrous exudate which can promote bacterial growth and infection. The goal of treatment at this stage is to remove the exudate and debris. Black wounds indicate the presence of necrotic or dead tissue which provides a medium for bacterial growth and proliferation.

A black wound requires cleaning and debridement of the area and is often encountered with full-thickness leg/foot ulcers and in patients with gangrene or deep burns. Rarely are wounds exclusively one color, and most manifest all three colors depending on the amount of necrotic tissue as well as systemic and local influences on the healing process (Acha, Serrano, Acha, & Roa, 2005; Eager, 1997; Fowler, Vesely, Pelfrey, Jordan, & Amberry, 1999; McGuiness, Dunn, & Jones, 2005).

## Wound Closure

Healthy wounds follow a logical progression of healing in a timely fashion. However, external factors such as trauma or compromised systems may cause complications and negatively affect the healing process. There are three types of surgical wound healing: primary closure, secondary closure, and delayed primary closure. Primary or "intention" closure refers to wounds which occur when full-thickness surgical incisions or acute wound edges are approximated and sutured together.

Primary closure is most often used when there is minimal skin loss and the acute wound edges can be approximated or apposed and aligned together. Secondary closure is used on wounds that are open, large, and full-thickness. Secondary wounds are left open following surgery and display soft tissue loss. The healing process with secondary wounds takes longer because the area is allowed to heal by production of connective tissue (scar). Delayed primary closure, or tertiary intention, occurs when the wound is initially left open for a short period of time followed by approximation and closure of the wound. Delayed primary closure most often occurs in complex wounds which may be contaminated or may develop infection during the acute phase of the healing process (Hermann, Bagi, & Christoffersen, 1988; Kuroyanagi, 2006; Melis, van Noorden, & van der Horst, 2006; Walters, Dombroski, Davidson, Mandel, & Gibbs, 1990).

In general, the normal healing process in a surgical wound should take approximately 4 weeks, at which point the area should display granular tissue and be covered with epithelial tissue. The wound healing process and rate of healing can be affected by the patient's age, underlying and associated systemic conditions, nutritional status, tissue perfusion, and vascularity. Infections within the wound also affect the healing process negatively, slowing collagen production. Dry wounds are at a disadvantage with regard to the rate of healing. Moist wounds heal at a quicker rate, as the moist environment facilitates epithelialization and reduces crust or scab formation. Epidermal cells require a moist surface to migrate across the wound surface. There are a wide variety of dressings that can facilitate the healing process and the reader is encouraged to explore the options available (Bolton & van Rijswijk, 1991; Hermans & van Wingerden, 1990; Poulsen, Freund, Arendrup, Nyhuus, & Pedersen, 1991).

# Phases of Normal Wound Healing

In a "normal" or healthy individual, the body's response to an injury is well ordered and sequenced, though the stages of repair may overlap. The healing process has been described as having either three or four phases, based on whether epithelialization is viewed as a distinct phase of repair or is included under the phase of proliferation. These phases of healing are not sequential, linear events, but are overlapping and dynamic. The initial phase of healing is the *inflammatory phase,* which initates the process of healing. The *proliferative phase* is characterized by histochemical changes initating fibroplasias and the re-epithelization of the wound. The *remodeling phase* is also referred to as the maturation phase and is characterized by continued fibroblastic activity and deposition of collagen synthesis and lysis leading to the final outcome of the tissue (Cooper, 1990; Hunt & Hussain, 1994; Kloth & McCulloch, 1995; Reed & Zarro, 1990).

## Table 3-1

### LOCAL AND SYSTEMIC INDICES OF INFLAMMATION

| Local Signs | Systemic Signs |
|---|---|
| Redness | Fever |
| Swelling | Leucocytosis |
| Heat | |
| Pain | |

## Phase I: Inflammatory

The inflammatory phase of healing is the body's initial response to an injury. Clotting and vasoconstriction (hemostasis) occur at the initial time of injury and decrease blood loss. The inflammatory response is both vascular and cellular and is the body's response to rid itself of bacteria, foreign matter, and dead tissue. The inflammatory response occurs quickly, and is associated with changes in skin color (red, blue, purple), temperature (heat), turgor (swelling), sensation (pain), and may include a loss of function. Acute inflammation begins immediately at the time of the injury. The acute inflammatory phase usually lasts for 24 to 48 hours and is completed within 7 days, though a subacute phase of inflammation may continue for approximately 2 weeks (Table 3-1) (Harding, 1990).

The initial response to an injury is characterized by vascular changes at the site of injury. Vasoconstriction occurs with platelet aggregation along the endothelium of the injured blood vessel. These platelets release vasoconstrictive, chemotactic, and growth promoting substances that facilitate the formation of fibrin clots, preventing excessive hemorrhage. The release of vasoactive substances, such as histamine and prostaglandins, as well as stimulation of local sensory nerve endings, causes a local reflex action leading to vasodilation and increased permeability (Bryant, 1977). This produces vasocongestion and leakage of the serous fluid into the wound bed, causing the wound to become erythematous, edematous, and warm with exudate. Vasodilation and leakage into the wound area continues for several days. Leukocytes or white blood cells (WBC) also migrate to the area. Neutrophils migrate through the blood vessel walls to phagocytose bacteria and other foreign contaminants. Leukocyte migration occurs within 20 minutes after the initial insult. Monocytes are converted into macrophages entering the tissue by day 2. Macrophages are critical for wound healing and engulf the bacteria and debris, cleaning the wound and breaking down necrotic tissue. Macrophages play an important role in the healing process—secreting growth factors and mediating the formation of blood vessels via angiogenesis. Chemical changes in the tissue are due in part to the histamine released by the mast cells and the prostaglandin which is released by the injured cell membrane (Hardy, 1989). The blood serum contains proteolytic enzymes which degrade necrotic tissue at the wound site and assist in cleaning the wound bed, further facilitating the healing process (Figure 3-2). The process of inflammation is vital to the healing process, and a balance must be achieved to ensure appropriate and timely healing (Table 3-2) (Schneider, Korber, Grabbe, & Dissemond, 2006).

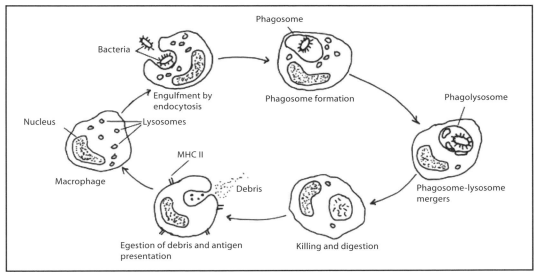

**Figure 3-2.** Phagocytosis by a macrophage. A bacterium, which may or may not be opsonized, is engulfed by the process of endocytosis. The bacterium is ingested in a membranous vesicle called the phagosome. Digestive granules (lysosomes) merge with phagosome, release their contents, and form a structure called the phagolysosome. The killing and digestion of the bacterial cell takes place in the phagolysosome. The macrophage egests debris while processing the antigenic components of the bacterium, which it returns to its surface in association with MHC II for antigen presentation to TH cells (Reprinted with permission from *Todar's Online Textbook of Bacteriology, www.textbookofbacteriology.net*).

## Phase 2: Proliferative

The proliferative phase of recovery has a number of different titles, including fibroplastic phase, granulation, and epithelialization phase. In the proliferative phase of healing, the area of damage is filled with new connective tissue and the wound is covered with new epithelium. The primary components of this phase of healing are granulation, epithelialization, and wound contraction. This process overlaps the inflammatory phase, continuing until the wound is healed. Epithelialization occurs through a series of events, including mobilization, migration, proliferation, and differentiation. Wound contraction is also occurring with the formation of red granulation tissue, which consists of newly formed collagen and blood vessels (Messer, 1989). Granulation tissue fills in the wound site. Wound contraction decreases the size of the affected area and begins approximately 5 days after the injury, peaking at approximately 2 weeks. The process of wound contraction closes the wound, resulting in a smaller area requiring repair by scar formation. Wound contraction should be complete approximately 2 to 3 weeks after the injury.

Wound contraction occurs through the action of myofibroblasts (Figure 3-3). Range of motion (ROM) exercises and functional activities assist in controlling contraction and ensure that the surrounding skin is supple and mobile. Myofibroblasts connect to the wound margins, pulling the epidermal layer inward and producing the characteristic picture frame beneath the skin (Langevin et al., 2006; Hardy, 1989). The shape of the picture frame predicts the speed of contraction, with linear wounds contracting rapidly, square or rectangular wounds contracting at a moderate pace, and circular wounds being the slowest to close and contract. Fibroblasts are the cells that are responsible

## Table 3-2

### SEQUENCE OF THE INFLAMMATORY RESPONSE

*Vasodilation occurs in response to tissue injury.*

Tissues become red and warm.

*Capillary permeability increases.*

Exudate flows into the injured tissues.
Tissues become swollen.
Blood clot forms.

*Leukocytes accumulate at the injury site (leukocytosis).*

Phagocytosis occurs

*Cellular repair begins.*

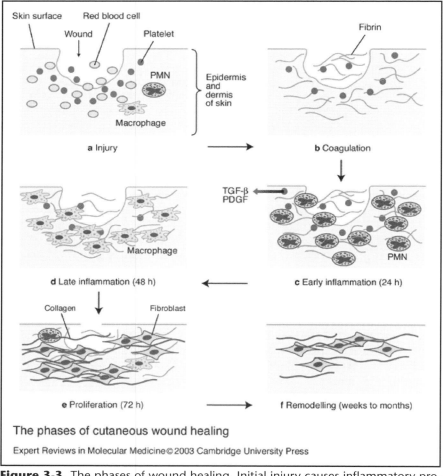

The phases of cutaneous wound healing

Expert Reviews in Molecular Medicine © 2003 Cambridge University Press

**Figure 3-3.** The phases of wound healing. Initial injury causes inflammatory process with vasodilation and increased capillary permability and exudate (Reprinted with permission from Cambridge University Press).

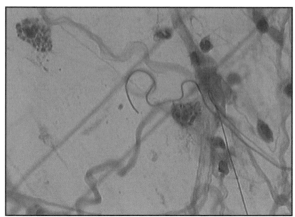

**Figure 3-4.** Loose connective tissue shows bundles of reddish collagen fibers, dark elastic fibers, and macrophages.

for fibroplasia and are stimulated by lactic acid, ascorbic acid, and other cofactors that stimulate the fibroblasts to synthesize collagen. Cross-linkage of the collagen tissue provides the wound with its tensile strength and durability. The tensile strength of remodeled skin is weaker and will never exceed 75% to 80% (Liao, Yang, Grashow, & Sacks, 2005; Schumann, 1982). Cellular activity in the second phase of repair consists of macrophage-stimulated collagen synthesis, formation of a network of blood capillaries, wound contraction, and wound epithelialization. The second phase of healing is completed when epithelialization has resurfaced the wound, a collagen layer has been formed, and initial remodeling is complete.

## Phase 3: Remodeling

The remodeling phase of wound healing has also been termed the maturation phase. The remodeling phase occurs approximately 2 weeks after the injury and may continue for up to a year or longer. The remodeling phase is characterized by a relative balance of collagen synthesis and collagen lysis, the formation and breakdown of collagen. The scar formed during fibroplasia is dense and disorganized. During remodeling, the scar may appear "rosier" than normal and is indicative that remodeling is occurring. This phase of remodeling normally provides the scar with its maximum tensile strength as well as changes in its appearance (Hardy, 1989). Scar tissue consists of disorganized collagen fibers laid down by the fibroblasts, randomly arranged, and different from the surrounding tissue (Figure 3-4). As the wound matures during remodeling, collagen lysis increases and the scar becomes more elastic, smoother, and the fibers stronger. If collagen synthesis exceeds collagen lysis, hypertrophic scarring, or keloid formation may occur. Keloid scars extend beyond the boundary of the wound and appear raised. Hypertrophic scars occur within the area of the wound and may eventually decrease in size and shape (Peacock, Madden, & Trier, 1970). One mechanism frequently used to control the development of hypertrophic or keloid scarring is the application of pressure garments. Wearing of pressure garments is continued until the process of remodeling is complete. As the process of remodeling continues, the collagen fibers are randomly oriented and arranged in a linear and lateral orientation. As the scar continues to mature and the process of collagen synthesis and lysis continues, these fibers assume some of the characteristics of the tissue they are replacing (Figure 3-5).

There are two primary theories which explain how collagen fibers become aligned: *induction theory* and *tension theory* (Gogia, 1995). Induction theory proposes that the

**Figure 3-5.** Abnormal healing process. Note extensor tendon adhesion and scar tissue limiting tendon gliding and decreasing active range of motion. Initial injury was caused by motor vehicle accident with road debris and infection.

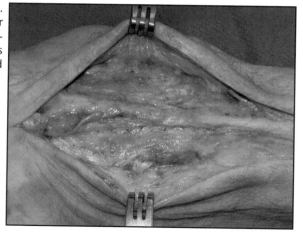

scar tissue attempts to mimic the characteristics of the tissue it is healing. Tension theory purports that internal and external stresses which are placed on the wound affect and align the fibers during remodeling. Tension theory is supported, to an extent, by several studies suggesting that adding tension during healing increases the tensile strength of soft tissue structures and bone, whereas immobilizing the area produces a loss of tensile strength and collagen fiber organization (Arem & Madden, 1976). Tension theory, in part, accounts for the use of dynamic splinting, serial casting, continuous passive motion (CPM) devices, positional stretching, neuromuscular electrical stimulation (NMES), and the use of silastic gel pads and compression garments in the treatment process (Table 3-3) (Hermans & van Wingerden, 1990; Sussman & Bates-Jensen, 1998).

## Factors Impacting Wound Healing

As remodeling continues, the bright pink color of the immature scar softens, flattens, and becomes white and soft. Full maturity for a scar may continue for up to 2 years. However, there are a number of factors that may affect the rate and outcome of normal healing. External and internal factors may delay or impair the healing process during any of the three phases of healing, and a balance is required to ensure appropriate healing. The presence of foreign objects or microorganisms also impairs the healing process. Common microorganisms which cause infections in wounds include *Pseudomonas eruginosa* and *Staphylococcus aureus*. Clinical signs of an infected wound include increased erythema, heat, edema, pus, increased body temperature, pain, purulent drainage, and an uncharacteristic odor. The risk of infection can be minimized through proper debridement procedures, cleaning, and dressing techniques. The presence of foreign bodies, necrotic tissue, and eschar also impairs the healing of the wound and may predispose the wound to bacterial infection. Surgical debridement of the eschar, necrotic tissue, or debris may minimize the adverse effects the foreign material may have on healing (Leininger, Rasmussen, Smith, Jenkins, & Coppola, 2006; Toporcer & Radonak, 2006).

Nutrition also plays a key role in the healing process, and a deficiency in any nutrient; vitamins A, C, and E; or trace metals, such as zinc or copper may impact the healing process (Berger & Shenkin, 2006; Pollack, 1979; Pollack, 1982). Systemic diseases such as diabetes mellitus, atherosclerosis, acquired immune deficiency

**Table 3-3**

## NORMAL WOUND HEALING AND REPAIR: SEQUENCE OF EVENTS

The wound healing process is a nonlinear sequence of events that overlap and begin the moment that the injury occurs and can continue for months and extend beyond a year. Remember time frames may vary with each patient and with co-morbidities or complications. This healing process occurs with both acute and chronic wounds. In chronic wounds, this process becomes disrupted and becomes either prolonged or incomplete with loss of normal tissue restoration.

### Inflammatory Phase (Immediately after injury to 2 to 5 days)

Hemostasis:
- Clot development

Epithelialization begins:
- Cell regeneration
- Vasoconstriction
- Platelet aggregation

Inflammation:
- Vasodilation
- Phagocytosis

### Proliferative Phase (2 days to 6 weeks)

Granulation:
- Fibroplasia-collagen fibers
- Neovascularization (angiogensis-cell budding)

Wound Contraction:
- Wound edges pull together from outer margins, inward.

Epithelilization:
- Scar formation
- Collagen fibers gather into large fibers (cross linked)

### Remodeling Phase (6 weeks to 2 years)

New collagen forms (synthesis-lysis balance)
Tissue differentiation
(Tensile strength of repaired tissue 2 years after injury is approximately 80%)

---

syndrome (AIDS), and other vascular diseases may also have a pronounced adverse effect on wound healing. Diabetes mellitus is a major cause of poor wound healing. Patients with poorly controlled diabetes have slower rates of healing, due in part to decreased circulation secondary to atherosclerosis, and diabetic neuropathy which decreases sensation in the extremities, particularly the lower extremity, which may lead to ulcerations at pressure points with weight-bearing. Patients using systemic medications such as steroids, nonsteroidal anti-inflammatory drugs (NSAIDS), chemotherapeutic agents, antibiotics, and anticoagulants will impact the normal healing process (Andreadis, 2006; Vince & Abdeen, 2006). The aging process and associated physiological changes which occur in the elderly slow the healing response. Delayed

Table 3-4

### FACTORS AFFECTING HEALING AND REPAIR

| Systemic Factors | Local Factors |
|---|---|
| Nutrition | Infection |
| Hematologic abnormalities | Adequacy of blood supply |
| Diabetes mellitus | Foreign bodies |
| Radiation therapy | Tissue hypoxia |
| Immunodeficiency | Repeated trauma |
| Age | Necrotic tissue |
| Medications | |

granulation and a decreased inflammatory response is more common in the elderly, along with a slow rate of epithelialization and a decreased tensile strength (Table 3-4) (Mulder, Brazinsky, & Seeley, 1995).

## Documentation

The involvement of the therapist in the management of open wounds and wound healing will depend on the clinical site, experience of the therapist, and involvement of other medical staff, such as nursing. Occupational therapists are often involved in the management of sprains, strains, and acute injuries and those practicing in orthopedics may be more deeply involved in the management of wounds and the healing process.

It is beyond the scope of this text to describe the wide variety and application of the types of dressings available. Therapists should be well versed in the indications and contraindications of each type of dressing, from gauze to hydrocolloids. Therapists requiring further information on dressings should review the number of excellent texts available on the subject.

The primary purpose of wound assessment is to obtain baseline information on what the wound looks like prior to treatment intervention. Additionally, clear and appropriate documentation demonstrates the effectiveness of the interventions to third party payers. The therapist should use a systematic approach when managing wounds. Questions such as: What caused the wound? Was it due to pressure, laceration, thermal (heat) or nonthermal (cold), chemical, or caused by a vascular impairment or disease process? Is the wound bleeding? (Review the medical record for the platelet count and to assist in determining clotting efficiency or if the patient is taking any medications, such as coumadin or heparin, that may impede clotting.) What is the extent and depth of the wound? Is it superficial, partial-, or full-thickness? Does it involve muscle, tendon, or bone? Is there foreign debris or dead necrotic tissue present? The presence of eschars may impede the healing process and facilitate wound infection. Does the wound show signs of a clinical infection (Figure 3-6)? Are there clinical signs such as increased erythema, edema, purulence, body temperature, pain, changes in the color of the exudate, or an uncharacteristic or foul odor? Clinicians should review any lab work for confirmation on cultures which may have been taken or for increased white blood cell count which may account for infections.

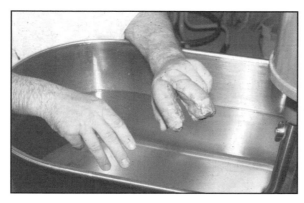

**Figure 3-6.** Traumatic injury to left index and middle finger. Note the suture line which has torn open secondary to the edema; also coloration of the wound and digital tips. Black color indicates tissue necrosis and must be debrided for healing process to occur.

When documenting a wound assessment, the therapist should include the following information:

1. Anatomical location and area of the wound

2. Size of the wound (length, width, depth)

3. Shape of the wound: draw the shape or use one of the many documentation patterns available

4. Presence of dead or necrotic tissue and its color (black, brown, yellow)

5. Description of the wound exudate (purulent pus, milky), serous (clean, yellowish), serosanguanous (pinkish)

6. Presence of any healthy granulation tissue at the base or epithelialization at the wound margins

7. Description of the surrounding intact skin: presence of erythema, heat, pain, edema

Determining an appropriate diagnosis and intervention occurs following the evaluation of the problem. The patient's potential prognosis and level of improvement is determined and aids in identifying appropriate interventions and technologies that will help achieve the stated goals (Doenges, Moorhouse, & Burley, 1995). Physical agent modalities have been demonstrated to be effective in influencing and impacting the healing process. In patients with open wounds, the use of hydrotherapy to cleanse and debride the wound may be effective. Electrical stimulation has been shown to assist in debridement as well as to facilitate epithelialization and contraction of the wound. Ultrasound has been used to promote wound healing during the proliferative and remodeling phases, and is used extensively in the management of soft tissue inflammation (Park & Silva, 2004; Petrofsky et al., 2005; Unger, Eddy, & Raimastry, 1991; Valdes, Angderson, & Giner, 1999). The use of continuous passive movement devices to assist with scar management and to promote healing is well documented, as is the use of early controlled mobilization through the application of dynamic splints though a concensus on the best strategy will require further research and study (Gelberman, Woo, Lothringer, Akeson, & Amiel, 1982; Peterson, Manske, Kain, & Lesker, 1986; Thien, Becker, & Theis, 2004; Woo et al., 1981).

# Summary

The wound healing process has been described as an overlapping cascade of events that include the three primary phases: *inflammation, proliferation*, and *remodeling*. An understanding of the healing process and the stages of recovery are vital for the therapist to aid in determining functional outcomes and to be able to influence the healing process through the potential application of physical agent technologies and interventions. Identifying an appropriate intervention and treatment plan to manage the wound and injury through debridement, facilitating healing through physical technologies, selection of appropriate dressings, and engaging an individual in developmentally and occupationally appropriate activities are all critical to facilitating an individual's return to normal occupational roles and performance (Figures 3-7 to 3-9).

# Case Study

M. J. is a 77-year-old female referred to occupational therapy following a fall that occurred at home in the early spring. Though there were no fractures, M.J. struck her face during the fall and landed on her right hand, rolling onto the extremity. M.J. is an active woman who lives alone, and enjoys gardening and canning the fruits of her labor in the fall. She is concerned over her inability to fully flex or extend the digits of her right hand and the stiffness that has developed in her wrist. Clinical evaluation reveals an alert, social female in no apparent distress. Primary complaint is of "stiffness and aching" in her right hand and wrist. Examination reveals edema and discoloration over the entire dorsal aspect of the hand. The skin is taut, with a purplish-blue color indicating a large hematoma. The right side of the patient's face also displays a large, dark purple-blue hematoma with areas of yellow. There is no drainage noted, but the extent of the hematoma and the associated edema are limiting the patient's active movement and prehension patterns. M.J. relates that she is able to dress herself and take care of her basic ADL needs, but is having difficulty with fastenings, manipulating objects using the right hand, higher level homemaking tasks such as cleaning, and activities requiring bilateral use of the hands.

Further evaluation of the patient included grip/pinch strength, prehension patterns, object manipulation, sensation, ADL components and measurements, determination of social support systems, and her adjustment to the injury. The treatment plan was established and included hydrotherapy to warm the tissue and increase blood flow, and for its cellular effects. During the whirlpool treatment, M. J. was encouraged to perform gentle exercises for muscle pumping and strengthening and to prevent edema in the dependent position. Following whirlpool, treatment using ultrasound was added to promote absorption of the hematoma. Because of the depth of the tissue involvement and size of the area, the hematoma took approximately 2 weeks to resolve. The treatment protocol for the ultrasound was 3 MHz, 0.5 W/cm$^2$, pulsed at 20% duty cycle for 6 minutes. A frequency of 3 MHz was selected due to the hematoma's location on the dorsal aspect of the hand and wrist, a superficial area. The nonthermal effects of the ultrasound were used to facilitate the biologic process of repair through its cellular effect of stable cavitation and/or acoustic streaming. Occupational activities preceded the physical agents, with M. J. engaging in a variety of activities facilitating active prehension patterns and use of the right hand and wrist.

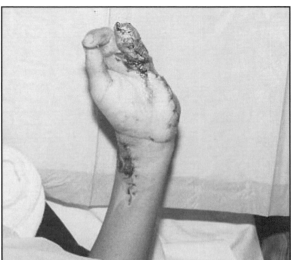

**Figure 3-7.** Normal wound healing. Initial injury to left hand secondary to traumatic ray amputation of #4, #5, and partial amputation of #3 digit. Patient's hand was caught in a power chain on a portable sawmill. Note tissue coloration, exudates and drainage, edema.

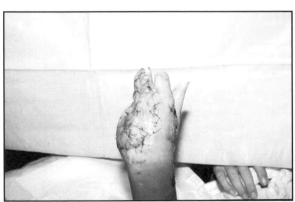

**Figure 3-8.** Dorsal view of same injury—traumatic ray amputation of left hand. Note skin grafting, sutures in place, edema and coloration of tissue.

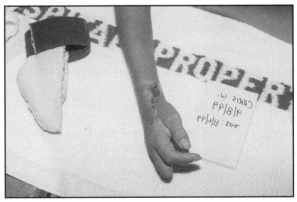

**Figure 3-9.** Ray amputation 5 weeks postinjury. Note decreased edema, coloration of healing tissue, wound margins. Soft protective splint to the left was fabricated to allow patient to participate in football and soccer, protecting the healing tissue.

# References

Acha, B., Serrano, C., Acha, J. I., & Roa, L. M. (2005). Segmentation and classification of burn images by color and texture information. *Journal of Biomedical Optics, 10*, 034014.

Andreadis, S. T. (2006). Experimental models and high-throughput diagnostics for tissue regeneration. *Expert Opinion on Biological Therapy, 6*, 1071-1086.

Ankrom, M. A., Bennett, R. G., Sprigle, S., Langemo, D., Black, J. M., & Berlowitz, D. R., et al. (2005). Pressure-related deep tissue injury under intact skin and the current pressure ulcer staging systems. *Advances in Skin & Wound Care, 18*, 35-42.

Arem, A. J., & Madden, J. W. (1976). Effects of stress on healing wounds: I. intermittent noncyclical tension. *Journal of Surgical Research, 20*, 93-102.

Benbow, M. (2006). Guidelines for the prevention and treatment of pressure ulcers. *Nursing Standard. 20, 52*, 42-44

Berger, M. M., & Shenkin, A. (2006). Update on clinical micronutrient supplementation studies in the critically ill. *Current Opinion in Clinical Nutrition and Metabolic Care, 9*, 711-716.

Bergstrom, N. (1994). Treatment of pressure ulcers. *Clinical Practice Guideline no. 15*. AHCRP Publication, N. 95-0652.

Bielecki, M., Skowronski, R., & Skowronski, J. (2006). Sacral pressure sores and their treatment. *Chirurgia Narzadow Ruchu i Ortopedia Polska, 71*, 51-56.

Bolton, L., & van Rijswijk, L. (1991). Wound dressings: Meeting clinical and biological needs. *Dermatology Nursing, 3*, 146-161.

Bryant, W. M. (1977). Wound healing. *Clinical Symposium, 29*, 1-36.

Chang, W. Y., Andrews, J., Carter, D. E., & Dagnino, L. (2006). Differentiation and injury-repair signals modulate the interaction of E2F and pRB proteins with novel target genes in keratinocytes. *Cell Cycle, 5*, 1872-1879.

Clark, F. A., Jackson, J. M., Scott, M. D., Carlson, M. E., Atkins, M. S., & Uhles-Tanaka, D., et al. (2006). Data-based models of how pressure ulcers develop in daily-living contexts of adults with spinal cord injury. *Archives of Physical Medicine and Rehabilitation, 87*, 1516-1525.

Cooper, D. (1990). The physiology of wound healing: An overview. *Chronic Wound Care*, 1-11.

Doenges, M. D., Moorhouse, M. F., & Burley, J. T. (1995). *Application of nursing process and nursing diagnosis*. Philadelphia, PA: FA Davis.

Eager, C. A. (1997). Monitoring wound healing in the home health arena. *Advances in Wound Care, 10*, 54-57.

Fowler, E., Vesely, N., Pelfrey, M., Jordan, S., & Amberry, T. (1999). Wound care for persons with diabetes. *Home Healthcare Nurse, 17*, 437-444.

Gelberman, R. H., Woo, S. L., Lothringer, K., Akeson, W. H., & Amiel, D. (1982). Effects of early intermittent passive mobilization on healing canine flexor tendons. *Journal of Hand Surgery, 7*, 170-175.

Gogia, P. (1995). *Clinical wound management*. Thorofare, NJ: SLACK Incorporated.

Harding K. G. (1990). Wound care: Putting theory into clinical practice. In D. Krasner (Ed.), *Chronic wound care: A clinical source book for health care professionals* (1st ed., pp. 24). Wayne, PA: Health Management Publications.

Hardy, M. (1989). The biology of scar formation. *Physical Therapy, 69*, 1014-1032.

Hermann, G. G., Bagi, P., & Christoffersen, I. (1988). Early secondary suture versus healing by second intention of incisional abscesses. *Surgery, Gynecology & Obstetrics, 167*, 16-18.

Hermans, M. H., & van Wingerden, S. (1990). Treatment of industrial wounds with DuoDERM bordered: A report on medical and patient comfort aspects. *Journal of the Society of Occupational Medicine, 40*, 101-102.

Hunt, T. K., & Hussain, M. (1994). Can wound healing be a paradigm for tissue repair? *Medicine & Science in Sports & Exercise, 26*, 755-758.

Kloth, L. C., & McCulloch, J. M. (1995). The inflammatory response to wounding. In J. M. MuCulloch, L. C. Kloth, & J. A. Feedar (Eds.), *Wound helaing: Alternatives in management* (2nd ed., pp. 3). Philadelphia, PA: FA Davis.

Krasner, D., & Weir, D. (1997). Recommendations for using reverse staging to complete the M.D.S.-2. *Ostomy Wound Management, 43*, 14-17.

Kuroyanagi, Y. (2006). Regenerative medicine for skin. *Japanese Journal of Geriatrics, 43*, 326-329.

Langevin, H. M., Storch, K. N., Cipolla, M. J., White, S. L., Buttolph, T. R., & Taatjes, D. J. (2006). Fibroblast spreading induced by connective tissue stretch involves intracellular redistribution of alpha- and beta-actin. *Histochemistry and Cell Biology, 125*, 487-495.

Leininger, B. E., Rasmussen, T. E., Smith, D. L., Jenkins, D. H., & Coppola, C. (2006). Experience with wound VAC and delayed primary closure of contaminated soft tissue injuries in Iraq. *Journal of Trauma, 61*, 1207-1211.

Liao, J., Yang, L., Grashow, J., & Sacks, M. S. (2005). Molecular orientation of collagen in intact planar connective tissues under biaxial stretch. *Acta Biomaterialia, 1*, 45-54.

McGuiness, W., Dunn, S. V., & Jones, M. J. (2005). Developing an accurate system of measuring colour in a venous leg ulcer in order to assess healing. *Journal of Wound Care, 14*, 249-254.

Melis, P., van Noorden, C. J., & van der Horst, C. M. (2006). Long-term results of wounds closed under a significant amount of tension. *Plastic and Reconstructive Surgery, 117*, 259-265.

Messer, M. S. (1989). Wound care. *Critical Care Nursing Quarterly, 11*, 17.

Mulder, G., Brazinsky, B., & Seeley, J. (1995). Factors complicating wound repair. In J. M. McCulloch, L. C. Kloth, & J. A. Feedar (Eds.), *Healing alternatives in management* (2nd ed., pp. 47-59). Philadelphia, PA: FA Davis.

National Pressure Ulcer Advisory Panel. (1989). Pressure ulcers: Prevalence, cost, and risk assessment: Consensus development conference statement. *Decubitus, 292*, 24-28.

Park, S. H., & Silva, M. (2004). Neuromuscular electrical stimulation enhances fracture healing: Results of an animal model. *Journal of Orthopaedic Research, 22*, 382-387.

Peacock, E. E., Jr., Madden, J. W., & Trier, W. C. (1970). Biologic basis for the treatment of keloids and hypertrophic scars. *Southern Medical Journal, 63*, 755-760.

Peterson, W. W., Manske, P. R., Kain, C. C., & Lesker, P. A. (1986). Effect of flexor sheath integrity on tendon gliding: A biomechanical and histologic study. *Journal of Orthopaedic Research, 4*, 458-465.

Petrofsky, J., Schwab, E., Lo, T., Cuneo, M., George, J., & Kim, J., et al. (2005). Effects of electrical stimulation on skin blood flow in controls and in and around stage III and IV wounds in hairy and non hairy skin. *Medical Science Monitor, 11*, CR309-16.

Pollack, S. V. (1982). Wound healing: A review. III. nutritional factors affecting wound healing. *Journal of Enterostomal Therapy, 9*, 28-33.

Pollack, S. V. (1979). Wound healing: A review. III. nutritional factors affecting wound healing. *Journal of Dermatologic Surgery and Oncology, 5*, 615-619.

Poulsen, T. D., Freund, K. G., Arendrup, K., Nyhuus, P., & Pedersen, O. D. (1991). Polyurethane film (opsite) vs. impregnated gauze (jelonet) in the treatment of outpatient burns: A prospective, randomized study. *Burns: Journal of the International Society for Burn Injuries, 17*, 59-61.

Read, J., & Watt, F. (1988). A model for in vitro studies of epidermal homeostasis: Proliferation and involucrin sysnthesis by cultured human keratinocytesduring recovery after stripping off the suprabasal layers. *Journal of Investigative Dermatology, 90*, 739-743.

Reddy, M., Gill, S. S., & Rochon, P. A. (2006). Preventing pressure ulcers: A systematic review. *Journal of the American Medical Association, 296*, 974-984.

Reed, B., & Zarro, V. (1990). Inflammation and repair and the use of thermal agents. In S. L. Michlovitz (Ed.), *Thermal agents in rehabilitation* (2nd ed., pp. 3). Philadelphia, PA: F.A.Davis.

Schneider, L. A., Korber, A., Grabbe, S., & Dissemond, J. (2007). Influence of pH on wound-healing: A new perspective for wound-therapy? *Archives of Dermatological Research, 298*(9), 413-420.

Schumann, D. (1982). The nature of wound healing. *AORN Journal, 35*, 1067-1077.

Shea, J. D. (1975). Pressure sore: Classification and management. *Clinical Orthopedics, 112*, 89-100.

Steenvoorde, P., Calame, J. J., & Oskam, J. (2006). Maggot-treated wounds follow normal wound healing phases. *International Journal of Dermatology, 45*, 1477-1479.

Sussman, C., & Bates-Jensen, B. (1998). *Wound care*. Gaithersburg, MD: Aspen Publishers.

Thien, T. B., Becker, J. H., & Theis, J. C. (2004). Rehabilitation after surgery for flexor tendon injuries in the hand. *Cochrane Database of Systematic Reviews* (Online), *4*, CD003979.

Toporcer, T., & Radonak, J. (2006). Vacuum assisted closure therapy—overview of lesson and applications. *Casopis Lekaru Ceskych, 145*, 702-7; discussion 707.

Unger P., Eddy, J., & Raimastry, S. (1991). A controlled study of the effect of high voltage pulsed current on wound healing. *Physical Therapy, 71,* 118-119.

Valdes, A. M., Angderson, C., & Giner, J. J. (1999). A multidisciplinary, therapy-based, team approach for efficient and effective wound healing: A retrospective study. *Ostomy/wound Management, 45,* 30-36.

Van Rijswijk, L. (1995). Frequency of reassessment of pressure ulcers, NPUAP proceedings. *Advanced Wound Care, 8,* 19-24.

Vince, K. G., & Abdeen, A. (2006). Wound problems in total knee arthroplasty. *Clinical Orthopaedics and Related Research, 452,* 88-90.

Wagner, F. (1981). The dysvascular foot: A system for diagnosis and treatment. *Foot Ankle, 3,* 64-122.

Walters, M. D., Dombroski, R. A., Davidson, S. A., Mandel, P. C., & Gibbs, R. S. (1990). Reclosure of disrupted abdominal incisions. *Obstetrics and Gynecology, 76,* 597-602.

Woo, S. L., Gelberman, R. H., Cobb, N. G., Amiel, D., Lothringer, K., & Akeson, W. H. (1981). The importance of controlled passive mobilization on flexor tendon healing. A biomechanical study. *Acta Orthopaedica Scandinavica, 52,* 615-622.

# PAIN THEORY AND PERCEPTION

## Learning Objectives

1. Define pain.
2. Discuss chronic and acute pain cycles.
3. Identify the biopsychosocial approach to pain perception.
4. Discuss the pain pathways.
5. List the types and theories of pain and pain management.
6. Describe the importance of assessing pain and its relationship to the clinical reasoning process.

## Terminology

| | |
|---|---|
| Biopsychosocial approach | Opiate-mediated theory |
| Chronic pain | Pain |
| Neurogenic pain | Pain perception |
| Neuromatrix theory | Referred pain |
| Nociceptors | Trigger point |

Pain is one of the most frequent ailments for which individuals seek medical attention. Pain is a multidimensional experience, and many of the patients treated by occupational therapists report pain as one of the components which may limit their ability to actively participate in their occupational roles and tasks. The physiological response to pain can also have an effect on an individual occupational performance skills as an outcome of pain may be muscle spasm and guarding or protecting the injured area. Pain is a multidimensional experience and has psychological, socioeconomic and physiological effects on the individual and community (Talo, Rytokoski, Hamalainen, & Kallio, 1996). Pain has been characterized as being chronic or acute. *Acute* pain, which lasts from seconds to days, has a biologic function, warning the individual of potential injury or that something is wrong. *Chronic* pain lacks the biological imperative of acute pain and is pain which recurs at intervals or persists and is of long duration. Chronic pain is often associated with anguish, apprehension, depression, or hopelessness. Pain that is perceived to be in areas other than where the nociceptors (pain receptors) were stimulated is known as referred pain. Low back pain has been described as acute, persistent, and chronic (DeRosa & Porterfield, 1992). This model is based on the nature of the symptoms, the patient's response to the symptoms, and the prescribed treatment strategies.

Most people have experienced nociceptive pain, which is typically related to a specific stimulus such as a hot or sharp sensation or the result of aching or throbbing that signals tissue irritation, impending injury, or an actual injury. Nociceptors are receptors located in the skin, viscera, cardiac, and skeletal muscle that receive and transmit painful stimuli. When nociceptors are activated in an affected area, signals are transmitted to the brain via the peripheral nerves and spinal cord. However, complex spinal reflexes may also be activated, which are followed by perception, cognitive, and affective responses, and possibly voluntary actions. Visceral pain is a subtype of nociceptive pain but tends to be sudden and often poorly localized, whereas somatic pain is more constant and well localized. Neuropathic pain can occur when there is an illness or injury in the peripheral nervous system (PNS) or central nervous systems (CNS). Neuropathic pain will present as burning, lancinating, or electric shock-like sensations and can be the result of nonpainful stimulus, such as light touch, as with persistent allodynia. Neuropathic pain may last for many months or even years after the damaged tissues have healed even though the pain signals no longer represent an ongoing or potential injury. Neuropathic pain is frequently chronic and treatment is often more complex. When an injury or illness occurs to the body, the damaged tissue will release intracellular chemical contents, such as histamine, serotonln, bradykinin, and hydrogen ions, that cause localized inflammation. Injury to the tissue causes a release of prostaglandin and bradykinin that sensitizes the nociceptors and causes a modification of the nerve's threshold. Nociceptors then release a neuropeptide known as substance P (pain) that sends the electrical impulse through the afferent fiber to the spinal cord. This response to an injury or infection initiates an orchestrated sequence of events and histochemical changes that begin the healing process in which the signs of inflammation include redness, swelling, increased local temperature, and pain.

## Theoretical Perspectives

There are a variety of theoretical perspectives of chronic pain, although the majority of the perspectives include the psychological factors of affective, behavioral, cognitive, situational, and sensory-physical (Crook, Milner, Schultz, & Stringer, 2002; Fordyce, 1976; Im, 2006). Theoretical perspectives on chronic pain have been categorized as *restrictive* and include mind-body dualism, psychological, radical operant behavioral, and radical cognitive. Other theoretical perspectives have been categorized as *comprehensive* based on the International Association for the Study of Pain (IASP): gate control, nonradical operant-behavioral, and cognitive-behavioral (McWilliams & Asmundson, 2007; Novy, Nelson, Francis, & Turk, 1995; Turner, Holtzman, & Mancl, 2006).

## Neuromatrix

The neuromatrix theory describes a theoretical framework in which the body-self is modulated by traditional sensory inputs as well as the stress system and cognitive functions of the brain. The body-self neuromatrix consists of the neurological network including the somatosensory, limbic, and thalmacortical components that subserve

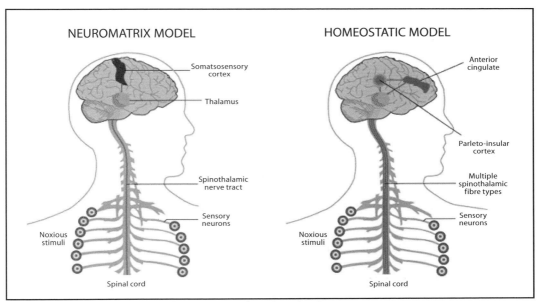

NEUROMATRIX MODEL

Somatsosensory
cortex

Thalamus

Spinothalamic
nerve tract

Sensory
neurons

Noxious
stimuli

Spinal cord

HOMEOSTATIC MODEL

Anterior
cingulate

Parleto-insular
cortex

Multiple
spinothalamic
fibre types

Sensory
neurons

Noxious
stimuli

Spinal cord

**Figure 4-1.** Neuromatrix and homeostatic theories of pain.

the sensory-discriminative, affective-motivational, and evaluative-cognitive aspect of an individual's pain experience. Each individual has a unique "neurosignature" output that determines the particular qualities and properties of the pain experience and behaviors. Inputs that impact this neuromatrix in an individual include sensory inputs from the cutaneous, visceral, and somatic receptors; visual and sensory inputs that influence the cognitive interpretation of the input or situation; phasic and tonic cognitive and emotional inputs from areas of the brain; intrinsic neural inhibitory modulation in brain function; and the activity of the body's stress-reglulation systems, which include cytokines and endocrine, autonomic, immune, and opioid systems. The neuromatrix theory proposes a unique, dynamic approach to pain and the associated outcomes seen by occupational therapists (Melzack, 1992; Melzack, 1999a; Melzack, 1999b; Melzack, 2001).

Recent advances in neuroscience have provided an additional perspective on pain theory and its functional implications. Pain is described as a multidimensional experience that occurs due to characteristic "neurosignature" patterns of nerve impuses, which are generated by a widely distributed neural network-the "body-self neuromatrix" in the brain. The neuromatrix theory of pain proposes that the output patterns of the body-self neuromatrix initiate perceptual, homeostatic, and behavioral responses after injury, pathology, or chronic stress (Figure 4-1). The neuromatrix theory purports that pain is produced by the output of a widely distributed neural network in the brain rather than by the sensory input evoked by injury, inflammation, or pathology. An individual's unique neuromatrix is genetically determined and modified by sensory experience, and is the mechanism which generates the neural pattern and produces pain. The output of the neuromatrix can be modified and is influenced by multiple factors, of which the somatic sensory input is one factor (Melzack, 1999a; Melzack, 2005).

# Gate Control and Opiate-Mediated Pain

Historically, pain was believed to be directly related to the amount of tissue damage; the more severe the injury, it was thought, the more severe the pain. During World War I, however, the components of the gate control theory began to be developed as physicians noted that some of the soldiers who were terribly disfigured had minimal if any pain. These initial concepts were further developed by Wall and Melzack during the 1960s with their gate theory of pain. Wall and Melzack postulated that modulation of periphal stimuli occurred in the dorsal horn of the spinal cord acting as a gate to the varying amounts of input from the large A-fibers that would close the gate; and small C-fibers that would tend to "open" the gate. Wall and Melzack's work was an impetus into the advancement of electrotherapeutic agents, as the use of electrical stimulation of sensory fibers could effectively decrease an individuals pain (Melzack, 1965).

Advances in imaging and neuroscience also led other researchers to explore the influence of pain-mediating chemicals produced by the body known as endogenous opiods. Endogenous opiods affect both the CNS and PNS through the interaction of specific chemoreceptors and pain-mediating substances. There are essentially three forms of opiods that have a pain-mediating effect: enkephalins, dynorphins, and beta-endorphins; each with a respective pain chemoreceptor binding site on the neurons. Enkephalin's are found in the dorsal horn and are released by spinal interneurons. These histochemicals are transmitted by C-fibers from the periphery to the dorsal horn. Beta-endorphins are located in the hypothalamus and are released into the bloodstream with stress (Kalliomaki et al., 2004; Kawakita et al., 2006; McMullan & Lumb, 2006; Perl, 1984; Zhang & Bao, 2006).

There are many definitions of pain and a variety of clinical phenomena experienced by our patients. Pain has been defined as the emotion that is the opposite of pleasure (Sweet, 1959), an "emotional experience" caused by tissue injury or described by the patient in terms of tissue damage, or both (Steinbach, 1968). The IASP defines pain as an unpleasant sensory or emotional experience which is associated with actual or potential tissue damage or which is described in terms of such damage (Hakim, 1995). Musculoskeletal pain is often the primary complaint of individuals reporting both acute and chronic pain, and is frequently seen in individuals with arthritis (Kazis, Meenan, & Anderson, 1983; Keefe & Egert, 2001). Pain occurs when there is a noxious event such as an injury or inflammation to an area of the body. This event or injury causes an excitation of nociceptors in somatic or visceral tissue.

Because pain is such a universal human experience and many of the patients treated by occupational therapists have pain, an understanding of the primary characteristics of pain and interventions that can affect the pain cycle is important. Chronic pain affects all facets of life and society; from its impact on the economy, employment, and health care systems, to the impact on an individual's functional performance in life roles and tasks. By actively treating pain in our patients through the technologies available to us, we are able to more fully integrate our patients into their primary roles and activities, improving outcomes and improving the quality of life.

# Biopsychosocial Approach

Pain perception is a multifaceted reaction based on anatomical, physiological, chemical, and psychological factors. These interrelated factors have led to the development of a biopsychosocial approach to the conceptualization and treatment of persistent pain. Biopsychosocial approaches view pain as a complex experience affected by sensory input, but also closely influenced and related to *behavioral, cognitive-affective*, and *environmental factors*. These three variables can influence and be influenced by changes in a competing set of variables. Variables that may influence an individual's perception and level of pain may include such factors as pain-related catastrophizing, perceived social support, pain beliefs, and pain coping. The biopsychosocial variables and approach provide a more comprehensive perspective on pain consistent with the underlying values of occupational therapy. The biopsychosocial model of pain posits that pain perception is influenced by the dynamic interactions among the biologic, psychosocial, and sociocultural factors. For example, a young, newly diagnosed patient with rheumatoid arthritis becomes withdrawn, depressed (a cognitive-behavioral variable), and is in denial (cognitive behavioral variable). She is resistant to help and is unwilling to take her medication which can decrease the disease activity and symptoms (a biological variable). Because of her lack of follow-through and resistance to treatment, she becomes dependent on her spouse, family, and friends (an environmental factor), limiting her occupational behaviors and roles. Because of the influence and dynamic interaction between these competing variables (cognitive-behavioral, biological, and environmental), the patient experiences high levels of pain (Fillingim, 2005; Keefe & Egert, 2001; McWilliams & Asmundson, 2007; Osborne, Jensen, Ehde, Hanley, & Kraft, 2007).

To effectively treat the patient with persistent pain, the therapist must recognize the influence and interactions of the factors underlying the biopsychosocial approach and develop strategies and interventions related to each area. The patient and his or her condition must be viewed holistically within their occupational context. Treating the symptom of pain with transcutaneous electrical nerve stimulation (TENS) or other technologies and interventions without addressing the underlying influence of the environmental, cognitive-behavioral, or biological variables and their interaction will result in less than adequate outcomes. A common intervention used to modify the perception of pain is TENS. TENS can play an important role in the treatment and management of pain, and can be an effective adjunct to conventional occupational therapy intervention. However, to fully enhance the patient's functional independence and outcomes, TENS should never be used in isolation or in place of traditional occupational therapy interventions without regard to the greater contextual psychosocial situation and dynamics.

## Pain Pathways

Pain is a multidimensional phenomenon that profoundly affects an individual psychologically, socioeconomically, and physiologically. Patients experiencing chronic or acute pain may be depressed, anxious, withdrawn, or irritable, and display a variety of maladaptive behavioral responses. Pain is a protective response and is the body's way of informing the individual that something is wrong or that there may be potential tissue damage. The body responds to trauma through a complex series of reactions, including those associated with the sympathetic response of the autonomic nervous system (ANS), the "fight-or-flight" response.

Nociceptors are receptors located in the skin, viscera, cardiac, and skeletal muscle that receive and transmit painful stimuli (Bonica, 1990; Sherrington, 1906). Nociceptors may also be affected by the release of endogenous pain-producing substances into the tissue, including potassium, serotonin, bradykinin histamine, prostaglandins, and substance P, which then cause a cascade of effects (Lariviere, McBurney, Frot, & Balaban, 2005; McMullan & Lumb, 2006; Zhang & Bao, 2006; Perl, 1984). Nociceptors are sensory receptors specific to pain that identify potential or actual tissue damage and are located in the skin, viscera, cardiac and skeletal muscles, and respond to different stimulus inputs. Nociceptors are sensitive and responsive to mechanical distortion, variations in the chemical components in the tissue fluid, and by thermal changes. These specialized receptors possess variable thresholds, some high, some low. Nociceptors respond to the stimulus and signal actual or potential damage to the tissue (Godfrey, 2005; Torebjork & Hallin, 1973; Zhang & Bao, 2006). Nociceptors carry the action potential by the primary afferent (sensory) neuron, either small myelinated A-delta fibers or small unmyelinated C-fibers. The small myelinated A-delta fibers conduct the impulses at a faster rate than the C-fibers and stimulation of them may cause a localized sharp "pricking" pain sensation. Stimulation of the unmyelinated C-fibers causes a dull, poorly localized burning sensation. Neural activity is carried by these two primary pathways to the higher centers in the brain. The A-delta and C-fibers terminate at various levels in the spinal cord in the dorsal horns. Wide dynamic range neurons and nociceptive-specific neurons receive input from the A delta and C-fibers, assisting in discriminating the type of pain. These wide dynamic range cells are also known as T (transmission) cells (Dubner & Bennett, 1983; Henry, 2004).

There are several ascending tracts (pathways) that transmit pain signals to the brain. Axons of the majority of the transmission cells cross over, ascending as the lateral spinothalamic tract terminating in the thalamus. This pathway terminates in the portion of the brain known as the somatosensory cortex and perceives pain information as sharp, discriminative, and localized. Other signals are carried by the spinoreticulothalamic pathway which terminates in the reticular formation of the brainstem and thalamus. Axons of this pathway also connect to the midbrain and to structures of the limbic system, basal ganglia and cerebral cortex. This pathway carries information that is perceived as diffuse, poorly localized somatic and visceral pain (Hanegan, 1992; Henry, 2004; Kalliomaki et al., 2004; McMullan & Lumb, 2006). Descending inhibitory fibers located in the higher brain centers release neurotransmitters, including norepinephrine, serotonin, and enkephalins, which moderate and affect the flow of afferent impulses. These inhibitory or descending tracts are activated by endogenous opioids and other neurotransmitters (Fields, Heinricher, & Mason, 1991; Gillman & Lichtigfeld, 1985; Charman, 1989).

# Types of Pain

Pain can be categorized as acute, chronic, referred, and can signal potential or actual tissue damage. Theories related to understanding pain, led to advances in clinical interventions to modulate pain. TENS has been used therapeutically for pain management for approximately 20 years. The IASP has defined pain as an unpleasant sensory and emotional experience associated with actual or potential tissue damage (Fedorczyk, 1997). Though the classification of pain may differ, there are two primary classifications of pain— acute and chronic— though some researchers identify referred pain as a third type. Dependent upon the etiology and clinical manifestations of the condition, each level or type of pain will require a unique therapeutic intervention.

Acute pain has been described as the pain most closely associated with tissue damage and nociception. Acute pain usually occurs with a rapid, sudden onset, and is considered a warning signal by the body that tissue damage or injury is about to occur, or has already occurred. There is most often an underlying etiology, and since acute pain signals tissue damage, use of therapeutic physical modalities would be indicated as part of the treatment approach to the condition (Travell, 1976).

Chronic pain is often poorly localized, with the underlying cause not being fully understood or clear to the patient or clinician. Chronic pain is often of long duration and pervades the individual's life more completely. Physical modalities and technologies are usually ineffective in consistently relieving pain in patients with chronic pain conditions. Persistent pain is pain which continues for long periods of time or is consistently recurrent. Persistent pain is all consuming, affecting all areas of the individual's occupational behaviors. Persistent pain is most effectively treated by limited use of physical agent technologies, with an emphasis placed on behavior modification techniques, patient education, medication, and general conditioning.

Referred pain is pain felt at a site different from the original source of the injury or disease. Irritable points in the muscle that referred pain were identified by Travell (1976) as "trigger points." A trigger point is a small, localized, hypersensitive area located in the muscle or fascia. Trigger points can be clinically located primarily through palpation. Patients will often be able to localize and identify trigger points when questioned. If the trigger point is stimulated by pressure, heat, or cold, the pain is referred to a remote site. A diagnostic criterion for trigger points includes tenderness in a hyperirritable spot within a palpable taut band, a local twitch response elicited by snapping palpation, and elicited referred pain with palpation. Patients with myofascial pain syndrome (MPS) will have myofascial trigger points located within taut bands of skeletal muscle fibers (Fernandez-de-Las-Penas, Alonso-Blanco, & Miangolarra, 2006; Fernandez-de-Las-Penas, Alonso-Blanco, Cuadrado, & Pareja, 2006; Hong, 2006). Trigger points can be stimulated by acute overload, overwork, fatigue, cooling, and through direct trauma to the

---

### SOURCES OF PAIN

- Peripheral neurogenic pain
- Peripheral nociceptive pain
- CNS-mediated pain
- Autonomic nervous system mediation of pain
- Affective motivational components

---

muscle. Patients will often report localized deep tenderness, which is often associated with a tight band of skeletal muscle or in the muscle fascia. The trigger point is identifiable as pain upon palpation or compression.

An understanding and identification of the sources of pain are components of effectively utilizing TENS and physical agent technologies. The IASP has identified five different sources of pain: *peripheral neurogenic pain, peripheral nociceptive sources of pain, central nervous system-mediated pain, autonomic nervous system mediation of pain*, and the *affective motivational component*. Peripheral neurogenic pain is caused by the involvement of the neural tissues resulting in mechanical and physiological changes in the body. Clinically, these changes are observed as limitation in movement, pain, paresthesias, or sensory changes. Peripheral nociceptive pain is accompanied by inflammation secondary to the release of chemical mediators such as prostaglandins, histamines, and bradykinins. Peripheral nociceptive pain sources are often the target of involved tissues, and may be mechanical in origin resulting in local dysfunction. The peripheral neurogenic and peripheral nociceptive sources of pain are those most often encountered by the clinician, and respond most successfully to therapeutic intervention and physical agent technologies.

If the pain is nociceptive or neuropathic, the next step is to evaluate the cause or specific source of the pain, and to determine if it is reversible. An ongoing or impending injury is considered nociceptive pain and accurate determination and treatment of the problem becomes a critical matter. The initial evaluation should determine what the fundamental pathology is; whether there is an underlying sprain, tear, fracture, infection, obstruction, or foreign body, and whether the inflammation is caused by an underlying arthritic or autoimmune disorder. However, myofascial pain may indicate there are abnormal acute or chronic muscle stresses. Clear, concise, and accurate differential diagnosis is crucial to clinical reasoning and in determining the appropriate intervention.

## Assessment of Pain

When evaluating a patient's complaint of pain, it is important to remember that pain is an experience, rather than a bodily function, and it must be placed within the greater contextual picture. An individual's psychological and mental factor as well as situational factors can either trigger or extinguish the pain experience. These additional factors can modify the individual's perception of pain through their influence on the spinal processing of pain through the descending inhibitory and facilitory neural pathways. Suffering should not be considered synonymous with pain as there may be different intensities of pain for similar injuries as well as differing degrees of suffering, distress and emotional impact on each individual. There may be daily, monthly, and seasonal patterns associated with pain that provide additional clues about the etiology of the pain. For example, a patient with arthritis may report that their pain is worse in the mornings or during cold, damp seasons. A patient with migraine headaches may report patterns associated with a variety of factors such as stress or menstrual cycling. It is crucial to ask about any aggravating or alleviating factors which may lead to exacerbation or even reduction of the pain. By understanding such activities, a more accurate diagnosis may be obtained, which will assist in refining the appropriate treatment intervention (Chen, Yu, & Wong, 2005; Evans, Shipton, & Keenan, 2005; Im, 2006; Oddson, Clancy, & McGrath, 2006; Stimmel, Crayton, Rice, & Raffeld, 2006; ten Klooster et al., 2006).

To accurately assess the nature and origin of the patient's pain, a thorough patient history should be a component of the evaluation that includes a description of the pain, how the pain developed, the location of the pain and whether it has spread, the pattern of the pain over time, the patient's level of function and impairment, any previous attempted treatments, and the patient's impression about the effectiveness previous treatments. The words and phrases that the patient uses to describe the pain can assist in determining the type of pain and its emotional impact on the individual. Associated symptoms such as nausea, sweating, flushing, or sensations of hot or cold in the affected area may indicate an autonomic or sympathetic component of the pain. Since individuals will have different perceptions about the intensity of pain, obtaining this information is very important to help gauge the impact of the pain and to monitor any changes (Fillingim, 2005; McLean, Clauw, Abelson, & Liberzon, 2005).

Having a primary understanding of pain-mediation principles facilitates the clinical reasoning process in determining the appropriate intervention for pain control and management. A complete evaluation that assesses pain and function, identifies movement abnormalities, and evaluates anatomical tissue structures assists in identifying realistic treatment goals and interventions. Pain is a very subjective experience, and clearly identifying the type, location, and sensation of pain in a patient can become problematic. Utilizing both subjective patient and objective descriptions of pain measures assists in determining the treatment approach, potential response to intervention, and clinical efficacy. Therapists must also assess the affective motivational component and sources of pain which may influence the evaluation, treatment, prognosis, and outcomes. There are a number of pain-related scales and instruments that are often specific to a particular discipline such as dental surgery (e.g., the Visual Analog Scale [VAS], the Dental Discomfort Questionnaire, etc.). Aside from the patient's subjective reporting of pain, there are two primary tools which can be used by clinicians to provide a more objective mechanism of reporting—the McGill Pain Questionnaire and VAS (Ceran & Ozcan, 2006; Chang, Chen, & Huang, 2006; Kievit et al., 2006; McWilliams & Asmundson, 2007; Pallant, Misajon, Bennett, & Manderson, 2006; Poole, Bramwell, & Murphy, 2006).

## McGill Pain Questionnaire

The McGill Pain Questionnaire (MPQ) is frequently utilized during the initial evaluation. It consists of three parts and includes body diagrams to assist the patient in identifying and locating the area of pain as well as determining whether the pain is internal, external, or both. The MPQ also includes a Pain Rating Index, which consists of a collection of words grouped into categories. The patient is given a standardized list of adjectives and asked to select the word that best describes the pain. The MPQ provides the patient with a method describing the pain and intensity of pain related to activity. Due to the ability to score the MPQ, it provides the clinician with a quantitative method of assessing pain in a patient. Sometimes the patient is also told to keep a diary of the pain, but this may be counterproductive because it can be a continual reminder of the pain (Byrne et al., 1982; Chang et al., 2006; Klepac, Dowling, & Hauge, 1981; Melzack, 1975; Yakut, Yakut, Bayar, & Uygur, 2006).

## Visual Analog Scale

There are several types of pain scales that can provide the clinician with primary information on the patient's response to pain. Utilizing a pain scale provides a mechanism to determine changes and patterns in the level and/or type of pain experienced by the patient. The VAS is the most frequently-used method to assess pain intensity and any changes that occur over time. The VAS provides the clinician with a quick and relatively accurate method for patients to rate their pain. Visual and analog scales have a 10 cm line marked on a paper with the descriptors: "Pain as bad as it could be" on the left, and "no pain" on the right side of the line (Figure 4-2). Patients are asked to mark along the line to indicate the amount or intensity of pain they are experiencing. This scale can be administered before and after treatment sessions, and the therapist measures the distance along the continuum to provide a method of rating the patient's response. Because of the ease of application, if used consistently, the VAS can assist the clinician in monitoring patient progress and response to treatment interventions (Table 4-1). The same assessment can be given verbally by asking the patient on a scale of 0 to 10, with 0 representing no pain and 10 being the worst pain level, to indicate how much pain he or she is experiencing. The FACES Assessment for Children offers a similar method for young patients as the scale displays cartoon-like pictures

**Figure 4-2.** Analog pain scales.

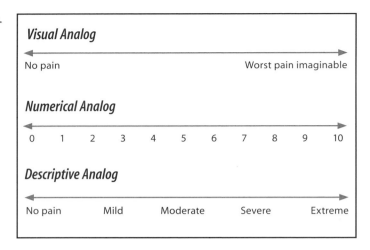

**Table 4-1**

## PAIN SCALE

| | |
|---|---|
| 10+ | Maximal pain |
| 10 | Very, very strong pain |
| 9 | |
| 8 | |
| 7 | Very strong pain |
| 6 | |
| 5 | Strong pain |
| 4 | Somewhat strong pain |
| 3 | Moderate pain |
| 2 | Weak pain |
| 1 | Very weak pain |
| 0.5 | Very, very weak pain |
| 0 | No pain at all |

Adapted from Borg, G. A. V. (1982). Psychological bases of perceived exertion. *Medicine & Science in Sports & Exercise*, 14, 377-388.

of faces in various degrees of distress, and the child is asked to choose the one that best represents the pain. The Wong-Baker FACES Pain Rating Scale was also developed to assess pain in children (Figure 4-3).

# Summary

An understanding and appreciation of pain in our patients provides the clinician with an additional clue in the clinical reasoning process. Pain is a component of many of the soft tissue injuries that can be treated with physical agent technologies. Along

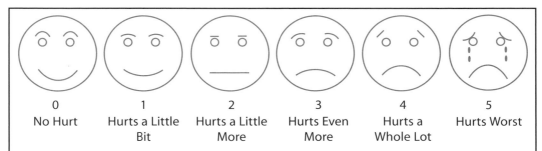

0 — No Hurt  
1 — Hurts a Little Bit  
2 — Hurts a Little More  
3 — Hurts Even More  
4 — Hurts a Whole Lot  
5 — Hurts Worst

**Brief word instructions**: Point to each face using the words to describe the pain intensity. Ask the child to choose the face that best describes own pain and record the appropriate number.

**Original instructions**: Explain to the person that each face is for a person who feels happy because he has no pain (hurt) or sad because he has some or a lot of pain. *Face 0* is very happy because he doesn't hurt at all. *Face 1* hurts just a little bit. *Face 2* hurts a little more. *Face 3* hurts even more. *Face 4* hurts a whole lot. *Face 5* hurts as much as you can imagine, although one doesn't have to be crying to feel this bad. Ask the person to choose the face that best describes how he/she is feeling.

Rating scale is recommended for persons age 3 years and older.

**Figure 4-3.** Wong-Baker FACES Pain Rating Scale (Adapted from Hockenberry, M. J., Wilson, D., & Winkelstein, M. L. (2005). *Wong's essentials of pediatric nursing.* [7th ed., p. 1259]. St. Louis, MO: Mosby).

with pain, the patient may display any number of occupational performance components, including altered sensation, edema, muscle guarding, weakness, or loss of movement.

Recognizing pain patterns associated with different sources of pain, and understanding the patient's altered biomechanics and musculoskeletal compensations will facilitate treatment outcomes and enhance appropriate occupational interventions.

# References

Bonica, J. J. (1990). *The management of pain, vols I and II*. Malvern, PA: Lea & Febiger.

Byrne, M., Troy, A., Bradley, L. A., Marchisello, P. J., Geisinger, K. F., & Van der Heide, L. H., et al. (1982). Cross-validation of the factor structure of the McGill pain questionnaire. *Pain, 13*, 193-201.

Ceran, F., & Ozcan, A. (2006). The relationship of the functional rating index with disability, pain, and quality of life in patients with low back pain. *Medical Science Monitor: International Medical Journal of Experimental and Clinical Research, 12*, CR435-9.

Chang, M. Y., Chen, C. H., & Huang, K. F. (2006). A comparison of massage effects on labor pain using the McGill pain questionnaire. *Journal of Nursing Research, 14*, 190-197.

Charman, R. A. (1989). Pain theory and physiotherapy. *Physiotherapy, 75*, 247-254.

Chen, W. Q., Yu, I. T., & Wong, T. W. (2005). Impact of occupational stress and other psychosocial factors on musculoskeletal pain among Chinese offshore oil installation workers. *Occupational and Environmental Medicine, 62*, 251-256.

Crook, J., Milner, R., Schultz, I. Z., & Stringer, B. (2002). Determinants of occupational disability following a low back injury: A critical review of the literature. *Journal of Occupational Rehabilitation, 12*, 277-295.

DeRosa, C. P., & Porterfield, J. A. (1992). A physical therapy model for the treatment of low back pain. *Physical Therapy, 72*, 261-9; discussion 270-2.

Dubner, R., & Bennett, G. J. (1983). Spinal and trigeminal mechanisms of nociception. *Annual Review of Neuroscience, 6*, 381-418.

Evans, S., Shipton, E. A., & Keenan, T. R. (2005). Psychosocial functioning of mothers with chronic pain: A comparison to pain-free controls. *European Journal of Pain (London, England), 9*, 683-690.

Fedorczyk, J. (1997). The role of physical agents in modulating pain. *Journal of Hand Therapy, 10*, 110-121.

Fernandez-de-Las-Penas, C., Alonso-Blanco, C., Cuadrado, M. L., & Pareja, J. A. (2006). Myofascial trigger points in the suboccipital muscles in episodic tension-type headache. *Manual Therapy, 11*, 225-230.

Fernandez-de-Las-Penas, C., Alonso-Blanco, C., & Miangolarra, J. C. (2006). Myofascial trigger points in subjects presenting with mechanical neck pain: A blinded, controlled study. *Manual Therapy, 12(1), 29-33.*

Fields, H. L., Heinricher, M. M., & Mason, P. (1991). Neurotransmitters in nociceptive modulatory circuits. *Annual Review of Neuroscience, 14*, 219-245.

Fillingim, R. B. (2005). Individual differences in pain responses. *Current Rheumatology Reports, 7*, 342-347.

Fordyce, W. E. (1976). *Behavior methods for chronic pain and illness.* St. Louis, MO: C.V. Mosby.

Gillman, M. A., & Lichtigfeld, F. J. (1985). A pharmacological overview of opioid mechanisms mediating analgesia and hyperalgesia. *Neurological Research, 7*, 106-119.

Godfrey, H. (2005). Understanding pain, part 1: Physiology of pain. *British Journal of Nursing (Mark Allen Publishing), 14*, 846-852.

Hakim, M. H. (1995). Pain and its measurement. *Hamdard., 38*, 86-90.

Hanegan, J. L. (1992). Principles of nociception. In M. R. Gersch (Ed.), *Electrotherapy in rehabilitation* (1st ed., p. 26). Philadelphia, PA: FA Davis.

Henry, J. L. (2004). Future basic science directions into mechanisms of neuropathic pain. *Journal of Orofacial Pain, 18*, 306-310.

Hong, C. Z. (2006). Treatment of myofascial pain syndrome. *Current Pain and Headache Reports, 10*, 345-349.

Im, E. O. (2006). A situation-specific theory of Caucasian cancer patients' pain experience. *ANS.Advances in Nursing Science, 29*, 232-244.

Kalliomaki, M. L., Pertovaara, A., Brandt, A., Wei, H., Pietila, P., & Kalmari, J., et al. (2004). Prolactin-releasing peptide affects pain, allodynia and autonomic reflexes through medullary mechanisms. *Neuropharmacology, 46*, 412-424.

Kawakita, K., Shinbara, H., Imai, K., Fukuda, F., Yano, T., & Kuriyama, K. (2006). How do acupuncture and moxibustion act? Focusing on the progress in japanese acupuncture research. *Journal of Pharmacological Sciences, 100*, 443-459.

Kazis, L. E., Meenan, R. F., & Anderson, J. (1983). Pain in the rheumatic diseases: Investigations of a key health status component. *Arthritis Rheum, 8*, 1017-1022.

Keefe, F. J., & Egert, J. (2001). A cognitive behavioral perspective on patients with cumulative trauma disorders. *Psychosocial aspects of musculoskeletal disorders in office work.* (1st ed.). Durham, NC: Taylor and Francis.

Kievit, W., Welsing, P. M., Adang, E. M., Eijsbouts, A. M., Krabbe, P. F., & van Riel, P. L. (2006). Comment on the use of self-reporting instruments to assess patients with rheumatoid arthritis: The longitudinal association between the DAS28 and the VAS general health. *Arthritis and Rheumatism, 55*, 745-750.

Klepac, R. K., Dowling, J., & Hauge, G. (1981). Sensitivity of the McGill pain questionnaire to intensity and quality of laboratory pain. *Pain, 10*, 199-207.

Lariviere, W. R., McBurney, D. H., Frot, M., & Balaban, C. D. (2005). Tonic, phasic, and integrator components of psychophysical responses to topical capsaicin account for differences of location and sex. *Journal of Pain, 6*, 777-781.

McLean, S. A., Clauw, D. J., Abelson, J. L., & Liberzon, I. (2005). The development of persistent pain and psychological morbidity after motor vehicle collision: Integrating the potential role of stress response systems into a biopsychosocial model. *Psychosomatic Medicine, 67*, 783-790.

McMullan, S., & Lumb, B. M. (2006). Spinal dorsal horn neuronal responses to myelinated versus unmyelinated heat nociceptors and their modulation by activation of the periaqueductal grey in the rat. *Journal of Physiology, 576*, 547-556.

McWilliams, L. A., & Asmundson, G. J. (2007). The relationship of adult attachment dimensions to pain-related fear, hypervigilance, and catastrophizing. *Pain, 127*, 27-34.

Melzack, R. (2005). Evolution of the neuromatrix theory of pain. the prithvi raj lecture: Presented at the third world congress of world institute of pain, barcelona 2004. *Pain Practice, 5*, 85-94.

Melzack, R. (2001). Pain and the neuromatrix in the brain. *Journal of Dental Education, 65*, 1378-1382.

Melzack, R. (1999a). From the gate to the neuromatrix. *Pain, Suppl 6*, S121-6.

Melzack, R. (1999b). Pain—an overview. *Acta Anaesthesiologica Scandinavica, 43*, 880-884.

Melzack, R. (1992). Phantom limb pain. *Patologicheskaia Fiziologiia i Eksperimental'Naia Terapiia, 4*, 52-54.

Melzack, R. (1975). The McGill pain questionnaire: Major properties and scoring methods. *Pain, 1*, 277-299.

Melzack, R., Wall, P. D. (1965). Pain mechanisms: A new theory. *Science, 150*, 971.

Novy, D. M., Nelson, D. V., Francis, D. J., & Turk, D. C. (1995). Perspectives of chronic pain: An evaluative comparison of restrictive and comprehensive models. *Psychological Bulletin, 118*, 238-247.

Oddson, B. E., Clancy, C. A., & McGrath, P. J. (2006). The role of pain in reduced quality of life and depressive symptomology in children with spina bifida. *Clinical Journal of Pain, 22*, 784-789.

Osborne, T. L., Jensen, M. P., Ehde, D. M., Hanley, M. A., & Kraft, G. (2007). Psychosocial factors associated with pain intensity, pain-related interference, and psychological functioning in persons with multiple sclerosis and pain. *Pain, 127*, 52-62.

Pallant, J. F., Misajon, R., Bennett, E., & Manderson, L. (2006). Measuring the impact and distress of health problems from the individual's perspective: Development of the perceived impact of problem profile (PIPP). *Health and Quality of Life Outcomes, 4*, 36.

Perl, E. R. (1984). Characteristics of nociceptors and their activation of neurons in the superficial dorsal horn: First steps for the sensation of pain. In L. Kruger, & J. C. Liebeskind (Eds.), *Advances in pain research and therapy* (6th ed., p. 23). New York: Raven Press.

Poole, H., Bramwell, R., & Murphy, P. (2006). Factor structure of the beck depression inventory-II in patients with chronic pain. *Clinical Journal of Pain, 22*, 790-798.

Price, D., D., & Harkins, S. W. (1987). Combined use of experimental pain and visual analogue scales in providing standardized measurements of clinical pain. *Clinical Journal of Pain, 3*, 1.

Sherrington, C., S. (1906). *The integrative action of the nervous system.* New York: Scribner.

Steinbach, R. A. (1968). *Pain—A psychophysiological analysis.* New York: Academic Press.

Stimmel, T., Crayton, C., Rice, T., & Raffeld, P. M. (2006). Pain perception as a function of self-focused rumination. *Perceptual and Motor Skills, 103*, 21-28.

Sweet, W. H. (1959). *Pain—Handbook of physiology, 1*, 14-19.

Talo, S., Rytokoski, U., Hamalainen, A., & Kallio, V. (1996). The biopsychosocial disease consequence model in rehabilitation: Model development in the finnish 'work hardening' programme for chronic pain. *Internationale Zeitschrift Fur Rehabilitationsforschung.Revue Internationale De Recherches De Readaptation, 19*, 93-109.

ten Klooster, P. M., Vlaar, A. P., Taal, E., Gheith, R. E., Rasker, J. J., & El-Garf, A. K., et al. (2006). The validity and reliability of the graphic rating scale and verbal rating scale for measuring pain across cultures: A study in egyptian and dutch women with rheumatoid arthritis. *The Clinical Journal of Pain, 22*, 827-830.

Torebjork, H. E., & Hallin, R. G. (1973). Perceptual changes accompanying controlled preferential blocking of A and C fibre responses in intact human skin nerves. *Experimentelle Hirnforschung. Experimentation Cerebrale, 16*, 321-332.

Travell, J. (1976). Myofascial trigger points: Clinical view. In J. J. Bonica, & D. G. Able-Fessard (Eds.), *Advances in pain research and therapy* (2nd ed., pp. 919). New York: Raven Press.

Turner, J. A., Holtzman, S., & Mancl, L. (2006). Mediators, moderators, and predictors of therapeutic change in cognitive-behavioral therapy for chronic pain. *Pain, 127*(3), 276-286.

Yakut, Y., Yakut, E., Bayar, K., & Uygur, F. (2006). Reliability and validity of the Turkish version short-form McGill pain questionnaire in patients with rheumatoid arthritis. *Clinical Rheumatology,...*

Zhang, X., & Bao, L. (2006). The development and modulation of nociceptive circuitry. *Current Opinion in Neurobiology, 16*, 460-466.

# Chapter 5

# CRYOTHERAPY

## Learning Objectives

1. List the biophysical and biophysiological changes that occur with cryotherapy.
2. Identify the indications, contraindications, and precautions for the application of cold agents.
3. Demonstrate the clinical reasoning involved in the application of cold agents.
4. Identify commonly used types of cold agents.
5. Describe application procedures for each cold modality.

## Terminology

| | |
|---|---|
| Conduction | Hemodynamic |
| Convection | Hyperemia |
| Cryoglobulinemia | Ice massage |
| Cryotherapy | Superficial cooling |
| Evaporation | Vapocoolant |

## Introduction

Cryotherapy or "cold" therapy is a common modality frequently used by therapists in the treatment of acute injuries or trauma, for decreasing spasticity, spasms, and in reducing edema. Cryotherapy is the application of any substance to the body resulting in a withdrawal of heat from the body, effectively lowering the temperature of the tissue. Cryotherapy has been used historically in medicine since the ancient Greeks, and derives its name from the Greek word for cold, "cryos." When used therapeutically, superficial cold techniques exert their effect on the tissue to depths of 1 to 2 cm. As with any other physical technology, cryotherapy is most effectively used as an adjunct or preparatory to the treatment process to facilitate occupational performance (Allen, 2006; Hubbard, Aronson, & Denegar, 2004).

# History

The ancient Greeks and Romans recorded applications of cold as treatment for a variety of health-related problems using naturally forming ice and snow as the modality. Cold modalities were used as early as the 1800s following surgery, a practice commonly used even today following orthopedic procedures or surgery. Today, the application of cold is a common and practical treatment for acute or subacute injuries and musculoskeletal conditions. Application of cold to the body produces many biophysiological changes and can relieve pain, decrease the inflammatory response and associated swelling that may occur following injury, and decrease bleeding or hemorrhage. Clinically, there are a number of specific indications for applying cold; these include the presence of edema, postexercise edema and pain, arthritic flare-up, acute bursitis or tendonitis, spasticity due to central or peripheral nerve damage such as strokes or spinal cord injuries, acute or chronic pain secondary to muscle spasm, and to maintain soft tissue elongation after exercise (Aiello, 2004; Allen, 2006; Gracies, 2001; Kuznetsov, Stiazhkina, & Gusarova, 2004). When used therapeutically, superficial cold application exerts an effect on the tissue to depths of 1 to 2 cm. As with any other physical technology, cryotherapy is most effectively used as an adjunct to the treatment process or preparatory to an occupational task or activity.

The application of cooling to the body has multiple effects, both systemic and localized. Applications of cold agents exert a number of biophysiological changes in the underlying tissue. Cold application has a hemodynamic effect on the circulation of the blood, as well as affecting neuromuscular and metabolic processes within the body. Cold agents reduce the local metabolic activity of underlying tissues, slow nerve conduction and, by its direct effect on muscle spindle activity, reduces muscle spasm and guarding. The therapeutic effect of icing can produce a physiological effect on tissues to a depth, of approximately 1 to 2 centimeters (cm). Application of cold can also influence trigger points associated with the myofascial pain that limits movement and function. Superficial thermal agents can inactivate trigger points and can be used effectively as a facilitative technique for stimulating movement in musculoskeletal rehabilitation (Kerschan-Schindl, Uher, Zauner-Dungl, & Fialka-Moser, 1998; Lehman, 1990).

# Conduction, Convection, and Evaporation

There are a number of techniques and methods of applying cold agents to tissue including ice massage, cold or ice packs, cold baths, cold compression units, and vapocoolantcoolant sprays. Transmission of cooling occurs through the primary mechanisms of conduction, convection, and evaporation. When the source of the cold is in direct contact with the tissue surface and there is a difference in the temperature between the source and the tissue surface, energy is transferred through conduction (Cohn, Draeger, & Jackson, 1989). *Conduction* involves heat transfer where there is an exchange of thermal energy between two materials in physical contact. For example, if a cold physical agent is applied to the skin, the transfer of heat is from the patient's extremity to the cooling agent, thereby reducing the temperature of the skin under the physical modality. At this point of contact, molecular activity is slowed and a specific physiologic response is achieved. *Convection* is the transfer of heat through the circulation of a specific medium consisting of a different temperature. In convection, heat transfer occurs through the contact of the body part between a circulating medium of another material consisting of a different temperature. In cryotherapy, this could occur through the application of a cool or tepid whirlpool where the cooler water is kept in motion around the body part. Another form of energy transfer is evaporation. *Evaporation* occurs when a liquid is changed to a gas. This change from liquid to gas requires energy in the form of heat to occur. In the use of vapocoolantcoolant sprays, the heat necessary to produce this change comes from the skin surface effectively cooling the tissue. The most common example of this is sweating, which is a way that the body cools itself.

In therapy, cold sprays such as fluori-methane or ethyl chloride have been used to reduce pain and muscle spasms. These vapocoolantcoolant (skin refrigerant) sprays are intended for topical application in the management of myofascial pain, restricted motion, muscle spasm, and for minor sports injuries. These sprays can be used over acupressure or trigger points, as well as along referred pain routes. Vapocoolantcoolant agents are sprayed directly onto the skin in a liquid state. The liquid absorbs heat from the skin facilitating the chemical reaction thereby cooling the skin. The effect is only at the most superficial depths of the skin and affects primarily the A nerve fibers. This can impact the pain and muscle spasm responses as described by the gate control theory. The amount of cooling depends on the "dosage" or length of time the cooling spray is applied. As with any thermal agent, the dosage is related to and varies with the duration of the application (Modell, Travell, Kraus, et al., 1952; Davies & Molloy, 2006; Sheehan, 1950; Travell, 1952; Zappa, Nabors, & Wise, 1991; Zappa & Nabors, 1992).

---

### METHODS OF HEAT TRANSFER

- Convection (cold whirlpool)
- Conduction (ice packs)
- Evaporation (cold sprays)

---

## Tissue Temperature Variation

Superficial cooling of the tissue lowers tissue temperature to varying degrees and is most often used with neuromuscular and musculoskeletal conditions, and following an acute injury. Superficial cold lowers the tissue temperature and can produce analgesia, decrease edema, reduce muscle spasm, and lower metabolic activity. Tissue temperature change and the associated biophysical effects of the cooling are related to the time of exposure, the method used to cool the tissue, and thermal conductivity of the tissue. Thermal conductivity refers to the rate at which the tissue transfers heat by conduction. The thermal conductivity of a material can be expressed in (cal/sec) or by (cm2 X °C/cm). The thermal conductivity of bone and muscle is approximately 0.0011 (cal/sec), while fat has a thermal conductivity of 0.0005 (cal/sec).

Deeper subcutaneous tissue such as muscles and joints will require a longer exposure to the cooling agent in order to affect biophysical changes in the tissue. Cooling of the tissue is dependent in part, on the type of tissue. The depth of the tissue will also influence the biophysical changes and length of time needed to cool the tissue. Thermal conductivity refers to the efficiency of a tissue to conduct heat. Muscle, which has high water content, conducts heat more efficiently than adipose or fat tissue, which acts as an insulator (Anderson & Martin, 1994; Ducharme & Tikuisis, 1991; Hatfield & Puch, 1951; Wolf & Basmajian, 1973). Therefore, obese patients may not achieve the same biophysical effects when cold is applied, requiring longer exposure time to the intervention. However, caution needs to be used when considering the length of exposure to the cold agent as changes in the skin's temperature occur very quickly. Damage to the skin and tissue may occur before the desired biophysical effects are achieved.

## Cryotherapy Effects

Application of cold can have hemodynamic, neuromuscular, and metabolic effects on the body. Tissue cooling when used as an adjunctive modality can contribute positively to the therapeutic effect by producing analgesia, reducing edema, decreasing muscle spasms, and reducing the metabolic activity of the cooled tissues (Lehmann, Masock, Warren, & Koblanski, 1970). The intensity and rapidity of analgesia is dependent upon the mechanism of application of the cooling agent. The application of a cryotherapy technique to the skin will result in a characteristic response in most patients. Cold application produces four distinct stages of sensation that lead to an anesthetic response. The initial stage of cooling is marked by an intense cold sensation with the skin reddening (hyperemia). This is followed by a "burning" sensation, followed by a "deep aching" feeling, finally leading to analgesia. This sensory process usually occurs within 10 to 20 minutes, depending upon the modality used.

There are a variety of methods for applying cold to targeted tissue. Cold treatment can be applied by means of commercially available ice packs, chemical gel packs, and cold packs. These products are prescribed for clinic as well as home use. Cold modalities can be made for home application by using a bag of ice chips, frozen chunks of ice (typically frozen in 5 to 12 ounce cups), or as an "ice slush" (one part alcohol and three parts water mixed and stored in a baggie). The type of cold modality you use depends upon the desired effect you wish to achieve.

Tissue temperature change and the subsequent biophysical effects of cooling are directly related to the time of exposure, the method used to cool the tissue, and the conductivity of the tissue. The therapeutic effect of icing exerts a physiological change on tissues to a depth of up to 2 cm. There is no set time period in which one progresses through the stages of tissue cooling leading to analgesia and will vary depending on a number of factors including the amount of adipose tissue, fluid, and location of the targeted tissue. Generally, individuals with thicker subcutaneous tissue require longer periods of time to achieve a therapeutic response whereas individuals who are thin require less time. Treatment times can range from as little as 5 minutes to upwards of 45 minutes depending upon the area treated, the depth of penetration to be achieved, and the cooling method employed (Anderson & Martin, 1994; Barber, 2000).

## Nerve Conduction Velocity

Application of cold has a direct effect on the nerves and nerve endings causing the analgesic effects through counter irritation and by reducing the metabolic activity of the tissue (Lehmann et al., 1970). All nerve fibers are impacted by the application of cold, but the small, myelinated pain fibers are the first to be affected by the cold. As the temperature is decreased, there is a concurrent reduction in the nerve conduction velocities along with a reduction in acetylcholine production. As the exposure to cold is lengthened, there is a concomitant increase in the recovery cycle of the nerve following excitation along with an increase in the refractory period. Changes in nerve conduction velocity can occur fairly rapidly, within 5 minutes of applying a superficial cooling agent. In "normal" individuals, cold application applied for 5 minutes will take approximately 15 minutes to reverse the effects of nerve conduction velocities. As the duration of application increases, there is a subsequent increase in the time it takes for the conduction velocities to recover. When cold is applied for 20 minutes, it will take approximately 30 minutes or more to recover normal nerve conduction velocity. The analgesic effect of cryotherapy can be used to the therapists' advantage by involving the patient in activities and occupations that may be limited due to pain. The analgesic effect of cold intervention may also decrease a patient's need for pain medication. This analgesic effect can also cause difficulties if the patient and therapist fail to monitor the amount of activity as the bodies' normal protective mechanism of pain sensation is compromised. Care must be taken to monitor the activity level to ensure that further trauma does not occur through overuse (Cohn et al., 1989; Conolly, Paltos, & Tooth, 1972; Levy & Marmar, 1993).

## Biophysiological Response to Cooling

When cold material is placed upon the skin, the immediate hemodynamic effect is constriction of the cutaneous blood vessels. This occurs through activation of the cold receptors that in turn stimulate the smooth muscle of the blood vessel walls to contract. Vasoconstriction continues as long as the duration of the cold application is less than 15 minutes. The initial effect of vasoconstriction occurs in the tissue where the cold is being applied. This cooling process inhibits the production of histamine and prostaglandins, which trigger the vasodilatation response of blood vessels. Concurrently, there is an increase of blood viscosity that results in a resistance to blood flow. The net effect of vasoconstriction is that the body attempts to compartmentalize the treatment area, limiting the amount of blood that is cooled as well as preventing warmer blood from being shunted into the area raising the temperature through the convective effect of blood flow (Conolly et al., 1972).

## Hemodynamic Effects

When cold is applied for periods of time longer than 15 minutes, the body may respond by vasodilation. Vasodilation is a reaction in which blood vessels increase in size. There are some inconsistencies related to the occurrence of cold-induced vasodilation, though it occurs with greater frequency in the distal extremities, the hands and feet, when cold is applied longer than 15 minutes and below 1°C (Levy & Marmar, 1993). The body's alternating response of vasoconstriction and vasodilation was coined the "hunting response." The "hunting response" has been described as a delayed vasodilation of arterioles following a period of cooling. If the cold technique is applied for long periods of time (greater than 15 minutes and when tissue temperatures reach 50°F [10°C]), the body may react by causing vasodilation for a short period of time (usually 4 to 6 minutes). Vasodilation in turn is followed by vasoconstriction for an additional period of time (usually up to 30 minutes). When this reaction occurs, it is called the "hunting response." Application of cold to tissue also decreases the amount of oxygen available to the tissue. Cooling of the tissue decreases oxygen-hemoglobin dissociation with a subsequent increase in oxyhemoglobin of the blood under the area of application. This, in part, causes the redness that is often seen when applying cold to tissue. Application of cold, which causes vasodilation, has a net effect of decreasing oxygen delivery to the targeted body part (Healy, Seidman, Pfeifer, & Brown, 1994; Webb, Williams, Ivory, Day, & Williamson, 1998).

Cold can also cause a decrease in edema in some patients. Following an acute injury, there is an increase in fluid and proteins and increased interstitial pressure, all contributing to edema in the affected tissue which further compromises the circulatory flow that leads to a secondary hypoxia. Cold application decreases the metabolic activity of the affected tissue, reducing the need for energy and oxygen requirements of the surrounding tissue, allowing them to survive without suffering from hypoxic damage (Knight, 1995). Application of cold causes vasoconstriction by sympathetic reflex and through cold's effect on the smooth muscle of the blood vessels. Reduction of edema appears to be most effective when combined with compression (Conolly et al., 1972; Licker, Schweizer, & Ralley, 1996; Sloan, Giddings, & Hain, 1988). Vasoconstriction of the arterioles and venules occurs following application of cold for 15 minutes or less. In patients with acute trauma, application of cold is most effective when combined with compression and elevation (Healy et al., 1994; Levy & Marmar, 1993). To lower the possibility of thermal damage to postoperative patients, application of a less intense cold 3 to 4 times daily for 20 to 30 minutes in combination with compression and elevation should be considered.

# Metabolic Effects

Cold affects the rate of metabolic reactions that are involved in the inflammatory and healing process. Application of cryotherapy decreases or slows the metabolic reactions that occur during inflammation and healing. Because of this, cold applications should be used judiciously. Cooling selected tissues can affect the healing process by delaying the production of metabolites that are needed for this process. Cooling also has the effect of interrupting the inflammatory process. This can in turn either impede the healing process or enhance it, depending upon the condition of the tissues involved.

Intra-articular enzymatic activity may be decreased following application of cold. Reduction of metabolic activity can reduce energy requirements which may facilitate and account in part, for colds effectiveness in the acute phase of injuries. Because of cooling's biophysical effects on the healing process, cold is the thermal intervention that should be used following an acute injury (24 to 72 hours). Applying cold to the area immediately following injury will decrease pain, inflammation, edema, and muscle spasm. Use of cryotherapy as part of the treatment protocol in treating musculoskeletal trauma and postorthopedic surgical swelling and pain is well documented. Benefits of applying cold after injury or surgery include a reduction in the need for pain medication, decreased pain, decreased edema, improved ROM, decreased spasm, reduction of exercise induced muscle soreness, and quicker return to activity (Hedenberg, 1970; Johnson & Leider, 1977; Journee & de Jonge, 1993; Kerschan-Schindl et al., 1998; Major, Schwinghamer, & Winston, 1981; Tachibana, 1987; Zankel, 1966).

## Muscle Tone

Muscle spasm can have a detrimental effect on occupational performance through the experience of pain and limited range of motion (ROM). A cooling agent can be applied over a muscle spasm in an effort to decrease the spasm. The cold temperature affects the muscle spindle mechanism as well as the sensory wrappings of the spindle thereby decreasing the spasm. The effect of cooling on spasticity appears to be due to a decrease in gamma motor neuron activity and a subsequent decrease in afferent spindle and Golgi tendon organ activity (Bell & Lehmann, 1987; Boes, 1962). With a decrease in muscle spasm, the patient may gain ROM and be better able to resume routine functional activities (dos Santos & de Oliveira, 2004).

Cryotherapy can also be used to temporarily decrease spasticity in patients with upper motor neuron lesions; while applications for 10 to 30 minutes or longer may decrease clonus and resistance to passive stretch. Longer applications of cold (e.g., up to 30 minutes) are more effective to decrease spasticity and should be considered. Spasticity requires a cooling period of between 10 to 20 minutes before spastic muscle decreases in tone facilitating movement. Spasticity reduction following prolonged cooling generally lasts for up to 1 hour, during which time occupational activities should be engaged (Kesiktas et al., 2004; Lee, Bang, & Han, 2002; Miglietta, 1973).

Cooling the tissue affects both spastic muscle as well as normal muscle tone. It is important to note, that if a hand or forearm segment is cooled to less than 80.6°F, grip strength and the ability for sustained muscle contraction will be reduced. With cooling of the upper extremity, most patients will experience a decrease in the ability to perform fine motor activities. Engaging individuals in occupations requiring fine motor dexterity may be problematic and frustrating for the patient. Measuring grip or pinch strength following superficial cooling of the tissue may also hamper accurate results. The use of cold packs or ice massage when combined with static positional stretch or contract-relax techniques is a very effective counter measure for muscle spasms. Generally, 10 to 20 minutes of cooling time should be enough to decrease the muscle spasm in most individuals, unless they are obese (Abuziarov, Chemeris, Abeuova, & Ibragimova, 1992; Allison & Abraham, 2001; Petrilli et al., 2004; Price & Lehmann, 1990).

## Edema

The treatment of edema that follows injury or disease is of paramount concern for therapists. When confronted with edema following acute musculoskeletal trauma, remember the mnemonic RICE, which stands for **r**est, **i**ce, **c**ompression and **e**levation. A cold modality should be the physical agent of choice for the first 24 to 48 hours following acute injury or surgery. Cryotherapy can be an effective intervention and can be used to control the development of edema, particularly when edema is associated with acute inflammation. The application of a cooling modality should be applied to the injured area for 20 to 30 minutes per 2 hour period for the first 6 to 24 hours after trauma. Ice packs are usually applied for up to 30 minutes and are helpful because they conform to body contours and produce comfortable and safe pain relief.

Cold application produces a vasoconstriction of blood vessels due to a sympathetic reflex response that affects the smooth muscles of the blood vessels. Vasoconstriction of the arterioles and venules occurs during the application of cold for 15 minutes or less. Cryotherapy decreases the intravascular fluid pressure by decreasing blood flow into the affected area and by increasing the blood viscosity. Cryotherapy also affects capillary permeability by decreasing histochemical release during the inflammatory phase of healing. Cooling is most effective at reducing edema when combined with compression. For postoperative patients, in order to decrease thermal damage to a surgical repair, applications of a less intense cooling agent 3 to 4 times daily for 20 to 30 minutes, combined with compression and elevation, would be beneficial (Barry, Wallace, & Lamb, 2003; Cohn et al., 1989; Dover & Powers, 2004; Gibbons, Solan, Ricketts, & Patterson, 2001; Holmstrom & Hardin, 2005).

> ## FACTORS INFLUENCING BIOPHYSIOLOGICAL EFFECTS OF COOLING
>
> - Time or length of exposure
> - Thermal conductivity of the tissue
> - Volume or area of tissue cooled
> - Type and depth of the targeted tissue
> - Type of cooling agent applied

# Applications

Cryotherapy is the recommended modality of choice immediately following an injury and during the acute inflammatory phase. There are a number of physiological responses that occur with application of cold. Cold will decrease swelling, bleeding, inflammation, and pain by decreasing the metabolism of the affected tissues. Cryotherapy can be used therapeutically in the treatment of injuries, pathology, and diseases. There are a number of indications for using cooling as an adjunctive modality to prepare your patient for involvement in occupation. The most common use of cryotherapy is in the treatment of acute injury or during the inflammatory process. The inflammatory process occurs approximately 24 to 48 hours postinjury. As mentioned previously, the anacronym RICE is effective in decreasing many of the effects of acute musculoskeletal trauma. Cooling of the tissue decreases the rate with which the chemical reactions occur that are associated with the acute inflammatory process. Decreasing affected tissue temperature causes vasoconstriction and increases the viscosity of the blood limiting interstitial fluid movement controlling bleeding and fluid loss following an acute injury.

Cold has a direct effect on the nerves and nerve endings and causes analgesia through counterirritation (as described in the gate control theory) by decreasing metabolic activity within the tissue. Small, myelinated pain fibers are first to be affected by the reduction in temperature resulting in analgesia. The reason for this may be explained by a decrease in blood flow to the targeted tissue thereby affecting the inflammatory process and ultimately curtailing edema formation. This results in a decrease in pressure on nerves and consequently a decrease in pain. The analgesic advantage is that the therapist can involve the patient in activities and occupations, which may have been limited due to the pain. However, care must be taken to prevent further injuries during this period as the pain threshold has been changed. Although the analgesic effect may decrease the need for pain medication, the therapist must monitor the patient's activity level to ensure that further trauma does not occur through overuse. A false sense of security due to pain relief can possibly lead to aggravating the original condition or lead to a new injury.

With a decrease in temperature, there is a concurrent decrease in nerve conduction velocities and a decrease in acetylcholine production. A decrease in nerve conduction velocity after 5 minutes of cooling will generally recover in individuals with normal circulation within about 15 minutes. After 20 minutes of cooling, reversing the effect on delayed nerve conduction velocity will take about 30 minutes or longer. This should be kept in mind during treatment and when assessments are being conducted. The inflammatory process lasts approximately 48 to 72 hours following an acute injury. As the area heals and the inflammatory process slows, the superficial temperature of the area should resolve and decrease. The surface temperature of the area can be a good indicator of the healing process. If the temperature of the area remains elevated, this may indicate an infection or may be indicative of more severe trauma, chronic overuse syndromes or inflammatory disease such as arthritis. In these cases, referral to the attending physician is warranted. As the inflammatory process resolves, application of cold should concurrently be discontinued to avoid impeding the second and third phases of the healing process and limiting histo-chemical and metabolic reactions.

---

### CRYOTHERAPY INDICATIONS

- During acute/subacute inflammation
- Acute pain (secondary to muscle spasm)
- Chronic pain (secondary to muscle spasm)
- Acute swelling
- Myofascial trigger points
- Muscle guarding
- Muscle spasm
- Acute muscle strain
- Acute ligament strain
- Acute contusion
- Bursitis
- Tenosynovitis
- Tendonitis
- Arthritic flare-up
- Spasticity
- Delayed onset muscle soreness (postexercise edema and pain)
- Postexercise to maintain soft tissue elongation

---

## Cold Agent Applications

There are a number of methods and techniques that clinicians can use to administer crotherapy. Cold packs, ice massage, cold-water immersion baths, cool whirlpools, ice towels, and vapocoolant sprays are the most commonly used cryotherapy agents used in the clinical setting. Each one is effective to meet the physiological and therapeutic objectives associated with the relief of pain and the decrease in the inflammatory process. The standard protocol of RICE is effective in decreasing the effects of acute musculoskeletal trauma. Patients will feel a variety of sensations when applying cold, the intensity and rapidity of the sensation may be dependent upon the mechanism of application used.

**Figure 5-1.** Size variations of commercially available cold packs. Select the appropriate size cold pack for the volume of tissue that you will be treating (Photo courtesy of Chattanooga Group).

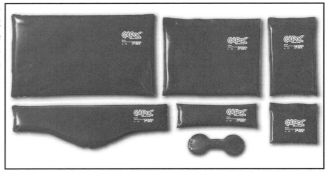

## Cold Packs

Cold packs are commonly used in cryotherapy. Cold packs are available commercially or can very easily be made at home using either a homemade alcohol pack, crushed ice in a plastic bag, or simply using a frozen bag of peas. Cold packs are an effective and inexpensive method for administering cold to an area. Selecting the type of cold pack to be used should be based on its ability to conform to the extremity or area to be treated (Figure 5-1). Use of cold packs is also advantageous as the therapist can target large or multiple areas for treatment and combine elevation and icing to facilitate edema reduction. When used for musculoskeletal injuries, the cold pack ideally should cover the entire muscle from origin to insertion though this is not always possible.

The cold pack can be applied directly to the area, it may be wrapped in a wet or dry towel, or it can be placed in a pillowcase and then applied (Figure 5-2). An insulating material should always be used when the ice pack is placed over a bony prominence. If a distal extremity such as a hand, wrist, or elbow is the targeted tissue, the extremity can be covered with an bandage wrap, compression wrap (such as Tubigrip [ConvaTec, Princeton, NJ]), or a stockinette, followed by the placement of wet or dry cloth towels or paper towels acting as an interface between the tissue and the cold pack. Bandage wraps or other elastic type wraps such as Coban tape (3M, St. Paul, MN) or cellophane can be used to maintain and hold the position of the cold pack on the area being treated. Cold packs can be left on for an average treatment time between 10 to 20 minutes with close monitoring of the skin to prevent tissue damage from too rapid or prolonged cooling.

During cold applications, be sure to closely monitor any bony prominences. If additional protection is needed to the body segment being treated, consider using stockinette, tubigrip, bandage wraps, or compression wraps under the cold pack. Leave the cold pack on for an average treatment time between 10 to 20 minutes and monitor the skin to prevent tissue damage from too rapid or prolonged cooling.

### Cold Pack/Ice Pack Clinical Application

You need to determine if a cold pack is the appropriate treatment for your patient. Identify any precautions or contraindications. Ask them if they have had previous cryotherapy treatment applications and review the procedure with them. Collect your supplies. You will need a damp towel and a cold pack. Conduct an assessment of the area to be treated. You will want to determine the status of light touch sensibility, circulation, presence of open wounds or rashes, skin irritation, and range of motion. Remove jewelry and clothing from the treatment area.

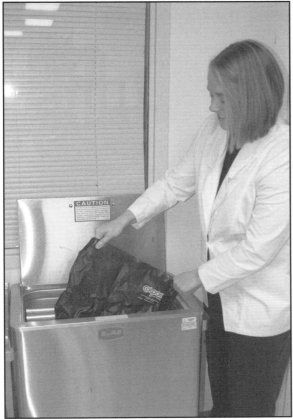

**Figure 5-2.** ColPac Chilling Unit (Chattanooga Group, Hixson, TN). The cold pack can be placed in a pillowcase. Skin condition should always be monitored to prevent tissue damage from overcooling (Photo courtesy of Chattanooga Group).

Keep the extremity well supported. Remember, bony prominences and those areas where pressure may occur will conduct the cold quicker than other areas. If necessary, drape the patient with towels or sheets to preserve patient's modesty and protect clothing.

1. Wrap the cold pack in a towel or pillowcase.

2. Inform your patient before your place the cold pack on the body segment. Wrap the cold pack in place and secure if necessary to prevent slippage. Set your treatment timer for 15 to 20 minutes (or the treatment time you determine as best for your patient 10 to 20 minutes total). Remember to monitor the patient's skin and response to the cold during this time period (Figure 5-3).

3. Ask your patient what they are subjectively feeling at the end of 2 minutes and again at 5 minutes. Make consistent visual checks of the treated area for any adverse effects or patient response. If the skin begins to develop welts or if the color of the extremity changes from red to an absolute white within the first 4 minutes, stop the treatment.

4. When the treatment is completed, remove the cold pack and dry the area with a towel. Remove draping material and assist patient with dressing if appropriate. Have the patient continue with the therapeutic intervention as outlined in the treatment plan.

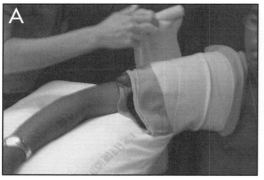
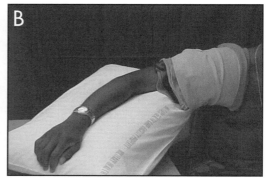

**Figure 5-3.** Cold pack application. Note the (A) protective covering and (B) the use of the bandage wrap to provide greater conduction of the agent.

## Ice Massage

Ice massage is the application of ice on the skin or targeted area of treatment and is most often used to anesthetize an area or to apply cold to a trigger point. Because the ice is applied directly to the skin, smaller, localized areas are more effectively treated. As with any cryotherapy application, the size of the area to be treated and the amount of adipose or fat tissue needs to be taken into consideration before applying the intervention. Ice cubes or water placed in a paper or styrofoam cup and frozen are the most frequently used methods of application, although commercial cryo-probes kept in the freezer are available. As always, care must be taken to prevent cryotrauma to the area being treated (van Linschoten & den Hoed, 2004; Isabell, 1992).

The patient should be positioned comfortably with the area to be treated exposed and draped with a towel to absorb the melting water. The ice cube or ice cup is slowly rubbed in small, rhythmical circles maintaining direct contact with the skin at all times. The patient should be informed of the stages of cold, burning, and aching, followed by "numbness" indicating analgesia. The patient should be repeatedly questioned to identify which stage of cooling is occurring. When the patient reports "numbness" or analgesia, it is generally safe to continue for approximately one more minute. Rarely should ice massage exceed 7 minutes in length, most often treatment should last from approximately 3 to 10 minutes depending on the size of the area being treated. Intermittent applications may enhance the therapeutic effect of ice in pain relief after acute soft tissue injury (Bleakley, McDonough, MacAuley, & Bjordal, 2006; Hocutt, Jaffe, Rylander, & Beebe, 1982; Hubbard & Denegar, 2004; Thorsson, 2001).

### Ice Massage Clinical Procedure

Ice massage is one of the most frequently applied physical agents used to anesthetize a relatively small area or to disrupt the pain cycle of a trigger point. It is most effective when the area of treatment is superficial, localized, and relatively small. As the ice cup melts during application, you will want to position your patient comfortably and drape the area with a towel to catch and absorb the melting ice.

To effectively perform ice massage, use of ice cups or frozen water popsicles are most often made by freezing water in small cups or Styrofoam cups or by applying a tongue depressor into a water cup before completely freezing. The stick is conveniently used as a handle when the cup is removed from the frozen water. Ice massage is performed by slowly rubbing or moving the modality in small, rhythmical circles maintaining direct contact with skin at all times (Figure 5-4).

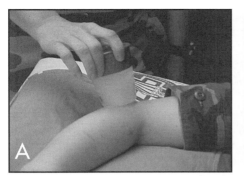
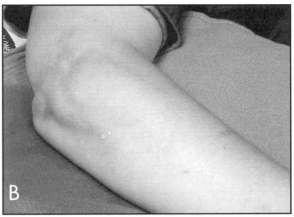
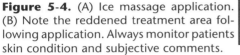

**Figure 5-4.** (A) Ice massage application. (B) Note the reddened treatment area following application. Always monitor patients skin condition and subjective comments.

The treatment regimen continues even after the patient reports that the treatment area is "numb," indicating an analgesic effect. "Numbness" generally occurs within a 3 to 10 minute time frame. Depending upon the size and area being treated and as a general rule, you do not want to apply an ice massage to exceed 10 minutes as frostbite and tissue damage may occur due to the intensity of the cold. Patients will usually experience numbness within a 3- to 10-minute time (Barrett & O'Malley, 1999; Ownby, 2006; Sevier & Wilson, 1999; Waters & Raisler, 2003; Zemke, Andersen, Guion, McMillan, & Joyner, 1998).

### Application Procedure

1. Define the patient's problem and have them help you to set the goal for this intervention. Decide if an ice massage is the most appropriate modality. Outline the contraindications and precautions relative to your patient and educate them to the procedure and answer any questions they might have.

2. The patient should be placed in a well-supported and comfortable position with the body part to be treated exposed. Remove jewelry and clothing from the area to be treated. If necessary, drape the patient with towels or sheets to preserve patient's modesty and protect clothing from melting ice.

3. Evaluate the area to be treated for light touch sensibility, circulatory status, and include pulses and capillary refill. Ensure that there are no open wounds or rashes and evaluate the body part or extremity for ROM.

4. To prepare the ice for application, pull it from its container and rub the ice with your hand to smooth any hard edges. Before you begin the ice massage, inform the patient that you are about to begin. If this is the first application, you can apply the ice massage for about 10 seconds, remove it, and ask the patient if they have any questions regarding the procedure. This will provide them with the initial sensory feedback and understanding of the procedure.

5. Begin rubbing the ice in back and forth and circular motions on the body segment being treated. You do not have to add extra pressure to the ice as you do not want to decrease any blood flow unnecessarily. Keep the ice moving up to 10 cm per second. If the ice is melting and running over areas that you do not want cooled, catch the run off with an extra towel.

6. After approximately 2 minutes, ask the patient how they are doing. Remember that there are four stages the patient will experience: an intense feeling of cold, a stinging/burning sensation, followed by an aching sensation leading to numbness. If after 4 to 5 minutes you notice the skin color turning from red to an absolute white, discontinue treatment. Note how long it takes for the patient to report analgesia or "numbness."

7. Continue with the ice massage until the desired outcome has occurred, but not longer than 10 minutes as a general rule. When the patient experiences analgesia and your treatment time is complete, discontinue the ice massage and dry the area.

8. Assess the area with a light touch to make sure anesthesia has been achieved. Discard the ice.

The patient is now ready to continue with your therapeutic intervention as outlined in the treatment plan.

## Cold/Ice Water Immersion Baths and Cool Whirlpool

Cold water baths or cool whirlpools are most often used for edema reduction and used in conjunction with string wrapping or compression wrapping and garments. These techniques are often effective and used for digital or hand injuries. An advantage to the use of cold or ice baths is the fact that there is complete contact of the cooling agent on the tissue being treated as the extremity is completely immersed in the water. Cool whirlpools can be effective as part of wound debridement, due to the agitation of the water, particularly in edemetous hand injuries. When used in upper extremity injuries, a disadvantage to the use of cold or ice baths and whirlpool, is the dependent position of the hand and extremity. To counteract the effects of the dependent position, patients should be advised to continue hand pumping and exercise throughout the treatment. Having the patient periodically elevate the extremity above the level of their heart with the pumping of the hand will help to facilitate venous return.

Treatment application depends upon the therapeutic goal, and the amount of adipose tissue present in the extremity. Therapeutic water temperatures may be between 35°F to 75°F, or 13°C to 18°C. Treatment duration is between 15 to 20 minutes, though colder temperatures will require a corresponding decrease in duration (Mizushima et al., 2006; Morton, 2006; Petrofsky et al., 2006).

## Ice Towels

Ice towels are another mechanism for draping the cold around the targeted area and can be made easily at home. They are also an economical way to apply cold to tissue. Ice towels may contain ice chips or shaving, or may be dipped in ice water, wrung out and wrapped around an extremity. Because the towels cool quickly, they will need to be changed frequently, often every 5 to 6 minutes. An advantage to the use of ice towels is the ability to circumferentially cover an extremity. Because of their ability to drape around and over the extremity, they may be more effective than other mechanisms at reducing spasticity. A drawback to ice towel application is that they melt quickly. As they melt they may be uncomfortable for the patient and therapist due to the melting water and inconvenience.

## Cold Compression Units

Cold compression units, such as the Cryotemp from Jobst Corporation (Toledo, OH) and the Game Ready system (Berkeley, CA), are refrigerated units that circulate cooled water and air over an extremity through a sleeve. These refrigerated units are similar in principle to the workings of a refrigerator or freezer cooling unit. The temperature can be adjusted by the therapist and can remain constant throughout the length of the treatment. The temperature of the water can be set between 10° and 25° C (50° to 77° F) effectively cooling the targeted area. The cooled medium is circulated through a sleeve or garment, which surrounds the targeted extremity. Cold compression units combine an edema compression pump with the advantages of cold and may be effective at edema reduction. Cold compression units are most often used following surgery to control postoperative inflammation and edema and to facilitate ROM. Following surgery, the compression sleeve is fitted over the affected extremity in the recovery room and the cold compression unit is sent home with the patient. The use of controlled compression units for postsurgery edema has been found to be more effective than the use of more conventional ice application alone. Cold compression units can also be used for treating a variety of musculoskeletal injuries. Most patients are able to tolerate 50°F for 15 to 20 minutes. A disadvantage to the use of cold compression units is the cost of the equipment. Care must also be taken with regard to the amount of pressure applied, and may be contraindicated for the treatment diagnosis (Barber, 2000; Barrett & O'Malley, 1999; Gibbons, 2001; Holmstrom, 2005).

Advantages of this technology are that it allows application of cold and compression simultaneously and can be easily and effectively controlled by the therapist or physician.

## Vapocoolant Sprays

Vapocoolant sprays were initially used in the treatment of trigger points. Janet Travell developed the "spray and stretch" technique used to facilitate elongation of muscle with passive stretch. There have been two commercially available sprays, ethyl chloride and Fluori-Methane (Gebauer Co., Cleveland, OH). Ethyl chloride is a local anesthetic but is flammable, and volatile, and may explode if heated or dropped. Flouri-Methane spray contained a fluorocarbon, which became banned in January of 1996 due to the Clean Air Act of 1990 limiting the release of fluorocarbons in the environment. One of the primary manufacturers has developed a new product, Gebauer's Spray and Stretch which replaced their earlier Fluori-Methane product and is nonflammable and nonozone depleting. Vapocoolant sprays contain a liquid, which is under pressure and provides a fine stream spray and cooling effect. This chemical is sprayed on the tissue coming into contact with the area of the skin being treated. Due to its chemical composition and properties, the chemical evaporates, cooling the skin for short periods of time. The rapid cooling acts as a counterirritant stimulus to cutaneous thermal afferents and causes a reduction in the resistance to stretch. The spray can be applied to a trigger point area, or to the entire length of the muscle in a sweeping, unidirectional motion with the muscle being positioned in a passive stretch (Modell, et al., 1952; Collure, 1976; Davies & Molloy, 2006; Kinawi, 1952; Lacour & Le Coultre, 1991; Newton, 1985). Vapocoolant sprays are used by many athletes and may be effective in the treatment of acute muscle spasms. However, their effectiveness may be relatively short lived (10 to 15 minutes), and the spray can be expensive (Gulick, Kimura, Sitler, Paolone, & Kelly, 1996; Isabell, Durrant, Myrer, & Anderson, 1992; Yackzan, Adams, & Francis, 1984; Zappa et al., 1991). In addition, the technique is very therapist dependent, requiring direct contact and support of the therapist throughout the intervention.

# Precautions

Cold is an effective intervention with physiological effects lasting several hours. Re-warming cooled tissue takes approximately 20 minutes. Though cold is relatively easy to apply and is indicated in a number of treatment conditions, care should always be used in its application. During and following cryotherapy application, it is important for the therapist to monitor the patient's skin condition and response closely. A cold gel pack should never be directly placed on the skin as the temperatures at the skin interface can be subfreezing. Application of the cold pack should never be for longer than 20 minutes. Application of cold for periods longer than 20 minutes or when improperly applied or monitored can lead to tissue damage or death due to freezing of the tissue. Improper application of cold can cause tissue death due to vasoconstriction, ischemia, and thromboses. Tissue damage can occur if tissue temperature is cooled to $15°$ C ($59°$ F). Frostbite occurs when the skin temperature drops to between -4° and -10° C ($39°$ to $14°$F) or lower. Extended application of cold to tissue may also cause temporary or permanent nerve damage or changes in nerve conduction. Aside from their volatility, caution should be used with vapocoolant sprays as they can freeze the skin on contact. When the patient reports "numbness" indicating analgesia, the patient's protective sensation is removed and the patient should be cautioned against overuse or reinjury to the area. In distal extremities such as hands, edema may result if cryotherapy is too severe, due in part to the increased permeability of the lymph vessels. (Dover, Borsa, & McDonald, 2004; Drez, Faust, & Evans, 1981; Keskin, Tosun, Duymaz, & Savaci, 2005; McGuire & Hendricks, 2006; Quist, Peltier, & Lundquist, 1996; Rudzki & Grzywa, 1978; Tsang, Hertel, & Denegar, 2003).

Cold should not be used in patients with specific cold-sensitivity such as cold urti-caria, cryoglobulinemia, and Raynaud's disease. Sensitivity to the cold may be indicated by the development of itching, hives, sweating, and the development of wheals with reddened borders and blanched centers. Patients with cold urticaria may also develop a massive histamine release and subsequent systemic reactions including increased heart rate, decreased blood pressure and syncope. Cryoglobulinemia is characterized by an abnormal blood protein, which forms a gel when it is exposed to cold. Patients with Raynaud's phenomenon may have episodes of pallor, cyanosis, rubor, numbness, tingling, or burning to the digits.

Cold should never be applied to areas of compromised circulation such as peripheral vascular disease or over an area with impaired circulation, in hypertensive patients, or to patients who have had frostbite in the area that is being treated. Application of cold to these conditions may exacerbate the condition due to vasoconstriction and increased blood viscosity. Cold should also not be applied over a deep open wound due to the negative effects of decreased circulation and metabolic rate, effectively slowing or delaying the healing process. Patients with impaired sensation or mentation also require careful monitoring. These individuals may be unable to indicate the level of cooling or sensation, and the therapist must closely monitor the patient's response and observe the skin for changes in color and effect.

# Contraindications

Cryotherapy or application of cold is generally considered a safe and effective treatment intervention. Cryotherapy is contraindicated for some conditions while caution should be used with others. As with any modality or treatment approach, if the patient's condition is worsening or not improving within two or three sessions, the treatment approach and intervention should be reconsidered. Cold therapy is contraindicated for any medical condition in which vasoconstriction will aggravate symptoms, such as impaired circulation, peripheral vascular diseases, hypersensitivity to cold, impaired sensation, open wounds or skin conditions (such as psoriasis), and infections. Some patients with hypersensitivity to cold can experience a histamine-like response evidenced by skin changes marked by slightly elevated patches, redness, or paleness and may be accompanied by itching and discomfort. Cooling agents should not be used with patients who have been diagnosed with cold urticaria, cryoglobulinemia, and Raynaud's disease (Kaplan & Garofalo, 1981; Shelley & Caro, 1962).

Cold urticaria is also called cold hypersensitivity or cold allergy. When cold is applied to the skin, a patient may experience adverse reactions, either during or after treatment. The more commonly experienced reactions include gentle to violent local skin reaction, such as wheals (a hive-like reaction). Some patients may develop various systemic reactions due to large release of histamine, such as sneezing, dysphasia, increased heart rate, decreased blood pressure, and syncope.

Cryoglobulinemia is a reaction to cold application whereby there is an abnormal collection of blood proteins that forms a gel in small vessels. This can result in a disruption of blood flow and possibly cause tissue ischemia. In a worst-case scenario, the patient may develop gangrene in the tissue or extremity. Raynaud's phenomenon, the more common idiopathic form of paroxysmal digital cyanosis, is due to a regional or systemic disorder. Raynaud's disease occurs in the distal extremities and is characterized by pallor, cyanosis, rubor, numbness, tingling, or burning sensation of the digits. This reaction can be precipitated by emotional upset or by cold and variations in temperature. Raynaud's phenomenon is most frequently seen in young women. The symptoms are bilateral and symmetrical in individuals with Raynaud's disease, but in those patients with Raynaud's phenomenon, the response generally occurs only in the cooled extremity. Raynaud's phenomenon and subsequent physiological reactions may also be associated with other syndromes such as carpal tunnel, thoracic outlet, or following traumatic injuries (Bentley-Phillips, Black, & Greaves, 1976; Dover et al., 2004; Leigh, Ramsay, & Calnan, 1974; Nadler, Weingand, & Kruse, 2004).

Never apply a cooling agent to someone with compromised circulation, peripheral vascular disease, hypertension, or a past history of frostbite. Circulatory conditions and impairments are often associated with peripheral vascular disease, trauma, or the healing process and are often accompanied by edema. It is important to determine the cause of edema and to distinguish between edema secondary to inflammation rather than that due to poor circulation. In general, inflammatory conditions causing edema are characterized by heat or redness to the area, whereas circulatory disorders may be distinguished by the coolness and pallor of the skin. Frostbite is a recognized danger when applying cold modalities and skin condition must be monitored. Incorrect application may also cause nerve palsy though they may resolve without any significant sequelae. Most of these complications can be avoided by not using ice for more than 30 minutes and by guarding superficial nerves in the area (Collure, 1976; Drez et al., 1981; Graham & Stevenson, 2000; Jonderko, Golab, Rosmus-Kuczia, & Nowicki, 1988; Keskin et al., 2005; Khajavi, Pavelko, & Mishra, 2004; McGuire & Hendricks, 2006; O'Toole & Rayatt, 1999; Quist et al., 1996; Wilke & Weiner, 2003).

**Table 5-1**

---

### CRYOTHERAPY PRECAUTIONS

- Monitor blood pressure, since cold can cause a temporary increase in systolic and diastolic blood pressure.
- Avoid use in patients with impaired circulation or hypersensitivity to cold.
- Avoid application directly over wounds that are 2 to 3 weeks postinjury.
- Avoid prolonged placement over superficial nerve.

  *Note: Always monitor patient's skin condition.*

---

# Documentation

Though cold is easily and safely applied, patients should always be monitored closely for reactions to the treatment. Any form of cryotherapy should never be used for longer than 1 continuous hour; skin condition and the patient's response should always be monitored. Documentation should include the treatment parameters, including duration, site of application, and the method used to apply the cold. Other considerations include the patient's subjective comments, subjective and objective response to the treatment and any changes or revisions to the patient goals. Any changes in the patient's occupational performance and abilities should also be documented (Table 5-1). Documentation must always comply with local, federal, and institutional regulations and requirements.

# Case Study

A 38-year-old right-hand dominant female has a primary complaint of pain in the left elbow with recent onset of 24 hours. She states that she "banged the outside" of her elbow against the doorframe when carrying groceries into her house. She reports "constant" pain in the elbow and rates the pain as a 6 to 7 out of 10, with magnification of the pain with use. She describes the pain as radiating down toward her fingers and she is unable to lift heavy objects. Medical history is unremarkable, she has no known allergies. No current medications. The patient is an active female who is employed as a cashier at a local retail store. Her occupational tasks require her to manipulate items across the price scanner and then place them into bags.

Examination of the elbow and the proximal posterior forearm reveal temperature variation, with the area warmer to the touch than the noninvolved side. Circumferential measurements are greater on the affected side. ROM measurements are WNLs, though movements are guarded and the patient does not use the extremity unless necessary. There is point tenderness over the lateral epicondylitis and pain associated with the wrist loaded in extension. Grip and pinch strengths are decreased secondary to pain. There is discoloration with bruising noted at the elbow where the impact occurred. Treatment goals are to decrease pain, improve pain-free ROM, and improve strength. Initial treatment protocol includes application of an ice pack to the affected area. The patient is also instructed in a home exercise program (HEP) of icing to the area to decrease the edema and inflammation. Three MHz ultrasound at 20% duty cycle at

$0.2W/cm^2$ for 6 minutes is also used as part of the treatment to decrease the inflammatory process and facilitate healing. Monitoring the patient's HEP and compliance is crucial to determine any changes to the goals and treatment protocol. Engagement in occupational activities requiring gentle flexion and extension to the elbow are also included in the protocol after the physical agents. Use of wrist splint and epi-strap will be considered as part of her initial evaluation and appropriate measurements taken. Alternative treatment intervention includes the use of iontophoresis with dexamethasone.

## Clinical Reasoning Questions

1. What precautions and contraindications should you be aware of with this patient and condition?

2. How would you monitor the patient's skin and response to application of cryotherapy?

3. What stage of healing is the patient exhibiting?

4. What other physical agents might be appropriate for this patient and condition?

5. When would you increase the level of activity and exercise resistance?

# References

Abuziarov, M. B., Chemeris, A. V., Abeuova, G. K., & Ibragimova, S. A. (1992). The generator of locomotor activity as the probable modulator of the afferent flow from the thermoreceptors of the skin fields of the flexor and extensor muscles. *Neurophysiology, 24*, 598-604; discussion 633-635.

Aiello, D. D. (2004). The hot and the cold of it. *Rehab Management, 17*, 18-23.

Allen, R. J. (2006). Physical agents used in the management of chronic pain by physical therapists. *Physical Medicine and Rehabilitation Clinics of North, 17*, 315-345.

Allison, S. C., & Abraham, L. D. (2001). Sensitivity of qualitative and quantitative spasticity measures to clinical treatment with cryotherapy. *International Journal of Rehabilitation, 24*, 15-24.

Anderson, G. S., & Martin, A. D. (1994). Calculated thermal conductivities and heat flux in man. *Journal of the Undersea and Hyperbaric Medical Society, 21*, 431-441.

Barber, F. A. (2000). A comparison of crushed ice and continuous flow cold therapy. *American Journal of Knee Surgery, 13*, 97-101; discussion 102.

Barrett, S. J., & O'Malley, R. (1999). Plantar fasciitis and other causes of heel pain. *American Family Physician, 59*, 2200-2206.

Barry, S., Wallace, L., & Lamb, S. (2003). Cryotherapy after total knee replacement: A survey of current practice. *Journal for Researchers and Clinicians in Physical Therapy, 8*, 111-120.

Bell, K. R., & Lehmann, J. F. (1987). Effect of cooling on H- and T-reflexes in normal subjects. *Archives of Physical Medicine and Rehabilitation, 68*, 490-493.

Bentley-Phillips, C. B., Black, A. K., & Greaves, M. W. (1976). Induced tolerance in cold urticaria caused by cold-evoked histamine release. *Lancet, 2*, 63-66.

Bleakley, C. M., McDonough, S. M., MacAuley, D. C., & Bjordal, J. (2006). Cryotherapy for acute ankle sprains: A randomised controlled study of two different icing protocols. *British Journal of Sports Medicine, 40*, 700-5; discussion 705.

Boes, M. C. (1962). Reduction of spasticity by cold. *Journal of the American Physical Therapy Association, 42*, 29-32.

Cohn, B. T., Draeger, R. I., & Jackson, D. W. (1989). The effects of cold therapy in the postoperative management of pain in patients undergoing anterior cruciate ligament reconstruction. *American Journal of Sports Medicine, 17*, 344-349.

Collure, D. W. (1976). Cold injury from skin refrigerants. *Journal of the American College of Emergency Physicians, 5*, 814.

Conolly, W. B., Paltos, N., & Tooth, R. M. (1972). Cold therapy—an improved method. *Medical Journal of Australia, 2*, 424-425.

Davies, E. H., & Molloy, A. (2006). Comparison of ethyl chloride spray with topical anaesthetic in children experiencing venepuncture. *Paediatric Nursing, 18*, 39-43.

dos Santos, M. T., & de Oliveira, L. M. (2004). Use of cryotherapy to enhance mouth opening in patients with cerebral palsy. *Special Care in Dentistry, 24*, 232-234.

Dover, G., Borsa, P. A., & McDonald, D. J. (2004). Cold urticaria following an ice application: A case study. *Clinical Journal of Sport Medicine, 14*, 362-364.

Dover, G., & Powers, M. E. (2004). Cryotherapy does not impair shoulder joint position sense. *Archives of Physical Medicine and Rehabilitation, 85*, 1241-1246.

Drez, D., Faust, D. C., & Evans, J. P. (1981). Cryotherapy and nerve palsy. *American Journal of Sports Medicine, 9*, 256-257.

Ducharme, M. B., & Tikuisis, P. (1991). In vivo thermal conductivity of the human forearm tissues. *Journal of Applied Physiology, 70*, 2682-2690.

Gibbons, C. E., Solan, M. C., Ricketts, D. M., & Patterson, M. (2001). Cryotherapy compared with robert jones bandage after total knee replacement: A prospective randomized trial. *International Orthopaedics, 25*, 250-252.

Gracies, J. M. (2001). Physical modalities other than stretch in spastic hypertonia. *Physical Medicine and Rehabilitation Clinics of North America, 12*, 769-92, vi.

Graham, C. A., & Stevenson, J. (2000). Frozen chips: An unusual cause of severe frostbite injury. *British Journal of Sports Medicine, 34*, 382-383.

Gulick, D. T., Kimura, I. F., Sitler, M., Paolone, A., & Kelly, J. D. (1996). Various treatment techniques on signs and symptoms of delayed onset muscle soreness. *Journal of Athletic Training, 31*, 145-152.

Hatfield, H. S., & Puch, L. G. (1951). Thermal conductivity of human fat and muscle. *Nature, 168*, 918-919.

Healy, W. L., Seidman, J., Pfeifer, B. A., & Brown, D. G. (1994). Cold compressive dressing after total knee arthroplasty. *Clinical Orthopaedics and Related Research, 299*, 143-146.

Hedenberg, L. (1970). Functional improvement of the spastic hemiplegic arm after cooling. *Scandinavian Journal of Rehabilitation Medicine, 2*, 154-158.

Hocutt, J. E.,Jr., Jaffe, R., Rylander, C. R., & Beebe, J. K. (1982). Cryotherapy in ankle sprains. *American Journal of Sports Medicine, 10*, 316-319.

Holmstrom, A., & Hardin, B. C. (2005). Cryo/Cuff compared to epidural anesthesia after knee unicompartmental arthroplasty: A prospective, randomized and controlled study of 60 patients with a 6-week follow-up. *Journal of Arthroplasty, 20*, 316-321.

Hubbard, T. J., Aronson, S. L., & Denegar, C. R. (2004). Does cryotherapy hasten return to participation? A systematic review. *Journal of Athletic Training, 39*, 88-94.

Hubbard, T. J., & Denegar, C. R. (2004). Does cryotherapy improve outcomes with soft tissue injury? *Journal of Athletic Training, 39*, 278-279.

Isabell, W. K., Durrant, E., Myer, W., & Anderson, S. (1992). The effects of ice massage, ice massage with exercise, and exercise on the prevention and treatment of delayed onset muscle soreness. *Journal of Athletic Training, 27*, 208-217.

Johnson, D. J., & Leider, F. E. (1977). Influence of cold bath on maximum handgrip strength. *Perceptual and Motor Skills, 44*, 323-326.

Jonderko, G., Golab, T., Rosmus-Kuczia, I., & Nowicki, L. (1988). Changes in the skin and oral temperature during local cryotherapy of rheumatoid arthritis with extremely cold air: Prevention of congelation. *Przeglad Lekarski, 45*, 426-428.

Journee, H. L., & de Jonge, A. B. (1993). Ultrasound myography: Application in nerve conduction velocity assessment and muscle cooling. *Ultrasound in Medicine & Biology, 19*, 561-566.

Kaplan, A. P., & Garofalo, J. (1981). Identification of a new physically induced urticaria: Cold-induced cholinergic urticaria. *Journal of Allergy and Clinical Immunology, 68*, 438-441.

Kerschan-Schindl, K., Uher, E. M., Zauner-Dungl, A., & Fialka-Moser, V. (1998). Cold and cryotherapy. A review of the literature on general principles and practical applications. *Acta Medica Austriaca, 25*, 73-78.

Kesiktas, N., Paker, N., Erdogan, N., Gulsen, G., Bicki, D., & Yilmaz, H. (2004). The use of hydrotherapy for the management of spasticity. *Neurorehabilitation and Neural Repair, 18*, 268-273.

Keskin, M., Tosun, Z., Duymaz, A., & Savaci, N. (2005). Frostbite injury due to improper usage of an ice pack. *Annals of Plastic Surgery, 55*, 437-438.

Khajavi, K., Pavelko, T., & Mishra, A. K. (2004). Compartment syndrome arising from use of an electronic cooling pad. *American Journal of Sports Medicine, 32*, 1538-1541.

Kinawi, M. M. (1952). Ethyl chloride spray in the treatment of fibrositis, myositis and allied conditions. *Journal of the Egyptian Medical Association, 35*, 705-710.

Knight, K. (1995). *Cryotherapy in sport injury management.* Champaign, IL: Human Kinetics, 3-18, 59-71, 77, 107-130, 175-177, 217-232.

Kuznetsov, O. F., Stiazhkina, E. M., & Gusarova, S. A. (2004). Cryomassage--effective method in rehabilitation medicine. *Voprosy Kurortologii, Fizioterapii, i Lechebnoi Fizicheskoi Kultury; Voprosy Kurortologii, Fizioterapii, i Lechebnoi Fizicheskoi Kultury, 1*, 43-48.

Lacour, M., & Le Coultre, C. (1991). Spray-induced frostbite in a child: A new hazard with novel aerosol propellants. *Pediatric Dermatology, 8*, 207-209.

Lee, S. U., Bang, M. S., & Han, T. R. (2002). Effect of cold air therapy in relieving spasticity: Applied to spinalized rabbits. *Spinal Cord : The Official Journal of the International Medical Society of Paraplegia, 40*, 167-173.

Lehman, J. F. (1990). *Therapeutic heat and cold.* Baltimore, MD: Williams & Wilkins.

Lehmann, J. F., Masock, A. J., Warren, C. G., & Koblanski, J. N. (1970). Effect of therapeutic temperatures on tendon extensibility. *Archives of Physical Medicine and Rehabilitation, 51*, 481-487.

Leigh, I. M., Ramsay, C. A., & Calnan, C. D. (1974). Cold urticaria-"desensitisation." *Transactions of the St. John's Hospital Dermatological Society, 60*, 40-42.

Levy, A. S., & Marmar, E. (1993). The role of cold compression dressings in the postoperative treatment of total knee arthroplasty. *Clinical Orthopaedics and Related Research, (297)*, 174-178.

Licker, M., Schweizer, A., & Ralley, F. E. (1996). Thermoregulatory and metabolic responses following cardiac surgery. *European Journal of Anaesthesiology, 13*, 502-510.

Major, T. C., Schwinghamer, J. M., & Winston, S. (1981). Cutaneous and skeletal muscle vascular responses to hypothermia. *The American Journal of Physiology, 240*, H868-73.

McGuire, D. A., & Hendricks, S. D. (2006). Incidences of frostbite in arthroscopic knee surgery postoperative cryotherapy rehabilitation. *Arthroscopy: The Journal of Arthroscopic & Related Surgery: Official Publication of the Arthroscopy Association of North America and the International Arthroscopy Association, 22*, 1141.e1-1141.e6.

Miglietta, O. (1973). Action of cold on spasticity. *American Journal of Physical Medicine, 52*, 198-205.

Mizushima, T., Obata, K., Katsura, H., Yamanaka, H., Kobayashi, K., & Dai, Y. et al. (2006). Noxious cold stimulation induces mitogen-activated protein kinase activation in transient receptor potential (TRP) channels TRPA1- and TRPM8-containing small sensory neurons. *Neuroscience, 140*, 1337-1348.

Modell, W., Travell, J., Kraus, H., et al. (1952). Relief of pain by ethyl chloride spray. *New York State Journal of Medicine, 52*, 1550-1558.

Morton, R. H. (2006). Contrast water immersion hastens plasma lactate decrease after intense anaerobic exercise. *Journal of Science and Medicine in Sport, Nov 20*.

Nadler, S. F., Weingand, K., & Kruse, R. J. (2004). The physiologic basis and clinical applications of cryotherapy and thermotherapy for the pain practitioner. *Pain Physician, 7*, 395-399.

Newton, R. A. (1985). Effects of vapocoolants on passive hip flexion in healthy subjects. *Physical Therapy, 65*, 1034-1036.

O'Toole, G., & Rayatt, S. (1999). Frostbite at the gym: A case report of an ice pack burn. *British Journal of Sports Medicine, 33*, 278-279.

Ownby, K. K. (2006). Effects of ice massage on neuropathic pain in persons with AIDS. *Journal of the Association of Nurses in AIDS Care, 17*, 15-22.

Petrilli, S., Durufle, A., Nicolas, B., Robineau, S., Kerdoncuff, V., & Le Tallec, H. et al. (2004). Influence of temperature changes on clinical symptoms in multiple sclerosis: An epidemiologic study. *Annales De Readaptation Et De Medecine Physique: Revue Scientifique De La Societe Francaise De Reeducation Fonctionnelle De Readaptation Et De Medecine Physique, 47*, 204-208.

Petrofsky, J. S., Lohman, E.,3rd, Lee, S., de la Cuesta, Z., Labial, L., & Iouciulescu, R., et al. (2006). The influence of alterations in room temperature on skin blood flow during contrast baths in patients with diabetes. *Medical Science Monitor: International Medical Journal of Experimental and Clinical Research, 12*, CR290-5.

Plotkin, S. (1998). Clinical comparison of preinjection anesthetics. *Journal of the American Podiatric Medical Association. 88*(2), 73-79.

Price, R., & Lehmann, J. F. (1990). Influence of muscle cooling on the viscoelastic response of the human ankle to sinusoidal displacements. *Archives of Physical Medicine and Rehabilitation, 71*, 745-748.

Quist, L. H., Peltier, G., & Lundquist, K. J. (1996). Frostbite of the eyelids following inappropriate application of ice compresses. *Archives of Ophthalmology, 114*, 226.

Rudzki, E., & Grzywa, Z. (1978). Desensitization in cold-induced urticaria. *Przeglad Dermatologiczny, 65*, 311-313.

Sevier, T. L., & Wilson, J. K. (1999). Treating lateral epicondylitis. *Sports Medicine (Auckland, N.Z.), 28*, 375-380.

Sheehan, F. T. (1950). Acute stiff neck; treatment with ethyl chloride spray. *Medical Technicians Bulletin, 1*, 7-8.

Shelley, W. B., & Caro, W. A. (1962). Cold erythema. A new hypersensitivity syndrome. *Journal of the American Medical Association, 180*, 639-642.

Sloan, J. P., Giddings, P., & Hain, R. (1988). Effects of cold and compression on edema. *Physical Sports Medicine., 16*, 116-120.

Tachibana, S. (1987). Distribution of motor nerve conduction velocities in the ulnar nerve--a control study, its clinical application and limitations. *No to shinkei. Brain and Nerve, 39*, 807-815.

Thorsson, O. (2001). Cold therapy of athletic injuries. current literature review. *Lakartidningen, 98*, 1512-1513.

Travell, J. (1952). Ethyl chloride spray for painful muscle spasm. *Archives of Physical Medicine and Rehabilitation, 33*, 291-298.

Tsang, K. K., Hertel, J., & Denegar, C. R. (2003). Volume decreases after elevation and intermittent compression of postacute ankle sprains are negated by gravity-dependent positioning. *J.Athl Train., 38*, 320-324.

van Linschoten, R., & den Hoed, P. T. (2004). Diagnostic image (172). A man with blisters after the use of a cold pack. cryotrauma caused by frozen cold pack. *Nederlands Tijdschrift Voor Geneeskunde, 148*, 134.

Waters, B. L., & Raisler, J. (2003). Ice massage for the reduction of labor pain. *Journal of Midwifery & Women's Health, 48*, 317-321.

Webb, J. M., Williams, D., Ivory, J. P., Day, S., & Williamson, D. M. (1998). The use of cold compression dressings after total knee replacement: A randomized controlled trial. *Orthopedics, 21*, 59-61.

Wilke, B., & Weiner, R. D. (2003). Postoperative cryotherapy: Risks versus benefits of continuous-flow cryotherapy units. *Clinics in Podiatric Medicine and Surgery, 20*, 307-322.

Wolf, S. L., & Basmajian, J. V. (1973). Intramuscular temperature changes deep to localized cutaneous cold stimulation. *Physical Therapy, 53*, 1284-1288.

Yackzan, L., Adams, C., & Francis, K. T. (1984). The effects of ice massage on delayed muscle soreness. *American Journal of Sports Medicine, 12*, 159-165.

Zankel, H. T. (1966). Effect of physical agents on motor conduction velocity of the ulnar nerve. *Archives of Physical Medicine and Rehabilitation, 47*, 787-792.

Zappa, S. C., & Nabors, S. B. (1992). Use of ethyl chloride topical anesthetic to reduce procedural pain in pediatric oncology patients. *Cancer Nursing, 15*, 130-136.

Zappa, S. C., Nabors, S. B., & Wise, C. (1991). The use of ethyl chloride anesthetic spray before invasive procedures performed on pediatric oncology patients. *Journal of Pediatric Oncology Nursing, 8*, 87-88.

Zemke, J. E., Andersen, J. C., Guion, W. K., McMillan, J., & Joyner, A. B. (1998). Intramuscular temperature responses in the human leg to two forms of cryotherapy: Ice massage and ice bag. *Journal of Orthopaedic and Sports Physical Therapy, 27*, 301-307.

# Chapter 6

# THERMOTHERAPY
## SUPERFICIAL HEAT AGENTS

## Learning Objectives

1. Define thermotherapy.
2. Differentiate between conduction and convection.
3. Discuss the relationship between heat application and occupational performance.
4. Discuss the factors that influence tissue temperature elevation.
5. Discuss the biophysiological effects of heat.
6. Identify the indications for and precautions or contraindications of using superficial thermal agents.
7. Demonstrate clinical reasoning in the selection of superficial thermal agents.
8. Discuss the clinical application of hydrotherapy, fluidotherapy, hot pack, contrast bath, and paraffin.

## Terminology

| | | |
|---|---|---|
| Conduction | Heat dosage | Systemic effects |
| Convection | Local effects | Thermotherapy |
| Dependent limb position | Superficial thermal agents | |

## Introduction

Superficial thermal agents transfer energy either to or from body tissue that is located "superficially." Transfer of energy between the superficial agent and the tissue occurs due to a temperature gradient. The application of therapeutic heat to the body is known as thermotherapy. The mechanisms of heating tissue are classified as being superficial or deep, dependent on the depth of penetration into the underlying tissue. Heat can be transferred to the tissue through three primary mechanisms, radiation, conduction, or convection. Therapeutic ultrasound (which utilizes sound energy to produce a thermal effect in tissue) and diathermy devices (which use electrical or magnetic currents) are considered deep heating agents. Hot packs, heating pads, fluidotherapy (Chattanooga Group, Hixson, TN), and paraffin baths are examples of superficial heating agents (Health tips. hot vs. cold treatment, 2002; Aiello, 2004). Therapeutic ultrasound will be discussed in a later chapter.

# Thermal Heat Transfer

The application of heat to the body as a means to achieve a relaxing, soothing response has been acknowledged for centuries. The ancient Greeks believed the sun's radiation had natural therapeutic qualities that could treat illnesses. The Greek word for sun is "helio," and is used to form compound words such as heliotherapy (defined as "using the sunlight for the treatment of diseases"). During the 20th century, thermotherapy was a general term used to categorize the means of applying heat superficially that would cause a biophysiological response when treating certain pathologic conditions. In rehabilitation today, the application of thermal agents are most often used to achieve an increase in cell metabolism, blood flow, and soft tissue elasticity by elevating and sustaining tissue temperatures between 104° to 113° F. Clinically, application of superficial heat increases the tissue temperature varying degrees and has been used clinically to increase the extensibility of collagen tissue, decrease muscle spasm, decrease pain, increase metabolic rate, and for the subjective "comfort" many patients experience (Lehmann, Masock, Warren, & Koblanski, 1970; Lehmann, Dundore, Esselman, & Nelp, 1983; Lin, 2003).

# Methods of Heat Exchange

Superficial heating agents, or thermotherapy, are frequently used by occupational therapists in clinical practice. Superficial heat modalities have been defined as the therapeutic application of any modality to the skin resulting in an increase in skin and superficial subcutaneous tissue temperature. Superficial heat is contraindicated during the first 24 to 36 hours following an acute injury if hemorrhage and edema are noted. During the subacute phase of healing, superficial heat can be applied to facilitate the healing process. It is important for the therapist to consider the position of the extremity during the application of superficial heat agents as dependent positions of the extremity may ultimately contribute to edema. There are two primary methods of thermal heat transfer used by occupational therapists: *conduction* and *convection*. A third form of heat exchange, radiation, is used less frequently by occupational therapists.

## Conduction

Conduction involves an exchange of energy between two materials that have two different temperatures. When an area with higher temperature comes into contact with an area with lower temperature, it will result in the transfer of energy to the area with the lower temperature and raise its temperature until both areas are equally heated. For example, if a thermal physical agent such as a hot pack is applied to the skin to achieve a specific physiologic response, the heat will transfer from the agent to the patient's extremity, and thereby, increase the skin temperature. The degree of temperature variance between the thermal agent that will be applied, and the

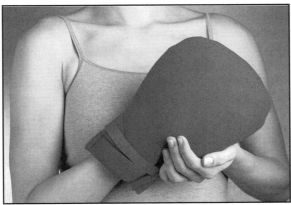

**Figure 6-1.** Therma-Wrap provides hot or cold therapy for relief of pain related to musculo-skeletal injuries (Photo courtesy of Chattanooga Group).

underlying tissue where heat is being transferred is an important characteristic that must be taken into consideration by the therapist. If the transfer of the heat from the thermal agent to the tissue is too slow, the desired therapeutic effect may not be achieved. Conversely, if heat is transferred too rapidly, it could burn the patient. Understanding the balance between the physiological condition of the patient's tissue and the temperature variance is critical for the safe application of any thermal agent. Commonly used physical agents used to transfer heat through conduction include hot packs, paraffin baths, heating pads, chemical heat wraps (Figure 6-1), and ThermaCare HeatWraps (Procter & Gamble, Cincinnati, OH) (Akin, Price, Rodriguez, Erasala, Hurley, & Smith, 2004; Ottawa Panel, 2004).

## Convection

Convection is the conveyance of heat by the movement of heated particles over an extremity. When heated air or water molecules move across the body part being treated, a temperature variation will result due to the higher temperature created by the air or water. As the molecules move across the body part, temperature variation occurs because the higher temperature of the air or water will transfer to the lower temperature of the patient's extremity (Aiello, 2004). This process of molecular movement is in contrast to conduction because the medium is continuously moving over the body part and the warm thermal elements are constantly coming into contact with the area being treated. With conduction, the same material remains in constant contact of the area being treated and as the material begins to cool, its efficiency decreases. PAMs utilized to transfer heat through convection include fluidotherapy and whirlpool baths (Figure 6-2).

## Radiation

Transfer of energy through radiation involves the movement of the radiant energy through the air from a warmer source to a cooler one. An example of a radiant form of heat, are the "heat lamps" frequently seen in restaurants where the food is placed after being cooked in order to keep it warm. Clinically, infrared lamps were used to heat specific areas of the body and to increase the temperature of the tissue. These were placed over the body part being treated and did not come into contact with the individual's skin or tissue. This form of heat agent is not commonly used in occupational therapy.

**Figure 6-2.** Whirlpool application for debridement. Whirlpool uses convection. Therapeutic temperature for whirlpool debridement is "tepid" or approximately 98° F.

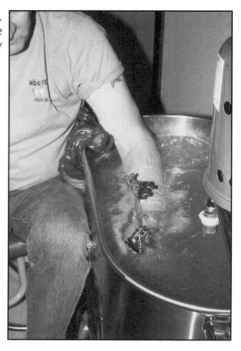

# Basic Principles

A primary reason for applying a heat agent is to increase the temperature of soft tissue to a specific therapeutic range so that a certain physiological response will be achieved. The application of heating agents will cause biophysiological responses such as increase of blood flow, rate of cell metabolism, oxygen consumption, capillary permeability, inflammation, and muscle contraction velocity. Conversely, heat agents will decrease the fluid viscosity, pain, and muscle spasm (by decreasing the pain and ischemia) (Matsumoto, Kawahira, Etoh, Ikeda, & Tanaka, 2006; Tao & Bernacki, 2005).

When the temperature of soft tissue is increased between a range of 104° to 113° F, it can have a positive therapeutic affect on the patient. If the soft tissue is heated to a level less than 104° F, then the cell metabolism will not be stimulated adequately enough to achieve a therapeutic response. If the same tissue is heated to a temperature level greater than 113° F, then catabolism and cell death will usually occur. Factors that will affect the extent of achieving a specific biophysiological response in tissue include the intensity of the heat, the modality being used to apply the heat, the length of exposure time, and the overall surface area that is involved. These factors must be taken into consideration by the therapist prior to applying a superficial heat modality and to avoid achieving a systemic rather than localized reaction. Superficial heating agents usually will penetrate the skin between 1 to 2 centimeters (cm). At a depth of 1 cm, the soft tissue temperature will elevate by 6°, whereas at a depth of 2 cm, the temperature will only elevate by 2° (Borrell, Parker, Henley, Masley, & Repinecz, 1980; Lehmann & deLateur, 1990a).

Applying a superficial heat agent preparatory to engagement in occupational activities can prepare the tissue for the activity. Greenburg noted that engagement in an activity increased blood flow to the tissue and that combining heat and activity increased blood flow even more when contrasted to either heat or activity alone (Greenberg, 1972). Animal studies, however, have been equivocal and have concluded that changes in blood temperature do not contribute to the hyperemic effect of limb warming is no more effective at promoting limb flow than exercise alone (McMeeken & Bell, 1990). Many of the patients occupational therapists treat, particularly those with musculoskeletal impairments, may benefit from superficial heat agents in order to facilitate occupational performance and activity.

Mobilization procedures require less force to elongate the tissue and improve viscoelasticity when superficial heat is applied before the procedures, and temperature elevation without stress does not improve the therapeutic extensibility of tissue deformation (Conroy & Hayes, 1998; Robertson, Ward, & Jung, 2005). Utilizing heat and therapeutic occupation facilitates deformation of the tissue, more effectively resulting in tissue elongation and deformation. For some diagnoses and conditions frequently seen by occupational therapists, application of heat may be advantageous to the target tissue, facilitate occupational performance, and support more effective outcomes.

## Physiological Response to Temperature Variation

An understanding of the physiological responses to tissue temperature variation before using a thermal agent is necessary to appropriately and effectively select the correct method and agent. Physiological changes to the tissue are safe and effective when they involve a subcutaneous tissue temperature increase between 0°F to 14°F (deLateur, Stonebridge, & Lehmann, 1978; Lehmann, Warren, & Scham, 1974). Physiological response in the underlying tissue is dependent on three primary factors, the rate that the temperature is added to the tissue (the intensity), the duration of tissue temperature elevation (how long the tissue is heated), and the area or volume of the tissue exposed (Hecox, Andemicael-Mehreteab, Weisberg, & Sanko, 2006). Thermal temperatures are considered either mild or vigorous. A mild application of heat occurs when the tissue temperature elevation is less than 40°C or 104° F. A vigorous dose of heat is considered when the temperature of the tissue is elevated between 40° to 45°C (104° to 113° F) and cell catabolism and tissue damage occurring when tissue temperatures are elevated beyond that level (Lehmann & deLateur, 1990b).

An important factor that influences the physiologic response of a superficial thermal agent is its *conductive nature*. The impact of conduction on the underlying tissue can be partially regulated by the therapist through the use of different application procedures or techniques. For example, by increasing or decreasing the coupling media, such as using layered towels with hot packs, can either provide additional insulation to prevent overheating of the tissue or increase the heat by using a damp towel. Positioning of the hot packs by draping the hot packs over the body part or extremity and securing them with hook-and-loop fasteners can ensure there will be a tighter fit of the area being heated and increase the conductive effect. Resting the body part on top of the hot pack may also influence the conduction of the heat into the tissue and must be taken into consideration.

The amount of adipose tissue and the location of the tissue will also influence the amount of heat transferred. Adipose tissue acts as an insulator and does not facilitate the conduction of heat to deeper structures. Patients with increased amounts of fat may require a different form of heat such as ultrasound in order for therapeutic temperatures to be reached below the fat layer. Deep structures or muscles generally do not demonstrate increases in tissue temperature unless the thermal agent is applied for a longer period of time, usually 20 minutes or longer. However, more superficial tissue such as that in the hand or on the dorsal aspect of the forearm will heat more readily due to the lack of insulating adipose or underlying tissue. If tissue temperatures elevate to levels greater than desired these factors and their influence on heat transfer must be taken consideration as well as the rate at which the heat is being delivered.

A mild dose of heat with a minimal change in tissue temperature may be sufficient to provide the patient with more of a sensory response of warmth, rather than a primary physiological change to the tissue. Patients frequently ask about "treatment" they can "do at home" when being treated for musculoskeletal conditions. Application of warm water soaks, low temperature heating pads, hot water bottles, and others are often safe, effective home interventions that can be recommended for a mild or moderate warm, sensory response. A vigorous dose implies a marked increase in blood flow with a tissue temperature rise of 107° to 113° F (Hecox et al., 2006). This dosage may be beneficial to ischemic conditions and is typically used when heat is indicated and increasing edema in the treatment area is not a concern. Tissue temperature elevation beyond 113° F can be unsafe and may cause tissue damage. It is crucial to educate patients with sensory paresthesias to monitor their skin condition when applying any heat agent in the clinic or at home, and inform them to use caution when around flame or high temperature appliances such as stoves or ovens so that burning or tissue damage doesn't occur. Special care and instruction is crucial if these individuals will be using any form of home program involving the application of heat to the tissue.

When heat is applied, the vascular protective response of vasodilation occurs. When the temperature of an area is elevated, there is an increase in the blood flow to the region, with cooler blood flowing into the area to dissipate some of the heat produced. The blood flow to the treatment area acts as a convective agent, attempting to reduce the heating of the tissue. If the heat is applied too rapidly, the excess heat is not dissipated quickly enough and tissue temperature elevation occurs with stimulation of the nociceptors and potential tissue damage (Baker & Bell, 1991). The convective effect of the blood assists in the regulation and removal of heat from the body. If the temperature of the tissues rises faster than the body can dissipate the heat, tissue temperature increases. This becomes unsafe at temperatures exceeding 113° F, and damage to the tissue may occur (Ersala, Rubin, & Tuthill, 2001; Krusen, 1950).

---

## BIOPHYSIOLOGICAL RESPONSE OF HEAT

*Increases*

- Blood flow
- Rate of cell metabolism
- Oxygen consumption
- Capillary permeability
- Inflammation
- Muscle contraction velocity

*Decreases*

- Fluid viscosity
- Fluid viscosity
- Pain
- Muscle spasm (by decreasing pain & ischemia)

# Biophysical Effects

There are four primary effects of superficial heat agents: *analgesic, vascular, metabolic,* and *extensibility.* These physiological responses provide the basis for heat application when therapeutic levels of heat are used.

## Analgesic Effect

The analgesic effect of heat involves reducing pain symptomatology. The application of heat acts selectively on free nerve endings, tissues, and peripheral nerve fibers—either directly or indirectly—reducing pain and elevating pain tolerance (De Jong, Hershey, & Wagman, 1966; Schmidt, Ott, Rocher, & Schaller, 1979). The vascular effects of heat can aid in pain relief and in decreasing muscle spasm. The vascular effects of heat application can aid in pain relief and decrease the muscle spasms that a patient may be experiencing. Since the blood flow will increase as a result of the heat, the outcome will be the removal of the local muscle metabolites and the reduction of the muscle spindle's sensitivity to stretch with subsequent pain and frequently muscle spasm. It also should be noted that most muscle tissue will not be directly affected by superficial heating modalities since they lie too deeply. When a decrease in pain occurs there is likely to be a concurrent improvement in functional ability and occupational performance.

## Vascular Effect

When a thermal agent is applied to an area of the body, the immediate response will be an increase of blood flow to the area being treated. As the tissue temperature increases, the blood vessels will dilate in response; blood vessels that are more superficial will dilate greater than the deeper blood vessels. Although the increased blood will act as a mechanism to counteract the increased temperature, the additional flow will also bring an extra supply of oxygen, nutrients, and antibodies to the affected area.

## Metabolic Effect

When there is an increase of the body temperature, metabolic activity will increase because of the cellular response. For example, if the temperature increases 10° F, the cells' metabolic rate will increase two-fold. Associated with the metabolic increase is a demand for additional oxygen as well as the creation of metabolites (as a by-product of cell metabolism). The increase in blood flow will also provide additional oxygen and cause the removal of the cells' by-products through venous return. A 6° to 14° F tissue temperature rise facilitates the release of substances, such as histamines and prostaglandins into the bloodstream, resulting in vasodilation and increased blood flow. This increase in blood flow reduces ischemia, muscle spindle activity, and tonic muscle contractions, thereby reducing pain (Lehmann et al., 1974; Lehmann & deLateur, 1990b; Samborski et al., 1992). The metabolic effects of heat can aid in pain relief and tissue repair. Increased blood flow and oxygen within the tissue bring greater numbers of antibodies, leukocytes, nutrients, and enzymes to injured tissues. Pain is also reduced by the removal of byproducts of the inflammatory process. Nutrition is enhanced at the cellular level and cellular repair occurs. Metabolites associated with chronic swelling and fibrotic joint changes are also reduced due to the application of heat to localized tissue (Abramson, Mitchell, Tuck, Bell, & Zays, 1961; Halvorsen, 1990; Hillman & Delforge, 1985; Wedlick, 1967).

## Extensibility Effect

Heat applications that are placed on soft tissue can assist in increasing the collagen extensibility. Raising tissue temperatures between 104° to 113° F for approximately 10 minutes will also facilitate soft tissue extensibility when combined with stretch. The elevation of the tissue temperature and the viscoelasticity of the connective tissues promotes elongation of the connective tissue following heat and stretch (Reid, 1992; Sapega, Quedecfeld, & Moyer, 1981). Application of heat to the targeted area may be useful for stretching cutaneous scar tissue, superficial joint capsules, and tendons. The connective tissue response involves an improvement in the properties of collagen and the extensibility of tissue when combined with passive or active mobilization and engagement in occupation. Joint stiffness is reduced and range of motion (ROM) may be improved.

For most musculoskeletal or neuromuscular conditions, all phases of wound healing, except the initial inflammatory stage, may benefit from the various forms of heat application. Therapeutic dosages used clinically include moderate to vigorous forms of heat. Clinical interventions should be able to provide the desired dosage based on temperature selection and conduction factors.

# Evaluation

The initial evaluation and patient interview is a crucial element of the clinical reasoning process. The patient interview is necessary to determine acuity of the injury or condition as well as to identify any potential precautions or contraindications that may preclude the use of thermotherapy.

---

### EVALUATION CONSIDERATIONS INCLUDE

- Past medical history
- Pregnancy
- Skin condition: color, temperature, sensitivity, dryness, and overall integrity
- Current medications and any known allergies

---

# Indications

Many of the musculoskeletal and neuromuscular conditions and disorders that are commonly seen by clinicians will benefit from superficial heat application. Heat can be used to decrease pain and stiffness, improve ROM and flexibility, increase tendon excursion, improve synovial viscosity, and promote healing and relaxation.

---

## CONDITIONS THAT BENEFIT FROM HEAT INCLUDE

- Stiff joints
- Subcutaneous adhesions
- Contractures
- Chronic arthritis
- Subacute and chronic inflammation/cumulative trauma
- Trauma/wounds (judiciously used whirlpool or hydrotherapy)
- Neuromas
- Sympathetic nervous system disorders
- Muscle spasms

---

# Precautions

Most thermotherapy applications are safe and effective when applied appropriately and cautiously. The occupational therapist must take the necessary precautions to assure that the heat treatment is a safe adjunct to the therapeutic program. Increased edema is a primary drawback of heat application, and proper positioning of the extremity and modality as well as any mobilization techniques must be considered to counteract any adverse effects. The therapist should be cautious when treating patients with other associated conditions, such as diminished sensation and compromised circulation as these may cause burning or tissue damage. The clinician should monitor the patient's response to the heat agent at all times by asking the patient for any subjective feedback as well as visually checking the skin condition if the modality allows. Subjective comments related to any negative effects should be immediately addressed and the heat agent removed or the application modified to ensure that there is no burning of the tissue. Overt physiological signs, such as respiration, blood pressure, and skin color, should be monitored as well. Application of heat should be discontinued if local signs related to the effects of heat overexposure, such as increased redness, petechiae, and blistering are noted. When superficial heat applications are recommended as part of a home treatment program, it is crucial that the patient be instructed in the proper application of the modality as well as being able to identify potential adverse reactions to the application and astute enough to discontinue the treatment.

# Contraindications

Determining whether to use heat as an adjunct to treatment often depends on the intensity of the heat modality under consideration and the patient's circulatory status and sensitivity to temperature variations. Heat should not be used with those patients who have appreciable circulatory impairment or in the presence of undetermined edema or during the acute, inflammatory phase of healing. Heat is typically used for its local effects though there are systemic effects that occur from a localized application of heat. Heat is dissipated from local tissue due to the convective action of the circulating blood. In individuals with circulatory impairment, the body is unable to efficiently rid itself of heat as efficiently as those who are healthy. The patient may experience an increased heart rate from the systemic effects of the heat application as well.

Superficial heat agents should not be used with the following conditions:

➤ Impaired sensation (superficial, skin graft, scar, or inability to determine temperature changes)

➤ Patients with poor thermal regulation

➤ Tumors/cancer

➤ Acute inflammation, including acute edema

➤ Deep vein thrombophlebitis

➤ Pregnancy—full immersion (the systemic effects of circulating blood on a fetus are unclear, superficial application over an extremity can be used)

➤ Bleeding tendencies

➤ Infection

➤ Primary repair of tendon or ligament

➤ Advanced cardiac disease

➤ Semicomatose or impaired mental status (or patients with speech and language difficulties, they may not be able to inform or understand the therapists directions)

➤ Rheumatoid arthritis (vigorous dosages of heat may facilitate proteins that act as catalysts to increase enzyme activity, exacerbating joint inflammation) (Schmidt et al., 1979)

# Modality Selection

Superficial heat agents should serve as an adjunctive modality that will prepare patients for involvement in purposeful occupations. The indications when using superficial thermal agents include, but are not limited to, the treatment of stiff joints, subcutaneous adhesions, soft tissue contractures, chronic arthritis, subacute and chronic inflammation, cumulative trauma, wounds, neuromas, and sympathetic nervous system disorders.

Modality selection will depend on a number of factors, based in part on the patient's diagnosis and condition, the findings on the initial evaluation, and the goals of the assessment. Appropriate selection of thermotherapy is related to the objective of superficial heat use, the location and surface area of the involved structure, the desired dosage or tissue temperature, and the desired depth of penetration. Other considerations include whether moist or dry heat is desired, positioning of the extremity in a (non) dependent or intermittently dependent position, and whether active or passive patient participation is desired. Consideration of whether the condition being treated is acute, subacute, or chronic is also necessary and is a vital component of the initial assessment. If depths greater than 1 cm are desired, ultrasound may be indicated (Michlovitz & Wolf, 1990). The effect that the heat application will have upon tissue will depend on the temperature of the application site and the type of modality used (Borrell et al., 1980; Lehmann & deLateur, 1990b). Common applications of heat used by occupational therapists include whirlpool baths or hydrotherapy, fluidotherapy, hot packs, paraffin wax, contrast baths, and warm water soaks.

## Table 6-1

### EFFECTIVE WHIRLPOOL TEMPERATURES

| Water Temperature | | Clinical Condition |
|---|---|---|
| 104° (Never exceed a temperature greater than 110° F) | HOT! Monitor patient closely for systemic and skin. | Soft tissue extensibility, chronic conditions, localized areas |
| 99° to 104° F | Very warm to hot | Pain, osteoarthritis, rheumatoid arthritis (nonacute) |
| 92° to 96° F | Neutral warmth | Wounds, chronic wounds, decubitus, peripheral vascular disease, circulatory disorders |
| 79° to 92° F | Tepid | Exercise, full body immersion, active movement |

# Clinical Applications

## Whirlpool Bath/Hydrotherapy

Whirlpool bath or hydrotherapy can be used when a mild, moderate, or vigorous dosage of moist heat is desired. The body part being treated is immersed into a tank of water that is agitated by a jet of water and air via an electric turbine. This form of hydrotherapy is most often used as a part of wound care, though there are other benefits to the use and application of water. One of the properties of water is buoyancy, which helps in producing a gravity-eliminated environment. This environment can be therapeutic for graded active mobilization of an affected body part such as a patient with a wrist fracture which has been immobilized for several weeks. An advantage to the use of whirlpool bath is that the therapist is able to see and have immediate access to the body part being treated. Water temperature can be controlled and set to the desired temperature (Table 6-1).

For wound debridement, a warm temperature is sufficient in order to prevent edema and its concurrent difficulties. The amount of water agitation can be controlled and can be adjusted to act as a soft tissue massage and/or a resistance for exercise. If wounds or excessive skin dryness or maceration are present (commonly seen after cast removal), a whirlpool bath can be used for cleaning and debridement, which further aids in the healing process. The use of hydrotherapy as a means of mechanical debridement will help remove necrotic and devitalized tissue, exudates, and dirt or foreign contaminants in the wound bed itself. Chronic ulcers or wounds are the type of injury most often treated for debridement using whirlpool, and should be placed in the whirlpool in neutrally warm water (92° to 96° F) for approximately 10 to 20 minutes. As with any open wound, care should be used to prevent aggressive agitation of the water that might shear off or mechanically debride new tissue growth. Use of an antimicrobial agent should be added to the water to prevent infection from contaminants and the whirlpool should be thoroughly cleaned after each use (Bohannon,

1985; Niederhuber, Stribley, & Koepke, 1975; Solomon, 1985). Whirlpool baths allow the patient to participate in a variety of active movements while in the whirlpool and thus may be prevent some of the difficulties associated with more passive forms of heat application (see Figure 6-2).

A disadvantage in using whirlpool bath is the dependent position of the extremity within the whirlpool bath. This dependent position—the hand/arm below the level of the heart—may cause an increase in edema. If edema is a concern, it may not be desirable to maintain the extremity below the level of the heart. To counteract this, the patient should be instructed to intermittently elevate the body part, such as the hand, and raise it above shoulder level. If feasible, this should be complemented by pumping or "fisting" the hand several times in succession (active flexion and extension of the fingers). If the water is being used for exercise, tepid water temperatures (79° to 92° F) should be used to prevent fatigue. This temperature is also used when the patient will be immersed completely in a tank or therapy pool. A hot whirlpool (99° to 104° F) is effective for decreasing pain and/or to increase the extensibility of soft tissue. Whirlpool temperatures should never exceed 110° as the higher temperature will cause cell catabolism and burns. Always make sure that your whirlpool has a thermometer in the water which is accurate and easily read. Optimal length of treatment is approximately 15 to 20 minutes.

A disadvantage to using whirlpool is the time required for set up and cleaning of the tank in order to avoid cross contamination and infection. This process may be too time consuming in busy clinics. Whirlpool baths are an effective modality to use with open or chronic wounds, status post fracture (where stiffness and excessive skin dryness is present), inflammatory conditions (with tepid water), peripheral vascular disease, and peripheral nerve injuries.

## Fluidotherapy

Fluidotherapy can provide a variety of dosages of dry heat. Analgesic effects can be obtained with lower temperatures and other physiological effects are achieved at higher temperatures. Fluidotherapy uses fine particles suspended in a hot air stream to heat the extremity (Borrell et al., 1980). The fine particles are made of ground cellulose from corn husks. The temperature of the circulating air is controlled by a thermostat on the machine. This type of treatment can be used on the distal extremities, primarily the hands and feet (see Figure 6-2). An advantage of using fluidotherapy is the ease of implementation and the consistency of the temperature of the circulating air. Fluidotherapy provides heat, a sensory effect useful for desensitization, and pressure oscillations that may decrease edema. The machine can be purchased with either single or dual accessibility, features which allow the therapist access to the patient's extremity while in the unit, allowing for passive ROM, joint mobilization, and manipulation. The accessibility feature also allows the treatment of up to two patients at a time. The force of the air and particles circulating within the machine can be graded via the blower speed. The force of the blower speed allows for mobilization to take place during the treatment process. Many therapists use fluidotherapy for the desensitization effect that it provides with abnormally hypersensitive areas. Benefits of fluidotherapy have been reported for pain, ROM, wounds and acute injuries, swelling, and increasing blood flow. Any open wounds, lesions, or infections must be covered with a protective dressing prior to inserting the extremity into the entry port to prevent cross contamination of the media or the wound.

A potential disadvantage of fluidotherapy is that the extremity is maintained in the dependent position. The clinician must be prudent in using this modality, particularly

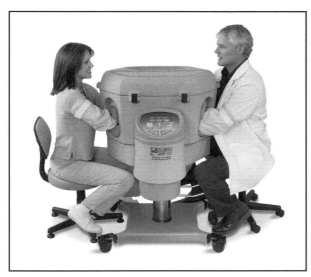

**Figure 6-3.** Fluidotherapy. Note additional ports for therapist to access to the extremity for mobilization, exercise, or manipulation (Photo courtesy of Chattanooga Group).

if edema is evident. If edema is a concern, fluidotherapy should be used with the patient engaging in functional movement of the extremity, using a pumping action of the hand to counteract any adverse effects of the heat dosage. A second issue relates to housekeeping duties. If a high volume of patients are treated throughout the day, particles from the machine often end up on the floor and may become slippery. It is also recommended that the media be replaced on a consistent basis dependent upon the amount of use (Figure 6-3).

The first step in using fluidotherapy is to pre-heat the unit to 105° to 118° F. The blower speed should be adjusted to provide the desired air and particle flow within the machine. The body part being treated should be clean and free from jewelry. Open wounds should not be placed in the unit. If any small open wounds or lacerations are present, the therapist needs to make sure they are adequately covered before treatment begins. The length of treatment is typically 20 minutes.

## FLUIDOTHERAPY CLINICAL CONSIDERATIONS

### Advantages

- Unit is easy to operate and move, and does not require towels or plumbing fixtures
- Heat can be evenly distributed over entire area being treated, including when wound is properly bandaged and covered with plastic
- Adjustments to airflow will allow effective intervention to treat hypertension
- PROM, AROM, and AAROM are possible during application

### Disadvantages

- Only applicable to distal extremity
- Hands must be in a dependent position
- Treatment can be messy and become a safety issue
- Unit is relatively expensive to purchase

**Figure 6-4.** Hot pack application. Note layers of toweling to protect the underlying tissue. The blue Nylatex strap (New York, NY) can be used to tighten down the hot pack providing greater conductivity to the tissue. Always monitor patients skin condition to avoid burns!

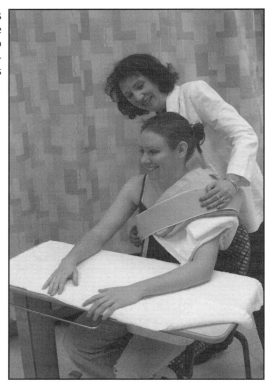

## Hot Packs

Hot packs transfer heat through conduction and are one of the most commonly used heat modalities in clinics. The thermal application is effective up to a depth of 1 cm and can elevate the subcutaneous soft tissue temperature nearly 39° F. Although heat can extend to a depth of 3 cm, it will not have the same therapeutic effect as at lesser depths (Draper et al., 1998; Greenberg, 1972). Hot packs consist of a silica gel medium covered by a canvas pouch and are kept in a thermostatically controlled cabinet containing water. The temperature maintained within the hydrocollator is between 165° and 175° F and is high enough to kill any bacteria that may collect on the canvas pouch. When the hot pack has been properly heated, the high temperature rate can be maintained for 30 to 45 minutes after removing the pack from the hydrocollator. Hot packs are typically used to provide moderate or vigorous doses of moist heat and come in a variety of sizes. Depending on the area that will be treated, hot packs can effectively treat larger areas of the body and are able to form over body contours such as the shoulder or neck. The temperature of the hot pack is typically between 104° to 113° F when it is removed from the hydrocollator. Hot packs are cooler than water because of the properties that make up the various materials of this heat agent (Figure 6-4). Generally, a new hot pack will require 2 hours of immersion in the hydrocollator unit to achieve its therapeutic temperature and effect. After each application, it will require approximately 30 minutes to reheat the pack before it can again reach a therapeutic temperature level.

Hot packs are generally easy to use and require minimal maintenance. The water in the hydrocollator tank should be monitored for temperature and depth, with water added as needed to completely cover the hot packs. The temperature of the water should be documented on a weekly basis to ensure that the effective therapeutic range is not exceeded. The hydrocollator unit can be drained and cleaned as needed. Because of the high temperature of hot packs, any direct contact with the skin will result in immediate pain and potential damage (including burns) to the soft tissue. Consequently, a coupling medium should be placed between the hot pack and skin that consists of at least six layers of dry Turkish towels. These towels are also beneficial in creating air pockets that can serve as added insulation. When treating a patient, dry towels should always be utilized as the coupling medium because heat will transfer at a more rapid rate if the heated towels are damp. Many clinics use a combination of a commercially-available terrycloth hot pack cover (that is the equivalent of approximately three layers of towels) combined with an additional number of towels. Because hot packs cool fairly rapidly when removed from the hydrocollator unit, they are somewhat "safer" to use as they will become increasingly cooler as the treatment time progresses. In addition, they are easy to remove, thereby facilitating skin checks and the ability to be quickly removed by either the patient or therapist if they become too hot. Hot packs are considered a "passive" form of treatment since patients are not actively involved during the application. However, a positional sustained stretch of the tissue being treated can be accomplished during the heating process if necessary. Hot packs are beneficial in helping to reduce pain and muscle spasms and to improve connective tissue extensibility (Michlovitz & Wolf, 1990; Perret, Rim, & Cristian, 2006; Robertson et al., 2005).

A disadvantage to using hot packs is that the larger size hot packs can be heavy and are contraindicated if too uncomfortable for the patient. Additionally, the area being treated is covered, making it difficult for the therapist to visually monitor the patient's skin integrity. Depending on the treatment site and the size of the hot pack, extra padding may be required if the patient is placing undue pressure over a bony prominence or body part (Michlovitz & Wolf, 1990).

The general instructions for hot pack application are as follows:

- ➤ The hot pack should be removed from the tank using tongs to prevent burning of the therapist's hands. The excess water should be allowed to drain into the tank and the hot pack quickly placed into the hot pack cover.

- ➤ The hot pack is wrapped in several layers of cloth toweling and/or commercial hot pack covers to prevent burns.

- ➤ Be aware that pressure from positioning will cause conductive heating. To decrease conduction, reposition body part and add additional toweling. To improve conduction, further secure hot pack with Thera-Band or toweling over the body part being treated (e.g., shoulder).

- ➤ Treatment length is approximately 20 minutes.

- ➤ Allow hot pack to reheat for at least 30 minutes before using it again.

- ➤ Check the patient's status and ask the patient how the treatment feels after the first 5 minutes of treatment.

- ➤ Remove the hot pack and towels to check the skin for signs of burning, excessive redness, or blistering.

- ➤ Clinical note: If there is evidence of overheating, discontinue treatment immediately and briefly apply a cold pack to stop the overheating response.

➤ At the end of the 20-minute treatment session, remove the hot pack and towels and again ask the patient how the treatment session felt.

➤ When inspecting the skin, the treated area should appear slightly red and be warm to the touch.

➤ The hot pack should then be placed in the hydrocollator and reheated for 30 minutes before using it again.

---

## HOT PACK CLINICAL CONSIDERATIONS

### Advantages

- Easy to use
- Require minimal maintenance (with a hydrocollator)
- Provide moderate and vigorous doses of heat
- Various size and shapes
- Passive form of treatment since patients are not involved during application
- Can incorporate heat treatment into intervention program
- Body segment can be placed into sustained positional stretch

### Disadvantages

- After hot pack has been applied, the skin cannot be observed
- Patient may not be able to tolerate treatment and weight
- Weight can accelerate rate of heat being transferred
- Passive treatment may not allow AROM during the heating period

---

## Contrast Bath

Contrast bath involves alternating placement of an extremity between water that has been either heated or cooled so that the extremity alternates between periods of vasoconstriction and vasodilation (Figure 6-5). Contrast baths are frequently used to decrease edema in an extremity and to improve peripheral blood flow and decrease edema. Concurrently, contrast baths may also reduce pain and stiffness and aid in the healing process (Lehmann & deLateur, 1990b). Contrast baths provide mild to moderate levels of heat and are frequently used to control subacute or chronic inflammation and for some musculoskeletal conditions. It is important to monitor the patient's reaction to the extremes of temperature variation due to the autonomic reaction which can occur, affecting blood pressure and heart rate. This issue is particularly important for those patients who will be using contrast baths as part of a home program to decrease or control their symptoms. The clinical intention of contrast baths is to facilitate a "pumping" type action through the alternating vasoconstriction and vasodilation. However, there is little to support this theory, and it may be that there is more of a superficial capillary response as the larger, deeper blood vessels do not constrict or dilate since the effect is more superficial (Morton, 2006; Myrer, Draper, & Durrant, 1994; Petrofsky et al., 2006; Stanton, Bear-Lehman, Graziano, & Ryan, 2003; Smith & Newton, 1994).

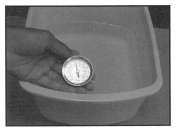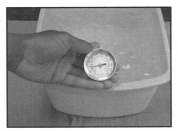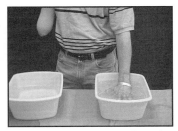

**Figure 6-5.** Contrast bath applications. Note temperature variations in the contrasting tubs. The patient alternates placing the extremity between the warm water and the cold water. This application is frequently used for the treatment of edema.

Application and treatment utilizing contrast bath involves alternating the affected extremity between warm and cold water. This can be accomplished by filling two containers with water, one with warm water between 100° to 110° F and one with cold tap water, typically at a temperature between 50° to 70° F. Although various protocols exist, the general guidelines are to have the patient immerse the part being treated in warm water for 10 minutes. After 10 minutes in warm water, the patient should place the body part in cold water for 1 minute. The patient then returns to warm water for 4 minutes and then cold water for 1 minute. This 4:1 cycle is completed two additional times. When a contrast bath is used as a superfical heat agent, the patient should end the treatment in 4 minutes of warm water, providing 30 minutes of total treatment (Lehmann & deLateur, 1990). Other variations suggest placing the extremity in the hot bath for a relatively short period initially and then gradually increase the length of time in the hot water during subsequent treatment sessions. Most of the recommended ratios are either 3:1 or 4:1 and may begin with cold. Depending on the condition and goals, the treatment can be modified and may include ending in the cooler water. As with any thermal modality, it is important to monitor the patient's skin condition during and following the application, as well as pulse, respiration and blood pressure (Smith & Newton, 1994).

## Warm Water Soak

Warm water soaks can be used when mild or moderate dosages of heat are indicated. This type of thermotherapy provides circumferential heat to the fingers and allows the patient to mobilize the hand and fingers while soaking in order to improve ROM and decrease subacute and chronic edema. This form of hydrotherapy is ideal for a home program. The temperature is typically initiated at 99° to 110° F. The water is in a container that the person's extremity can fit into. A 15 to 20 minute immersion is generally indicated. If edema is a concern, the patient may be instructed in controlling this by actively moving the part being treated while in the dependent position (for example flexing and extending the fingers), or to intermittently elevate the extremity above her heart. As with any home program, the patient should be instructed to monitor the temperature of the water to prevent potential burns.

## Paraffin Bath

The paraffin bath provides moderate to vigorous dosages of heat to a localized area and smaller joints. Paraffin baths have been shown to be an effective modality with arthritic patients as well as with systemic sclerosis (Helfand & Bruno, 1984; Robinson et al., 2002; Sandqvist, Akesson, & Eklund, 2004). Paraffin is primarily used to decrease stiffness and improve ROM. It is frequently used to treat chronic arthritic conditions and also offers pain control. Healed amputations, arthritis, and strains/sprains are just a few conditions that may benefit from paraffin. It is important to monitor the temperature of the paraffin using a thermometer to prevent thermal burns before application. The paraffin bath must be thermostatically controlled to ensure patient safety. The heated storage unit contains a mixture of paraffin and mineral oil. The temperature of the paraffin is typically between 118° to 135° F (Malick & Kasch, 1984), but should be kept at approximately 126° F for upper extremity use. Paraffin has a lower specific heat than water so the paraffin will feel cooler to the patient than water at the same temperature. Mineral oil contained in the paraffin lowers the melting point and allows for ease of removal of the paraffin from the body part. A ratio of approximately 6 parts wax to 1 of mineral oil provides an optimum mix for ease of use and to lower the effective melting point of the wax.

A primary advantage of paraffin is that it allows for an even distribution of heat to the treatment surface, which is effective in reducing stiffness and pain. This form of heat also reduces the viscosity of the synovia, reducing the stiffness associated with arthritis. When using paraffin with rheumatoid arthritis, it is imperative that one refrain from administering a vigorous heat dosage. The temperature of the paraffin should be maintained at the lower range. The provision of paraffin is easy, efficient, and rather inexpensive. Passive or positional stretching of joints can be accomplished with an elastic-type wrap. This form of treatment can be used in conjunction with the paraffin to maximize the benefits of mobilizing connective tissue.

The disadvantage of paraffin is that it cannot be easily used on all body parts. Although paraffin does gradually cool after being applied, there is no mechanism to control the temperature of the paraffin once it is applied to the skin. Because it is difficult to regulate the temperature, the risk of burns is substantially higher than other forms of heat. Paraffin should not be used with open wounds or over joints which are acutely inflamed. Paraffin maintains a therapeutic temperature for approximately 20 minutes (Michlovitz & Wolf, 1990).

Paraffin can be applied in a variety of ways, including wrap/gloving, immersion, dip, brush, and pouring methods. The most common form used in clinics is the "dipping" method (Figure 6-6). It is crucial that before any of the methods of application are applied, the therapist check the temperature of the paraffin and assess the patient's skin condition and sensation. The body part should always be thoroughly washed before any application, particularly the "dip" method. Any rings and jewelry should be removed before using paraffin.

## Wrap/Gloving Technique

This method may be the most popular method of paraffin application by the occupational therapist. The therapist should first observe the temperature of the paraffin unit's thermometer for safety, demonstrate the technique, and then ask the patient to slowly place her fingertips into the paraffin. The patient is then instructed to immerse the part into the bath while avoiding contact with the bottom and the sides of the paraffin unit. The patient's hands should be slightly flexed and abducted to facilitate patient comfort. The patient should be instructed to maintain the position of the hand to prevent the paraffin from cracking the layers and potentially causing burns as higher temperature paraffin will flow underneath the initial layers and become trapped causing increased temperatures. Once this first dip is completed, the patient is instructed to immediately remove the extremity and allow it to air dry for a few seconds prior to

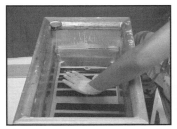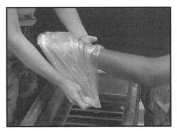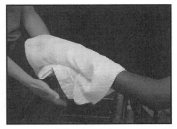

**Figure 6-6.** Dip method of paraffin. Note thermometer in top left corner. The initial dip should extend the highest up the forearm. Always check the temperature of the paraffin before placing patient's extremity in the paraffin to ensure that it is at a therapeutic level and will not burn the patient.

immersing once again. The dip process, referred to as "gloving," is repeated approximately 10 times depending on the patient's tolerance to the heat. The therapist then wraps the part in a large plastic bag and a cloth towel is wrapped around to serve as an insulating layer retaining the heat. The extremity should be placed in a comfortable position, preferably elevated to prevent edema from occurring. Typical treatment time lasts 20 minutes. At the conclusion of treatment, the paraffin should be removed and discarded.

### Immersion Technique

At an elevated therapeutic temperature of 125° to 135° F, this technique will provide a vigorous dosage of heat. The patient dips an initial layer of paraffin on their hand till it solidifies. The patient then immerses and leaves her hand in the paraffin bath for approximately 10 to 20 minutes. It is vital that the patient's skin condition is monitored to prevent burns from occurring.

### Dip Immersion Technique

Depending on the therapeutic temperature of the paraffin, this will provide a moderate or vigorous dosage of heat. This involves the gloving method noted earlier. Instead of wrapping the body part as the final step, the area being treated remains within the paraffin bath (Figure 6-6).

### Brush Technique

This process involves using a paint brush and brushing eight to 10 coats of paraffin onto an area that cannot be dipped, such as the lateral epicondyle at the elbow area. The treated area is wrapped with towels for approximately 20 minutes. A moderate dosage of heat can be obtained.

### Pouring Technique

This process involves carefully pouring the paraffin over the targeted area. The pouring technique can be used for many of the same reasons that brushing was used for. It may also be indicated when treating the hand, especially if the patient is unable immerse her hand into the bath.

Following any of the paraffin techniques, the wax should be removed over the tank and discarded. The paraffin in the tank should be replaced whenever it is noted to be soiled. Many patients will consider purchasing a home paraffin unit, particularly those with chronic arthritic conditions and pain. These units are relatively inexpensive and maintain the paraffin mixture at approximately 125° F. Patients should be cautioned to use a meat or candy thermometer to monitor the actual temperature of the paraffin before using the home equipment.

---

## Paraffin Clinical Considerations

- The patient should always wash their hands prior to dipping their hand in the paraffin.

- ALWAYS check the temperature of the paraffin before using it with a patient to ensure appropriate temperature.

- The patient's initial dip should be the deepest, with each subsequent dip slightly less to prevent the paraffin from getting underneath the existing layers and burning the patient's skin.

- The patient should avoid moving their hand once the initial layers have set up. Cracks in the paraffin may cause the hotter temperature paraffin to come in contact with the skin and burn the patient.

- The paraffin tank should be cleaned when it becomes soiled. This will be most noticeable at the bottom of the tank.

---

# Summary

Superficial thermal agents can be an effective adjunct to occupational therapy treatment. Though these modalities and interventions are commonly used in occupational therapy practice, there is a degree of risk such as burning the patient, which needs to be taken into consideration. Monitoring both the therapeutic temperature of the interventions before applying them and monitoring the patient's skin should be a primary concern for the therapist throughout the procedure. Engagement in purposeful occupation is the primary therapeutic medium of occupational therapists and superficial thermal agents an adjunct to occupation. As clinicians, we have the challenge of appropriately integrating thermal agents into clinical practice. Though widely used and accepted, therapists must be competent and proficient with thermal agents to safely and effectively use them in clinical practice. Superficial heat agents facilitate tissue healing and extensibility, and decrease pain by impacting the neurovascular, neuromuscular, and metabolic processes of the body. For many patients, thermotherapy can prepare them for active engagement in the therapeutic occupation.

# Case Study

Doug is a 33-year-old father of three young children. He incurred a traumatic injury to his dominant right hand while working at a local hospital within the maintenance department. He sustained musculoskeletal, vascular, and nervous tissue injuries, in addition to amputation of his third and fourth distal phalanges. One week following surgery, Doug was referred to occupational therapy for wound management and dressing, ROM (as tolerated), and splinting.

Initially, treatment consisted of whirlpool at a tepid temperature of approximately 90° F. Mild agitation was allowed. This process was favorable to cleaning the hand and wounds and also facilitated the healing process. Within the subacute stage of healing, approximately 3.5 weeks postsurgery, the wounds closed and greater ROM was warranted. Whirlpool continued to be the modality of choice due to the minimal edema that was present. The physiological effects of mild heat coupled with the intermittent ability of countering the effects of edema with elevation and active ROM were the determinants for modality selection at this phase. Immediately following superficial heat application, therapeutic occupations were implemented. During the subacute stage, skin integrity continued to improve, edema was considerably decreased, and all aspects of the musculoskeletal injuries were healed.

Fluidotherapy was determined to be the thermal agent of choice, providing moderate to vigorous doses of heat while allowing Doug to actively mobilize his hand and fingers during treatment. He also benefited from the desensitization effects of the modality which normalized his hyperesthesia. The dependent position of the extremity during the 20 minute treatment was no longer a concern. Finally, as Doug participated in functional job simulated activity, he recognized the positive thermal benefits of heat to the persistent stiffness that he was experiencing. Paraffin was then used prior to his engagement in therapeutic occupation. The thermal effects of paraffin were complemented by a sustained passive composite finger flexion stretch that was obtained with Coban wrap (3M, St. Paul, MN) as a part of treatment.

Superficial thermal agents allowed Doug to maximize his participation and performance in treatment and he quickly returned to his position within the maintenance department without restrictions. Doug's scenario demonstrates how occupational therapy intervention (from the most acute stages to return to work) can provide remedial and compensatory treatment such that an individual can fully return to his or her occupational roles.

## Clinical Reasoning Questions

1. What clinical complications can occur with this type of injury?

2. What other physical agents might be appropriate to use with this patient?

3. What would happen to the healing tissue if aggressive agitation was used during the whirlpool?

4. What stage of healing is this patient progressing through?

5. What is occurring at a cellular level with the application of the physical agents?

6. What precautions and contraindications should you be aware of with this patient?

# References

Abramson, D. I., Mitchell, R. E., Tuck, S. Jr., Bell, Y., & Zays, A. M. (1961). Changes in blood flow, oxygen uptake and tissue temperatures produced by the topical application of wet heat. *Archives of Physical Medicine and Rehabilitation, 42*, 305-318.

Aiello, D. D. (2004). The hot and the cold of it. *Rehab Management, 17*, 18-23.

Akin, M., Price, W., Rodriguez, G., Jr, Erasala, G., Hurley, G., & Smith, R. P. (2004). Continuous, low-level, topical heat wrap therapy as compared to acetaminophen for primary dysmenorrhea. *Journal of Reproductive Medicine, 49*, 739-745.

Baker, R., & Bell G. (1991). The effect of therapeutic modalities on blood flow in the human calf. *Journal of Orthopaedic and Sports Physical Therapy, 13*, 23.

Bohannon, R. (1985). Whirlpool versus whirlpool rinse for removal of bacteria from a venous stasis ulcer. *Physical Therapy, 62*, 402-406.

Borrell, R. M., Parker, R., Henley, E. J., Masley, D., & Repinecz, M. (1980). Comparison of in vivo temperatures produced by hydrotherapy, paraffin wax treatment, and fluidotherapy. *Physical Therapy, 60*, 1273-1276.

Conroy, D. E., & Hayes, K. W. (1998). The effect of joint mobilization as a component of comprehensive treatment for primary shoulder impingement syndrome. *Journal of Orthopaedic and Sports Physical Therapy, 28*, 3-14.

De Jong, R. H., Hershey, W. N., & Wagman, I. H. (1966). Nerve conduction velocity during hypothermia in man. *Anesthesiology, 27*, 805-810.

deLateur, B. J., Stonebridge, J. B., & Lehmann, J. F. (1978). Fibrous muscular contractures: Treatment with a new direct contact microwave applicator operating at 915 MHz. *Archives of Physical Medicine and Rehabilitation, 59*, 488-499.

Draper, D. O., Harris, S. T., Schulthies, S., Durrant, E., Knight, K. L., & Ricard, M. (1998). Hot-pack and 1-MHz ultrasound treatments have an additive effect on muscle temperature increase. *Journal of Athletic Training, 33*, 21-24.

Ersala, G., Rubin, J., & Tuthill, T. (2001). The effect of topical heat treatment on trapezius muscle blood flow using power doppler ultrasound. *Proceedings, Annual Conference and Exposition of the American Physical Therapy Association, June*, 20-21.

Greenberg, R. S. (1972). The effects of hot packs and exercise on local blood flow. *Physical Therapy, 52*, 273-278.

Halvorsen, G. (1990). Therapeutic heat and cold for athletic injuries. *Physical Sportsmedicine, 18*, 87.

Health tips. hot vs. cold treatment.(2002). *Mayo Clinic Health Letter (English Ed.), 20*, 3.

Hecox, B., Weisberg, J., Andemicael-Mehreteab, T., & Sanko J. (2006). *Integrating physical agents in rehabilitation.* 2nd ed. Upper Saddle River, NJ: Pearson, Prentice Hall.

Helfand, A. E., & Bruno, J. (1984). Therapeutic modalities and procedures. part I: Cold and heat. *Clinics in Podiatry, 1*, 301-313.

Hillman, S. K., & Delforge, G. (1985). The use of physical agents in rehabilitation of athletic injuries. *Clinics in Sports Medicine, 4*, 431-438.

Krusen, E. (1950). Effects of hot packs on peripheral circulation. *Archives of Physical Medicine and Rehabilitation, 31*, 145.

Lehmann, J. F., & deLateur B. (1990a). Therapeutic heat. In J. Lehman, & B. deLateur (Eds.), *Therapeutic heat and cold* (4th ed., pp. 417-457). Baltimore, MD: Williams & Wilkins.

Lehmann, J. F., & deLateur, B. J. (1990b). *Therapeutic heat and cold.* Baltimore, MD: Williams & Wilkins.

Lehmann, J. F., Dundore, D. E., Esselman, P. C., & Nelp, W. B. (1983). Microwave diathermy: Effects on experimental muscle hematoma resolution. *Archives of Physical Medicine and Rehabilitation, 64*, 127-129.

Lehmann, J. F., Masock, A. J., Warren, C. G., & Koblanski, J. N. (1970). Effect of therapeutic temperatures on tendon extensibility. *Archives of Physical Medicine and Rehabilitation, 51*, 481-487.

Lehmann, J. F., Warren, C. G., & Scham, S. M. (1974). Therapeutic heat and cold. *Clinical Orthopaedics and Related Research, (99)*, 207-245.

Lin, Y. H. (2003). Effects of thermal therapy in improving the passive range of knee motion: Comparison of cold and superficial heat applications. *Clinical Rehabilitation, 17*, 618-623.

Malick, M., & Kasch, M. (Eds.). (1984). *Manual on management of specific hand problems.* Pittsburgh, PA: Hamarville Rehab Center.

Matsumoto, S., Kawahira, K., Etoh, S., Ikeda, S., & Tanaka, N. (2006). Short-term effects of thermotherapy for spasticity on tibial nerve F-waves in post-stroke patients. *International Journal of Biometeorology, 50*, 243-250.

McMeeken, J. M., & Bell, C. (1990). Effects of selective blood and tissue heating on blood flow in the dog hindlimb. *Experimental Physiology, 75*, 359-366.

Michlovitz, S., & Wolf, S. (Eds.). (1990). *Thermal agents in rehabilitation.* Philadelphia, PA: FA Davis.

Morton, R. H. (2006). Contrast water immersion hastens plasma lactate decrease after intense anaerobic exercise. *Journal of Science and Medicine in Sport/Sports Medicine Australia, (in press).*

Myer, J. W., Draper, D. O., & Durrant, E. (1994). Contrast therapy and intramuscular temperature in the human leg. *Journal of Athletic Training, 29*, 318-322.

Niederhuber, S. S., Stribley, R. F., & Koepke, G. H. (1975). Reduction of skin bacterial load with use of the therapeutic whirlpool. *Physical Therapy, 55*, 482-486.

Ottawa Panel. (2004). Ottawa panel evidence-based clinical practice guidelines for electrotherapy and thermotherapy interventions in the management of rheumatoid arthritis in adults. *Physical Therapy, 84,* 1016-1043.

Perret, D. M., Rim, J., & Cristian, A. (2006). A geriatrician's guide to the use of the physical modalities in the treatment of pain and dysfunction. *Clinics in Geriatric Medicine, 22,* 331-54; ix.

Petrofsky, J. S., Lohman, E., 3rd, Lee, S., de la Cuesta, Z., Labial, L., & Iouciulescu, R., et al. (2006). The influence of alterations in room temperature on skin blood flow during contrast baths in patients with diabetes. *Medical Science Monitor, 12,* CR290-5.

Reid, D. (1992). *Sports injury assessment and rehabilitation.* New York: Churchill Livingstone.

Robertson, V. J., Ward, A. R., & Jung, P. (2005). The effect of heat on tissue extensibility: A comparison of deep and superficial heating. *Archives of Physical Medicine and Rehabilitation, 86,* 819-825.

Robinson, V., Brosseau, L., Casimiro, L., Judd, M., Shea, B., & Wells, G., et al. (2002). Thermotherapy for treating rheumatoid arthritis. *Cochrane Database of Systematic Reviews (Online), (1),* CD002826.

Samborski, W., Stratz, T., Sobieska, M., Mennet, P., Muller, W., & Schulte-Monting, J. (1992). Intraindividual comparison of whole body cold therapy and warm treatment with hot packs in generalized tendomyopathy. *Zeitschrift Fur Rheumatologie, 51,* 25-30.

Sandqvist, G., Akesson, A., & Eklund, M. (2004). Evaluation of paraffin bath treatment in patients with systemic sclerosis. *Disability and Rehabilitation, 26,* 981-987.

Sapega, A., Quedecfeld, T., & Moyer, R. (1981). Biophysiological factors in range-of-motion exercise. *Physical Sportsmedicine, 9,* 57.

Schmidt, K. L., Ott, V. R., Rocher, G., & Schaller, H. (1979). Heat, cold and inflammation. *Zeitschrift Fur Rheumatologie, 38,* 391-404.

Smith, K., & Newton, R. (1994). The immediate effect of contrast baths on edema, temperature and pain in postsurgical hand injuries, *Physical Therapy, 74,* 157.

Solomon, S. L. (1985). Host factors in whirlpool-associated pseudomonas aeruginosa skin disease. *Infection Control, 6,* 402-406.

Stanton, D. B., Bear-Lehman, J., Graziano, M., & Ryan, C. (2003). Contrast baths: What do we know about their use? *Journal of Hand Therapy, 16,* 343-346.

Tao, X. G., & Bernacki, E. J. (2005). A randomized clinical trial of continuous low-level heat therapy for acute muscular low back pain in the workplace. *Journal of Occupational and Environmental Medicine /American College of Occupational and Environmental Medicine, 47,* 1298-1306.

Wedlick, L. T. (1967). The use of heat and cold in the treatment of sports injuries. *Medical Journal of Australia, 2,* 1050-1051.

# Chapter 7

# THERAPEUTIC ULTRASOUND AND PHONOPHORESIS

## Learning Objectives

1. Discuss the theory and principles of therapeutic ultrasound.
2. Explain the biophysiological changes which occur with ultrasound.
3. Compare and contrast clinical parameters used in therapeutic ultrasound, for thermal and nonthermal applications.
4. Discuss the clinical applications for the use of therapeutic ultrasound.
5. Identify contraindications and precautions for therapeutic ultrasound.

## Terminology

| | | |
|---|---|---|
| Acoustic streaming | Frequency | Phonophoresis |
| Beam nonuniformity ratio | Intensity | Phonophoresis |
| Cavitation | Longitudinal wave | Shear wave |
| Duty cycle | Nonthermal effect | Thermal effect |

Ultrasound is considered a deep heat modality that can be used as an adjunct to occupational therapy treatment in order to facilitate occupational performance. By definition, ultrasound is acoustic energy that is inaudible by the human ear due to a frequency greater than 20 kilohertz (kHz). The frequency band for medical ultrasound is 800,000 to 3,000,000 Hz (0.8 to 3 MHz). Clinicians have been using ultrasound with increasing frequency in order to facilitate the healing process, speed recovery, and to decrease pain (Kennedy, Ter Haar, & Cranston, 2003; Oh, Early, & Azar, 2005; Samosiuk, Miasnikov, & Klimenko, 1999; Uhlemann, 1993; Walmsley, 1988). Ultrasound has two primary purposes and effects, to heat deeper lying tissues and to heal tissue through its mechanical, nonthermal effects. Historically, occupational therapists have employed paraffin or hot packs to "heat" selected tissues though these modalities primarily affect superficial tissue and penetrate only to a depth of approximately 1 to 2 centimeters (cm) (McDiamid & Burns, 1987). Therapeutic ultrasound is an additional treatment method which can be a beneficial adjunct to the occupational therapy process and that can be used to selectively heat deeper, collagen-rich structures or to facilitate the healing process (Figure 7-1).

**Figure 7-1.** Vectra Genisys ultrasound unit (Photo courtesy of Chattanooga Group).

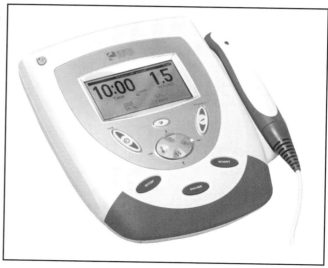

# Classification

Therapeutic ultrasound is a thermal modality that can be used to heat structures superficially (0 to 1 cm) or at greater depths (up to 5 cm). There is also a nonthermal component to ultrasound which facilitates tissue healing rather than causing a thermal or heating effect on the tissue. Ultrasound uses acoustic or sound energy which creates pressure waves which are transmitted into the underlying tissue. There are two primary frequencies available for use in the United States for therapeutic ultrasound, 1 MHz (1 million cycles/second), and an additional setting of 3 MHz. Therapeutic ultrasound produces tissue change through both a thermal and nonthermal effect and can be used as an adjunct to occupational performance. Thermal agents have two primary classifications: *superficial* and *deep*. Superficial thermal agents elevate tissue temperature to a depth of approximately 1 cm. Therapeutic ultrasound is considered a deep-heating thermal agent capable of elevating tissue temperatures to a depth of 5 cm or more (Draper, 1995). A frequency of 1 MHz will provide deeper penetration than 3 MHz. The sound energy dissipates in strength as it moves through tissue, becoming attenuated until it becomes dissipated (Figure 7-2).

Therapeutic ultrasound has two primary purposes: *to elevate tissue temperature* and *to provide nonthermal secondary cellular effects*. In order to safely and effectively use ultrasound in the treatment process, it is necessary to understand its history, principles, physiological effects, indications, and contraindications.

# History

Ultrasound consists of an acoustic energy and has been used in medicine for diagnosis and tissue destruction, and in physical medicine and rehabilitation to help restore and heal soft tissues. In 1880, Pierre and Jacques Curies discovered that certain crystals, such as quartz, lithium sulfate, and zinc oxide, generated an electrical charge when mechanically compressed. The Curies discovered that the crystals produce positive and negative electrical charges when they expand and contract, known

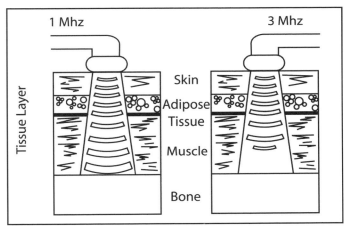

**Figure 7-2.** Ultrasound depth of penetration comparing 1 MHz and 3 MHz. Superficial areas are treated with a frequency of 3 MHz, deeper structures use a 1 MHz frequency.

as the piezoelectric effect. An indirect or reverse piezoelectric effect is the contraction or expansion of a crystal that occurs in response to electrical voltage being applied. The reverse piezoelectric effect is the production of mechanical energy secondary to the application of an electrical charge across the crystal. The polarity changes cause the crystal to oscillate and deform in response to the electrical current. Ultrasound uses the reverse piezoelectric effect to produce the high-frequency sound waves. The application of alternating current makes the crystal vibrate at the frequency of the electrical oscillation, generating a variety of frequencies (Williams, 1983).

The effects of ultrasound on biological systems were not well known until the sinking of the Titanic and World War I. During this period of technological advances, researchers were attempting to devise methods for detecting submarines which were sinking Allied shipping vessels and for underwater navigation. Researchers used a pulsed technology, or echo-location system, to locate or identify undersea objects. This hydrophone system was further refined during the intervening years between WWI and WWII and became SONAR (sound navigation and ranging), an active system used to echo-locate objects underwater and navigation system. When researchers were developing these devices to locate submarines and objects undersea, they found that when a piezoelectric transducer emitted ultrasonic waves into the ocean following excitation; the amplitude of the acoustic waves was often strong enough to kill marine animals and small fish. Researchers continued to explore the biologic effects on tissues exposed to these high-frequency sound waves during the 1930s and 1940s, with the application of ultrasound for medical treatment occurring in Germany and then in the United States (Buchtala, 1952; Kuitert & Harr, 1955). Researchers continued to explore the biologic effects on tissues exposed to these high-frequency sound waves during the 1930s and 1940s, with the intent of using ultrasound for medical treatment. Early researchers such as Paul Langevin noted the destruction of fish in the sea and pain in his hand when he placed it in a water tank insonated with high intensity ultrasound (Kuitert & Harr, 1955). The earliest experiments used ultrasound waves to destroy brain tissue in animals. By the 1940s some clinicians were using ultrasound as a "cure-all" remedy for a variety of treatments including eczema, asthma, arthritic pains, urinary incontinence, elephanthiasis, and even angina. There was concurrently, lacking research or scientific evidence to support these claims and the development of diagnostic ultrasound was hindered by subsequent cynicism and concern over these unfounded claims (Figure 7-3).

**Figure 7-3.** Ultrasound application in the 1940s. (A) Use in treatment of gastric ulcers. (B) Thermal use in arthritis.

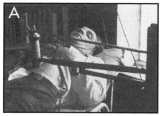
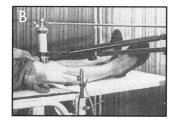

**Figure 7-4.** Various size sound heads varying from 1 cm up to 10 cm. Smaller size sound heads are used to treat smaller tissue areas such as hands and fingers.

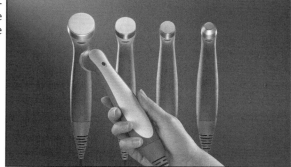

Although the initial research and work on ultrasound concentrated primarily on the thermal effects, more recent research has explored the nonthermal effects of ultrasound in the areas of tissue healing and administration of medication phonophoretically.

# Ultrasound Equipment

The basis for current ultrasound equipment was derived from the Curies' work on crystal oscillation and voltage polarization. The standard ultrasound unit consists of a power supply, oscillator circuit, transformer, coaxial cable transducer, and ultrasound applicator. Most often, therapeutic ultrasound units have a generator that uses alternating current as a power source, converting this electrical energy into ultrasonic energy. With therapeutic ultrasound machines, the crystal is located inside the applicator, which is called a *transducer*. The crystal consists of natural quartz or a synthetic material that vibrates by contracting and expanding in response to alternating current. Each crystal has a unique, naturally occurring vibration frequency to which the electronics of the ultrasound unit are matched. Because of this, ultrasound transducers are not interchangeable between units. Some of the current manufacturers, however, have solved this problem and are producing interchangeable sound heads (Figure 7-4).

The vibration of the crystal generates pressure waves that affect the tissue. The crystal deforms in response to the changes in the direction of the flow of the current and is proportional to the amount of voltage applied to the crystal. In therapeutic ultrasound, these pressure waves are transmitted to a small volume of tissue which causes the molecules to vibrate. Ultrasound travels poorly through air so a lubricant is used that allows the energy to be dispersed into the underlying tissue. The nonthermal aspects of ultrasound are primarily due to acoustic streaming, microstreaming, and cavitation, which alter the permeability of the cell membrane.

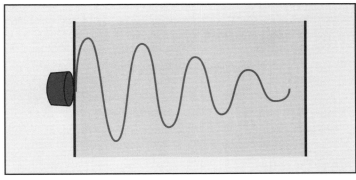

**Figure 7-5.** Decreasing ultrasound intensity in a longitudinal wave. Energy is transmitted, absorbed, reflected, and refracted depending on type of tissue and angle of wave.

# Physical Principles

In therapeutic ultrasound, the sound energy that is produced occurs as the electronics of the ultrasound machine, modifies the electrical energy and transmits it to the crystal located in the transducer of the sound head. These sound waves correspond to the frequency range of the ultrasound machine. The most common frequency for therapeutic ultrasound is 1 MHz (1 million Hertz), as well as 3 MHz. A frequency of 1 MHz is considered a "low" frequency which is most often used to treat deeper tissues, while a higher frequency of 3 MHz can be used to treat superficial tissues. Ultrasound energy occurs when alternating electrical current is applied to the crystal causing it to expand and contract in relationship to the amount of electrical current causing acoustical or "sound" waves. The sound waves created by the ultrasound unit can be visualized as being similar to waves in a pond created when a stone is tossed into the middle with the waves expanding away from the center until the energy is dissipated. The peak and trough of the sound waves mirror the phases of compression and rarefaction of the crystal. These sound waves are transmitted to the underlying tissue of the treatment area.

With the higher frequencies used in ultrasound, the sound waves are more "collimated," diverging less and traveling in a cylindrical beam with the flow of the molecules parallel to each other, or longitudinally. Due to the rapid generation of the sound waves, molecules in the wave's path are pushed back and forth by the alternating phases of successive waves. This type of wave—moving in one direction, compressing and decompressing the molecules in its way—is known as a *longitudinal (compression) wave*. The longitudinal wave continues to travel through the tissue until the energy is absorbed. Ultrasound can be transmitted, absorbed, reflected, and refracted depending on the type of tissue that the energy affects, and the angle of the wave (Figure 7-5) The rate at which the sound wave travels is dependent, in part, on the density of the molecules of the specific tissue. There is an inverse relationship between absorption and penetration. If the tissue molecules are widely dispersed, there is a low absorption of the sound energy, and the depth of penetration is greater. If the molecules of the tissue are close together or compressed, the rate at which the sound will travel will be less as the energy is absorbed because the molecules resist compression.

Because there is variability to human tissue, the sound wave will be attenuated to a certain degree. Attenuation refers to a decrease in the intensity of the energy which is due to either absorption of the energy by the tissue, or due to a scattering or dispersion of the sound wave due to reflection or refraction. Refraction occurs when the sound wave is redirected at an interface, continuing through the tissue in a different

Table 7-1

| ACOUSTIC IMPEDANCE LEVEL | |
|---|---|
| Tissue Type | Impedance (kg/m@sec x 10[6]) |
| Fat | 1.38 |
| Water | 1.5 |
| Blood | 1.61 |
| Muscle | 1.7 |
| Bone | 7.8 |

direction. Reflection occurs when the ultrasound strikes an area with different characteristics and impedances. Sound from the transducer which is transmitted into the air, will be reflected. The ultrasound energy also can be effectively transmitted through fat. At the interface of the tissue-bone, nearly all of the energy is reflected. The extent of the physical characteristics and difference between the tissues will affect the degree of reflection and refraction as well as the angle of return. If the reflected wave reverses course and returns toward the transducer on the same path it took into the tissue, it may interact with the sound waves that are traveling away from the sound head down into the tissue causing the energy to summate creating an area of intense energy in the tissue. When this summative effect occurs, it is known as a standing wave. Standing waves can be prevented from occurring by moving the sound head during treatment (ter Haar, Dyson, & Oakley, 1987). When the particle movement is at right angles to the propagation of the wave, a shear or transverse wave is created. This occurs in solid substances. Liquid substances, which have weaker intramolecular bonds, are less able to transmit the shear wave. Clinically, shear waves occur when a pressure wave reaches a bone with the wave being generated along the periosteum. This shear wave may cause heating of the outer covering of the bone (Arnheim, 1989).

Each tissue in the body has a different density, and each will transmit and absorb ultrasound according to its unique acoustical properties. Researchers have identified the acoustic absorption coefficient of various body tissues. Body fluids, such as blood and water, have the lowest impedance and acoustic absorption coefficient. Conversely, bone has the highest impedance and acoustic absorption coefficient, making it a good absorber of ultrasound energy (Lehman, Warren, & Guy, 1978; Piersol, Schwan, Pennell, & Carstensen, 1952). It is through understanding of the tissue healing process and appreciating the acoustic absorption properties of body tissues and their response, that therapeutic ultrasound becomes an important adjunct to the treatment process (Table 7-1).

# Energy Distribution

The therapeutic effect of tissue heating is due to the distribution of energy in the ultrasound field. The width or spread of the ultrasound is affected by the frequency and size of the crystal. The larger the sound head or transducer (and, therefore, the crystal), the greater the divergence of the energy field. The area of the transducer that produces the sound waves is known as the effective radiating area (ERA). A larger soundhead focuses or collimates the ultrasound energy beam while a smaller sound-

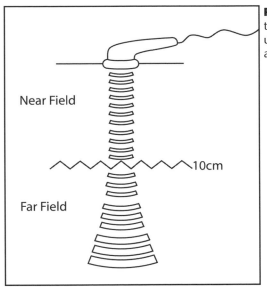

**Figure 7-6.** Ultrasound energy converges and the diverges. Length of the near field is based on ultrasound frequency and the effective radiating area (ERA) of the transducer.

head has a tendency to disperse the sound energy as it diverges from the soundhead. Ultrasound using a frequency of 1 MHz also causes greater divergence of the energy when compared to a 3 MHz frequency. There is also variation of the energy within the sound wave caused by a number of mechanisms, with peaks and troughs of the sound wave occurring in the near field and the far field with areas of higher intensities occurring within the sound beam (Figure 7-6). This variation in intensity of the sound energy is known as the beam nonuniformity ratio (BNR) and is indicated on the transducer by the manufacturer. The BNR is a ratio of the maximum intensity of the transducer to the average intensity produced across the face of the transducer. The BNR, in effect, describes the "highs and lows" of the sound energy of an ultrasound transducer.

The spatial peak intensity (SPI) is the maximum intensity appearing at any point in the beam. The spatial average intensity (SAI) is the average intensity over the area of the beam of energy. The intensity is higher in some areas of the ultrasound beam than others. The relationship between the SPI and the SAI is the BNR and is must be reported by the manufacturer for each ultrasound machine (Kimura, Gulick, Shelly, & Ziskin, 1998; Stewart et al., 1974). These higher intensity areas within the ultrasound beam are a primary cause for the "hot spots" which may occur during ultrasound application. These "hot spots" are prevented, in part, by keeping the sound head moving throughout the treatment. The therapist should make note of the BNR. Ideally, the lower the BNR, the more uniform the output with less potential for burning or discomfort.

## Intensity

Intensity describes the strength of the acoustic energy at the site of application. The spatial-averaged intensity is determined by measuring the acoustic power (Watts) of the applicator and dividing it by the ERA (sq. cm) of the transducer ($W/cm^2$). On most therapeutic ultrasound equipment, the intensity is identified as the power in "watts" (or as the spatial averaged intensity, $W/cm^2$). The intensity is the most significant factor in determining a tissue response. As a general rule, the greater the intensity, the greater the resulting tissue temperature elevation. It should be noted that the calibration and power output of the ultrasound machine may vary greatly which can adversely affect outcomes and patient comfort (Artho et al., 2002; Daniel & Rupert, 2003). Mechanical timers may also vary in their accuracy and should be tested for accuracy. If the actual output power and surface temperature varies, treatment effectiveness may be decreased and the possibility for damage or skin irritation may also occur, a consideration for those patients with sensory comprised skin (Kollmann, Vacariu, Schuhfried, Fialka-Moser, & Bergmann, 2005; Rivest, Quirion-de Girardi, Seaborne, & Lambert, 1987; Snow, 1982). The intensity of an ultrasound unit should always be decreased if the patient experiences discomfort at any time. Complaints of an "aching," "shooting," or "stabbing" pain are indications that the intensity should be decreased or the sound head should be moved more rapidly (Fyfe & Parnell, 1982). There are a wide variety of intensities that have been indicated for numerous conditions cited in the research, but there are no hard and fast rules that govern intensity selection. As such, patient response during the treatment application must be a consideration. A patient may feel deep warmth and heating during application of higher intensities; at this point, the intensity should be decreased in order to maintain a comfortable, gentle heating sensation (Draper, 1998). During the application of nonthermal ultrasound, however, the patient will likely not feel anything.

## Duty Cycle

The duty cycle is used to determine the overall amount of acoustic energy that a patient receives. This cycle also is a vital factor in determining the tissue response to the sound wave. The duty cycle is frequently seen as a percentage or ratio of the on-time of the pulse, the duration the unit is on, to the pulse period. A 50% duty cycle would provide twice as much acoustic energy as a 25% duty cycle since the on-time is twice as long. The temporal peak intensity is the maximum intensity of the sound wave during the on phase of pulsed ultrasound. The temporal average intensity is the intensity average over a given time span, which includes both on-and-off time (Hekkenberg, Oosterbaan, & Van Beekum, 1986).

> ### VARIABLES THAT MAY AFFECT THE DOSAGE OF ULTRASOUND DELIVERED TO TARGET TISSUE
>
> - Ultrasound frequency
> - Wavelength
> - Intensity
> - Effective radiating area of the transducer
> - BNR
> - Continuous or pulsed administration
> - Coupling medium used
> - Composition and structure of the targeted tissue
> - Movement and angle of the transducer
> - Frequency and duration of the application

Selection of continuous or pulsed ultrasound is $cm^2$ dependent on the pathology, the stage of wound healing and the amount of area to be treated (Stewart, Abzug, & Harris, 1980). Essentially, all current ultrasound machines can provide the ultrasound waves in either a *continuous* or *pulsed* mode.

During continuous ultrasound, the sound energy is being produced and transmitted without interruption. On some machines, continuous ultrasound may be labeled 100%, or continuous. Continuous ultrasound is most often used for a thermal or heating effect. Many ultrasound machines have preset pulsed duty cycles of 50%, 20%, and 10%. If the sound energy is periodically interrupted for short periods of time, the sound energy is described as being pulsed. During the period of time that the ultrasound energy is being interrupted (pulsed duty cycle), the overall average intensity of the ultrasound will be decreased. Because the ultrasound machine is not continuously delivering ultrasound energy, the overall effect is that there will be "less" energy being administered to the underlying tissue. As such, pulsed ultrasound reduces the overall heating of the tissue and is often used with lower intensities leading to a nonthermal or mechanical effect which is used clinically to facilitate soft tissue healing. Heating of the tissue can occur, however, in either continuous or pulsed ultrasound if the intensity is increased sufficiently in the higher ranges, while nonthermal effects occur when the intensity is lowered to 0.1 or 0.2 W/cm$^2$. Clinically, the therapist needs to determine whether the treatment is intended to "heat" or "heal" the tissue and select the appropriate intensities, duty cycles, and parameters based on the therapeutic goals.

# Physiological Effects

## Thermal or Continuous-Mode Ultrasound

The physiological effects of tissue heating are the same regardless of how the heat is applied. One of the primary advantages in using therapeutic ultrasound is the ability to target selected treatment sites and tissue. Superficial thermal agents can heat tissue to 1 cm, whereas low frequency ultrasound can penetrate selected tissues up to 5 cm. To achieve a thermal effect, intensities of 1.0 to 2.0 W/cm$^2$ are used in a continuous mode for between 5 to 8 minutes or longer. When ultrasound is used in a continuous mode for its thermal effect, it is considered a deep-heating modality. Patients and some occupational therapists often think that the ultrasound transducer produces heat and sends it to the tissue through conduction. In fact, the ultrasound beam does not itself transmit heat. Heat accumulates in the underlying tissue by the conversion of kinetic energy, which is absorbed from the sound wave in continuous-mode or high-intensity ultrasound. Energy is also absorbed from the ultrasound beam in proportion to the density of the tissue. Protein-dense structures such as scar tissue, joint capsules, ligaments, tendons, and bones are primarily composed of collagen fibers which accumulate heat readily and selectively absorb the ultrasound energy. Because of the propensity of protein dense structures to absorb the ultrasound, therapists can selectively heat dense or deep lying tissues (Binder, Hodge, Greenwood, Hazleman, & Page Thomas, 1985; Piersol et al., 1952; Robertson & Baker, 2001; Wells, 1977). Due to the extensive capillary network; muscles lose heat more quickly than these more dense structures and cool more quickly.

## Cavitation

Ultrasound causes a variety of responses at the cellular level due to its thermal or nonthermal biophysiological effects. It is up to the therapist to determine which effect is warranted based on the clinical condition and expected outcome. These thermal or nonthermal effects occur due to the interaction of the ultrasound energy at the cellular level. Ultrasound has the potential to cause two types of cavitation, stable and unstable. Cavitation is the formation and collapse of gas- or vapor-filled cavities in liquids, and occurs in relation to the compression and rarefaction cycles of the ultrasound. Cavitation causes an expansion and compression of these small gas bubbles which may be present in blood or tissue fluids located in the ultrasound beam's path. Cavitation occurs as a result of the pressure changes caused by the sound wave generation. Stable cavitation, which occurs as a result of pulsing the ultrasound energy, allows these bubbles to expand and contract in response to the ebb and flow of the ultrasound energy. Stable cavitation results in acoustic microstreaming, which allows for nonthermal, mechanical effects to occur at the cellular membrane.

Thermal effects of tissue heating can also occur due to cavitation. Micron-sized gas bubbles are present in the body fluids within the sound wave. With the application of higher intensity, these bubbles can reach a critical size and collapse, causing unstable cavitation. In unstable cavitation, energy is released into the surrounding tissue, causing an increase in temperature and damage to the tissue, blood cells, and other tissue located within the sound wave. Unstable cavitation occurs more frequently with 1 MHz ultrasound than with 3 MHz ultrasound, and can be avoided by using higher frequencies and avoiding the development of hot spots caused by the therapist failing to move the sound head consistently and developing standing waves.

A number of physiological effects occur in tissue when thermal modalities, including thermal ultrasound, are used. Clinically, thermal ultrasound is used to increase joint range of motion (ROM), facilitate tissue healing, decrease muscle spasm, decrease pain, and decrease chronic inflammatory process, decrease stiffness, decrease edema, and facilitate function (Casimiro et al., 2002; Citak-Karakaya, Akbayrak, Demirturk, Ekici, & Bakar, 2006; Ebenbichler et al., 1998; Morrisette, Brown, & Saladin, 2004). Because of the ability to selectively set the parameters for ultrasound, occupational therapists can effectively target specific tissues and structures to take advantage of the thermal effects of ultrasound in the healing process. Thermal ultrasound will increase soft tissue temperature as much as $0.2°$ C when administered at 1 W/cm$^2$ at 1 MHz; and by as much as $0.6°$ C using a frequency of 3 MHz (Figure 7-7). A lower intensity (approximately 3 times less) should be used during a 3 MHz application since much of the sound energy produced at will be absorbed superficially to a depth of approximately 1 to 2 cm deep, with higher energy levels concurrently causing a potentially greater increase in tissue temperature (Draper, Castel, & Castel, 1995).

## Nonthermal or Mechanical Ultrasound

When the heating effects of ultrasound are decreased by applying very low-intensity ultrasound or by pulsing it, cellular or mechanical changes occur. The physiologic effects of nonthermal ultrasound are often more significant to the therapist than thermal ultrasound in manipulating the wound healing process. Nonthermal ultrasound causes a destabilization of the cell membrane, causing increased cellular permeability, diffusion, and a cascade of second order effects. Use of pulsed or nonthermal ultrasound has been clinically shown to facilitate tissue repair (Dyson & Suckling, 1978; Ennis, Valdes, Gainer, & Meneses, 2006; Fyfe & Bullock, 1985). The nonthermal effects of pulsed ultrasound occur at the cell membrane due to mechanical vibrations causing cavitation, acoustic streaming, and micro-massage. The radiation force which occurs during the compression phase of pulsed ultrasound deforms the cell membrane, massaging the cell. Stable cavitation also occurs with the gas bubbles expanding and contracting in relation to the compression and rarefaction phases of the sound wave

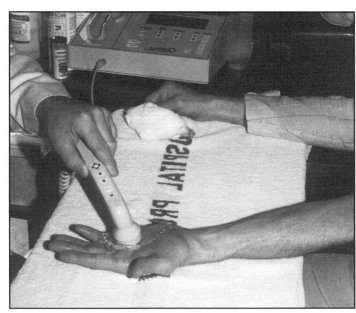

**Figure 7-7.** Transmission of ultrasound through homogenous tissue. The sound wave travels longitudinally into the underlying tissue-longitudinal wave.

(Apfel, 1989). This stable cavitation causes eddy currents in the fluid surrounding the vibrating bubbles, exerting a force and stress on nearby cells.

The unidirectional movement of the fluid within the pressure field is known as acoustic streaming and causes structural changes in the cell and an increase in cell permeability (Lehmann & Herrick, 1953). The destabilization of the cellular membrane allows the second-order effects of nonthermal ultrasound to occur. Changes in the cell membrane facilitate the diffusion of ions and metabolites, such as calcium ions and histamine across the cell. Calcium is a messenger for protein synthesis, while histamine is found in platelets within mast cells and granular leukocytes, and is influential in the vascular and cellular events of inflammation. Secondary effects of pulsed ultrasound include an increase of phagocytic activity of macrophages, an increase in the number and motility of fibroblasts with enhanced protein synthesis, increased granular tissue, and angiogensis facilitating wound contraction. Research has also indicated that low intensity pulsed ultrasound (LIPUS) can accelerate fracture healing in tibial, Colles, and scaphoid fractures and to increase the maturation of bone and decrease healing time (Chan, Qin, Lee, Cheung, Cheng, & Leung, 2006b; Claes, Ruter, & Mayr, 2005; Claes & Willie, 2007; Giannini, Giombini, Moneta, Massazza, & Pigozzi, 2004; Heckman, Ryaby, McCabe, Frey, & Kilcoyne, 1994; Ito, Azuma, Ohta, & Komoriya, 2000; Malizos, Hantes, Protopappas, & Papachristos, 2006; Mayr, Wagner, Ecker, & Ruter, 1999). High intensity, thermal ultrasound parameters could disrupt the bone healing process and should not be used.

Contrary to the popular belief that ultrasound is most effective for its thermal effects; the nonthermal secondary effects of pulsed ultrasound have a great impact on the wound healing process and may be more significant than the thermal effects. There continues to be some question as to the mechanism of action, though modulation of the extracellular matrix and histochemical factors have been cited as additional mechanisms of action (Bandow et al., 2007; Hill, Fenwick, Matthews, Chivers, & Southgate, 2005; Mukai et al., 2005). Ultrasound can facilitate resolution of the inflammatory phase of healing, and stimulate fibroblastic activity and maturation (Leung, Ng, & Yip,

2004). In contrast, high intensity ultrasound (1 MHz, 1.5 w/cm$^2$) can disrupt tissue repair and aggravate symptoms during the acute phase of healing, while LIPUS can facilitate bone healing (Busse, Bhandari, Kulkarni, & Tunks, 2002; Dudda, Pommer, Muhr, & Esenwein, 2005; Pilla et al., 1990). Use of ultrasound for healing of contusions or to facilitate skeletal muscle

> ## CLINICAL EFFECTS OF THERMAL ULTRASOUND
>
> - Increased tissue extensibility of collagen fibers of tendons and joint capsules
> - Decrease pain
> - Decrease joint stiffness
> - Increased blood flow
> - Decrease muscle spasm
> - Decrease chronic inflammation

regeneration is equivocal with further research needed to clarify parameters and clinical applications (Binder, Hodge, Greenwood, Hazleman, & Page Thomas, 1985; Markert, Merrick, Kirby, & Devor, 2005; Wilkin, Merrick, Kirby, & Devor, 2004).

In general, the effects of nonthermal ultrasound on tissue healing occur with short treatment durations and lower parameters of 0.1 and 0.2 W/cm$^2$ doses, pulsed at a 20% duty cycle. Effective fracture healing usually requires an application time of approximately 20 minutes. A frequency of 1 MHz will provide deeper penetration (up to 5 cm) than 3 MHz (1 to 2 cm). To best facilitate tissue repair, treatment sessions should be repeated every 24 to 48 hours.

## Applications and Indications

Ultrasound can be safely and effectively used to treat a variety of clinical conditions seen by the occupational therapist. Many of the therapeutic parameters and applications used in clinic settings have been based on clinical experience or anecdotal evidence and there is great variability. Much of the research in ultrasound is based on animal studies and there are no guarantees that clinical outcomes will be the same. Therapeutic parameters and research design in many studies is problematic as well. In addition, there may be variance in ultrasound devices and output which may affect treatment parameters and therapeutic effects (Artho et al., 2002; Merrick, Bernard, Devor, & Williams, 2003).

Further research to determine efficacy and consistency of therapeutic parameters is necessary to strengthen therapeutic use and application of ultrasound. The research does, however, provide a frame of reference and starting point for therapeutic application. As with any intervention, a thorough evaluation of the patient is required to identify problems and to set treatment goals. Ultrasound should not be used independently of other treatment approaches, and should be used to impact the healing process. Attention should be paid to the depth and anatomic location of the injury, the area and type of tissue that is to be treated, and any medical or surgical interventions which have taken place. Consideration of any potential precautions or contraindications is a necessary with ultrasound not being used in those cases. Clearly identifying the site and depth of the pathology is important because the desired depth of ultrasound penetration will in part determine the frequency. For example, in treating a patient with epicondylitis, the tissue is superficially located, and a frequency of 3 MHz would be more effective in achieving the therapeutic benefits of the ultrasound. When thermal effects are not warranted, for example in an acute or subacute condition or a superficial pathology located near a bony prominence, low intensities should be used.

One of the primary considerations for the therapist is to determine whether to stimulate the healing process through low intensity, pulsed ultrasound, or whether tissue heating is desired through high intensity, continuous ultrasound. This is where the therapist should consider whether the goal of treatment is to "heat" the tissue, or "heal" the tissue. The initial treatment should usually be of shorter duration than subsequent treatments, and acute conditions should be treated for shorter periods of time than chronic conditions. Smaller areas of tissue also require less treatment time than larger areas, particularly to achieve thermal effects (Michlovitz, 1996). Ultrasound may be used before initiating functional activity due to its pain-relieving effects. The sequence of ultrasound use in the treatment process is based in part on the identified goals, treatment approach, and desired outcomes determined from the evaluation.

## Tissue Lengthening

Most often, the goal of thermal ultrasound is to increase soft tissue length. How the tissue is stretched (positional stretch, splinting, functional activities, joint mobilization techniques) is less important than the fact that heated tissues should be stretched gently through the pain-free range soon after the application of ultrasound. When using any thermal heating agent, there is a short window-of-opportunity. The treated tissue stays heated for approximately 8 to 10 minutes, followed by a cool-down period. This means that any joint mobilization, passive or active stretch or manipulation of the tissue to increase extensibility should be performed during this time frame. A positional or static stretch is also possible while applying ultrasound for its thermal effects depending on the joint and structures being sounded (Draper & Ricard, 1995; Rose, Draper, Schulthies, & Durrant, 1996). During the remodeling phase of healing, the collagen fibers are further differentiating and aligning themselves along the lines of stress and function. Uncontrolled scar formation in the soft tissue, tendons, ligaments, or joint capsules can cause limitation of movement and joint contractures. Because of its ability to penetrate to deeper levels and due to the propensity of the scar tissue to respond to sound energy, ultrasound can be an effective method to heat these tissues. To increase tissue extensibility, continuous ultrasound at higher intensities such as 1.0 to 2.5 W/cm$^2$ will result in more vigorous levels of heat with application times between 5 and 10 minutes. Because of the short "window of opportunity" available before the tissue cools, implementing therapeutic interventions such as stretching, massage, joint mobilization, and others should be implemented during or immediately after sounding the tissue.

## Pain

Pain is a common adjunct to underlying conditions that occupational therapists will treat clinically. Ultrasound is most commonly used to treat a condition which has with it an associated component of pain. Many of the research studies where ultrasound was used for other conditions had a concurrent decrease in pain symptomology. Pain may be decreased in these individuals as the underlying diagnosis is treated. Conceptually, use of ultrasound may modify pain perception or transmission through the activation of free nerve endings when used with thermal ultrasound (Williams, McHales, & Bowditch, 1987). There have been a variety of conditions which have used ultrasound to decrease pain including shoulder pain, plantar fasciitis, bursitis, ankle sprains, reflex sympathetic dystrophy, lateral epicondylitis, myofascial trigger points, pelvic pain, and other soft tissue injuries (Okaro & Condous, 2005). Though there is no consistency regarding ultrasound parameters and mechanism of action as to the pain reduction, the primary treatment parameters for ultrasound intervention varied from 0.5 to 3.0 W/cm$^2$ with treatment times varying between 3 to 10 minutes with most using continuous ultrasound. There is wide variability of the therapeutic parameters for ultrasound to control pain and the underlying mechanism of action may be due to improving circulation, accelerating the phase of inflammation and healing of the soft tissues, or due to changes in nerve conduction velocity. The therapist should monitor the patient's progress and response and modify therapeutic parameters accordingly (Casimiro, 2002).

---

### PHYSIOLOGIC CHANGES WHICH OCCUR WITH TISSUE HEATING INCLUDE

- Increased metabolic rate
- Increased blood flow and tissue permeability
- Increased viscoelasticity of connective tissue
- Elevation of pain threshold
- Increased enzymatic reactivity, stimulating the immune system

---

## Inflammation

Ultrasound may be used to treat inflammatory conditions, both acute and chronic with the mechanism of action being increased blood flow facilitating healing, and for pain reduction through the heating mechanism. Some research has demonstrated improvement of function and decreased pain and tenderness with bicipital tendonitis, and therapeutic parameters of 1.0 to 2.0 W/cm$^2$ at a 20% duty cycle facilitate improvement in epicondylitis (Binder, Hodge, Greenwood, Hazleman, & Page Thomas, 1985; Green, Buchbinder, & Hetrick, 2003; Robertson & Baker, 2001). Pulsed ultrasound at 2.3 W/cm$^2$ has also been found to stimulate inflammation of acute ligament injury and should be a consideration in the treatment of acute inflammation of soft tissue injuries (Leung, Cheung, Zhang, Lee, & Lo, 2004; Leung, Ng, & Yip, 2004).

## Tissue Healing

There are a variety of studies that have indicated that ultrasound can facilitate tissue healing in vascular, dermal ulcers and in surgical skin incisions. There is conflicting evidence that ultrasound facilitates the healing of chronic wounds such as leg ulcers, diabetic foot ulcers or pressure sores. Reviews of randomized controlled studies on the treatment of these chronic wounds using ultrasound were equivocal though some researchers found that low-frequency, low-dose ultrasound could be helpful in cases not responding to conventional interventions  (Cullum, Nelson, Flemming, & Sheldon, 2001; Flemming & Cullum, 2000; Peschen, Weichenthal, Schopf, & Vanscheidt, 1997; Swist-Chmielewska et al., 2002). Other research by Dyson and Suckling (1978) found that pulsed ultrasound at 20% duty cycle to the wound margins facilitated the healing process. Effective therapeutic parameters appear to be at a 20% duty cycle, 0.8 to 1.0 $W/cm^2$ intensity at 3 MHz with the treatment applied for approximately 3 to 10 minutes (Baba-Akbari Sari, Flemming, Cullum, & Wollina, 2006; McDiamid, 1985).

Surgical incisions have also been treated using pulsed ultrasound using the parameters of 0.5 to 0.8 W/cm2 intensity, pulsed 20%, 3 to 5 times per week. Conceptually, it is thought that using pulsed ultrasound facilitates the process of angiogenesis or cell budding; a crucial component of the healing process leading to the formation of new circulatory loops in the injured tissue (Young & Dyson, 1990). Pulsed ultrasound has been demonstrated to increase the strength of the healing wound, as well as decreasing pain, and hematoma size in gynecological surgical wounds and episiotomies. Chronic, thickened, and painful scars secondary to episiotomy were successfully treated months and years after the surgery using pulsed ultrasound (Fieldhouse, 1979).

Therapeutic ultrasound in a pulsed mode has also been shown to promote tendon healing. Research has indicated that the use of ultrasound will increase the overall tensile strength of the tendons as well as improving ROM  and facilitating scar maturation. Ultrasound to facilitate tendon healing was applied immediately after the injury leading to the overall improvements. The majorities of studies have used a dose (between 0.5 to 1.5 $W/cm^2$) intensity continuous at a 1 or 3 MHz frequency for 3 to 5 minutes, and have been a mixture of animal and human studies. Ng and colleagues found that both low and high dose ultrasound accelerated the healing process of ruptured tendons in rats. They used an intensity of between 1.0 and 2.0 $W/cm^2$ for 4 minutes (Ng & Ng, 2003). Leung and his colleagues also found that pulsed ultrasound may enhance ligament repair through the histochemical changes that occur causing an increase in transforming growth factor beta-1 (Leung, Cheung, Zhang, Lee, & Lo, 2004). It is recommended that lower intensity doses may be more appropriate in order to prevent aggravating the inflammatory process and tissue.

Nonthermal ultrasound has also been demonstrated to reduce fracture healing time and stimulate bone growth in tibial diaphyseal fractures, in Colles' fractures and on distraction osteogenesis. The mechanism of action of nonthermal ultrasound appears to be through stimulation of osteoblastic cells during the healing process. (Heckman et al., 1994; Naruse, Miyauchi, Itoman, & Mikuni-Takagaki, 2003; Stein & Lerner, 2005) Low-dose ultrasound of 0.15 $W/cm^2$, 20% duty cycle, 1 MHz for 15 to 20 minutes daily has been shown to facilitate fracture healing and should be a consideration. There are currently commercial home units which can also be used for fracture healing.

## Selecting Thermal or Nonthermal

In general, acute conditions are best treated with lower-intensity dosages of between 0.1 and 0.5 $W/cm^2$. With intensity this low, the patient is unlikely to feel any warmth. Subacute conditions can be treated using a low-intensity dosage of 0.5 to 1.0 $W/cm^2$ and by increasing the duty cycle to 50% in order to provide more energy without an intense thermal or heat effect. For chronic conditions or to achieve a thermal change in the tissue, a setting of between 1.0 and 2.0 $W/cm^2$ should be used with a duty cycle of 100% (Table 7-2). The patient may experience some degree of warmth but should not report any pain, discomfort, or burning. If this occurs, the intensity should be reduced immediately and the sound head should be moved more quickly. An inadequate amount of ultrasound gel may cause an uncomfortable tingling sensation or vibration. Adding

## THERAPEUTIC EFFECTS OF ULTRASOUND

### Thermal

- Joint contracture
- Scar tissue
- Chronic conditions
- Chronic inflammation
- Increase tissue extensibility
- Pain modulation
- Increase blood flow
- Soft tissue heating
- Decrease muscle spasm

### Nonthermal

- Facilitate tissue healing and repair
- Increase protein synthesis
- Fracture or bone healing
- Acute injury or inflammation
- Acute injury or inflammation of peripheral nerves
- Open wounds, dermal ulcers, surgical skin incisions
- Plantar warts
- Myofascial trigger points

**Table 7-2**

### GUIDE TO INITIAL ULTRASOUND APPLICATION

|  | *Nonthermal* | *Mild Heating* | *Therapeutic Heating* |
|---|---|---|---|
| Inflammatory or Acute Care | 0.2 W/cm$^2$ 10 to 20% duty cycle |  |  |
| Proliferative or Subacute Phase |  | 0.2 to 0.8 W/cm$^2$ 50% duty cycle |  |
| Remodeling or Chronic Phase |  |  | 0.8 to 2.0 W/cm$^2$ 100% duty cycle |

additional gel or applying the ultrasound in water may reduce the patient's discomfort (Balmaseda, Fatehi, Koozekanani, & Lee, 1986; Draper, Sunderland, Kirkendall, & Ricard, 1993; Reid & Cummings, 1973) (Figure 7-8).

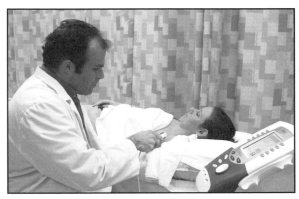

**Figure 7-8.** The applicator should be moved in a circular motion over the treatment area. Effective area which can be treated is equal to twice the size of the sound head.

The nonthermal effects of ultrasound, particularly when delivered at 20% duty cycle 0.2 W/cm$^2$, will provide the nonthermal, mechanical effects and will clinically facilitate tissue healing. Low intensity ultrasound will increase intracellular calcium, increase mast cell degranulation, increase chemotactic factor and histamine release, increase skin and cellular membrane permeability and increase the rate of fibroplasias. Because of the effect of nonthermal ultrasound on machrophage motility and effectiveness, nonthermal ultrasound should be considered during the inflammatory stage of healing.

Thermal ultrasound is commonly used to treat a variety of clinical conditions. Though the selection of thermal ultrasound is commonly determined by the necessity to heat tissue, there are also some of the nonthermal effects which occur concurrently. However, the thermal effects of ultrasound are used primarily for increasing tissue extensibility or for the reduction of pain. Thermal ultrasound parameters vary from 1.0 W/cm$^2$ to 2.5 W/cm$^2$ with a 100% duty cycle. Intensities at this level will provide a thermal, heating effect to the tissue and is commonly used to treat chronic conditions. Subacute conditions can be treated by using decreased intensity and decreasing the duty cycle. This will provide a greater amount of energy to the tissue, but the effects will be less thermal, a mild form of heating. Parameters between 0.3 to 0.9 W/cm$^2$ and 50% duty cycle would provide a less vigorous dose of ultrasound and less of a thermal effect while retaining the characteristics of the mechanical benefits. It should be noted that the research supporting ultrasound varies greatly and is limited by poor research design and a plethora of therapeutic parameters. The clinician needs to consider the stage of healing and determine the underlying cause of the condition—the differential diagnosis—to ensure that the correct parameters of ultrasound are selected. Further research will help to clarify clinical parameters and use of therapeutic ultrasound with specific diagnosis.

# Phonophoresis

Phonophoresis is the use of ultrasound to enhance the delivery of topically applied drugs, most frequently corticosteroids. Phonophoresis allows the application of medication through an essentially safe and painless technique similar to iontophoresis which uses a low level electrical current, however. It appears that phonophoresis actively transports the medication into the underlying targeted tissue through both a thermal and nonthermal mechanism. The medication used in phonophoresis has to cross the stratum corneum to reach the underlying area. Ultrasound, particularly thermal ultrasound, appears to increase the permeability of the stratum corneum allowing the medication to diffuse across it due to the higher concentrations and gradient pressure under the transducer.

Phonophoresis has been used clinically with great frequency as therapists attempt to impact the healing process. There have been inconsistencies regarding the effectiveness of phonophoresis in the research because of the variability in outcomes, due in part to the mechanism of delivery. Ultrasound in the form of phonophoresis has been shown to accelerate the tissue repair process and induce the transdermal delivery enhancing the percutaneous penetration of a variety of topical medications including hydrocortisone, and diclofenac gel although the mechanism remains unclear (Koeke, Parizotto, Carrinho, & Salate, 2005; Rosim, Barbieri, Lancas, & Mazzer, 2005). The variability of the treatment parameters: intensity, continuous vs. pulsed, frequency, duration, etc., often conflict. It is clear, however, that ultrasound exerts thermal, mechanical, and chemical effects on tissue. The primary factor often neglected or overlooked by clinicians is the type of transmission media utilized. Transmissivity of ultrasound is directly related to the conducting gel being utilized with wide variability noted. In comparing 19 media, Cameron and Monroe found only six that transmitted at 80% of water or greater, including: plain ultrasound gel (96%), ultrasound lotion (90%), mineral oil (97%), 0.05% betamethasone in ultrasound gel (88%), theragesic cream, 19% methyl salicylate (97%), and Lidex gel (Scottsdale, AZ), 0.05% fluocinonide (97%). None of the hydrocortisone powders or creams in any percentage transmitted well, and the most commonly used hydrocortisone creams in the clinic—1% or 10% hydrocortisone in a thick white cream base—did not transmit ultrasound at all, and are ineffective in therapeutic value. Dexamethasone sodium phosphate mixed with a sonic gel has been found to transmit ultrasound more effectively than hydrocortisone acetate and can be formulated by a pharmacist. The thick, white cream base consisting of 10% or 1% hydrocortisone transmits ultrasound poorly and should not be used (Table 7-3). The use of these preparations does not transmit the ultrasound effectively and the energy is subsequently reflected back into the transducer, which may cause overheating and damage of the transducer (Cameron & Monroe, 1992).

Many of the popular analgesic creams, such as Bio-Freeze (Performance Health, Export, PA) and Flexall (Chattem, Chattanooga, TN) are also used in the clinic as a coupling agent with the intention of decreasing pain perception. Some manufacturers have marketed their analgesic creams for use as an ultrasound couplant with the added benefit of decreasing pain through an analgesic effect (Myrer, Measom, & Fellingham, 2000). Research to date has been somewhat equivocal. Even when the mixtures are combined with ultrasound gel in a 50/50 ratio or even 80/20 ratio, their use may impede the vigorous heating which is desired and should be taken into consideration (Draper & Prentice, 2002).

Most of the medications commonly used with phonophoresis are anti-inflammatory medications, such as hydrocortisone, cortisol, or dexamethasone; analgesics, such as lidocaine; or nonsteroidal anti-inflammatory drugs (NSAIDs), such as diclofenac gel. Many of the medications used by therapists for phonophoresis are controlled substances and the therapist must have a prescription from the physician to use these medications. Therapists should check their state licensing board rules and regulations related to this issue as well as determining if there are institutional limitations in place. Before applying any medication it is also important to take into consideration the patients' reaction to these medications and whether they have any known allergies to the medication, as well as determining the interactive effects of any current medication they may be taking. A dressing such as plastic wrap that seals the area and pre-

## Table 7-3

### ULTRASOUND TRANSMISSION BY PHONOPHORESIS ACCORDING TO MEDIA

| Transmission Relative to Water (%) | Media/Products That Transmit Ultrasound Well |
|---|---|
| 97% | Lidex gel, fluocinonide 0.05% |
| 97% | Thera-Gesic cream (Mission Pharmaceutical, San Antonio, TX), methyl salicylate 15% |
| 97% | Mineral oil |
| 96% | Ultrasound gel |
| 90% | Ultrasound lotion |
| 88% | Betamethasone 0.05% in ultrasound gel |

*Media Products That Transmit Ultrasound Poorly*

| | |
|---|---|
| 36% | Diprolene ointment (Schering-Plough, Kenilworth, NJ), beta-methasone dipropionate 0.05% |
| 29% | Hydrocortisone powder 1% in ultrasound gel |
| 7% | Hydrocortisone powder 10% in ultrasound gel |

*Media/Product With Zero Transmissivity*

| | |
|---|---|
| 0% | Terra-Cortil ointment (Pfizer, New York, NY), hydocortisone 1% |
| 0% | Eucerin cream (Beiersdorf, Wilton, CT) |
| 0% | Hydrocortisone cream 1% |
| 0% | Hydrocortisone cream 10% |
| 0% | Hydrocortisone cream 10%, mixed with equal weight ultrasound gel |
| 0% | Myoflex cream (Morristown, NJ), triethanolamine salicylate 0.1% |
| 0% | Triamcinolone acetonide cream 0.1% |
| 0% | White petrolatum |

*Other*

| | |
|---|---|
| 68% | lidocaine hydrochloride (Chempad-L) |
| 98% | Polyethylene wrap |

Adapted from Cameron, M. H., & Monroe, L. G. (1992). Relative transmission of ultrasound by media customarily used for phonophoresis. *Physical Therapy, 72*(2), 145.

vents the escape of moisture should be applied after the treatment and may increase the effectiveness. Pretreating the skin with heat, moistening, or trimming long hair on skin should precede application of the phonophoresis. An intensity of 1.5 W/cm$^2$ should be used for both the thermal and nonthermal effects of the ultrasound with the application of low intensity ultrasound (0.5 W/cm$^2$) for treating open wounds or acute injuries. Ultrasound facilitates percutaneous penetration of the topical diclofenac gel, although the mechanism remains unclear; stimulates the acceleration of tissue repair processes and induces the transdermal delivery of hydrocortisone in a therapeutic concentration on the tendon (Byl, 1995; Cameron & Monroe, 1992; Koeke et al., 2005; Rosim et al., 2005).

# Application Procedures

Direct application of ultrasound to the tissue requires that a thin layer of couplant gel be applied to the area to ensure adequate contact between the ultrasound head and the tissue. Any air pockets between the applicator and tissue should be avoided with the sound head size selected based on the treatment area. Obviously, smaller treatment areas such as fingers, elbows, etc., would require a smaller sound head such as a 2 cm or possibly 5 cm size. Warming the ultrasound gel will not affect the therapeutic effects of the ultrasound since thermal effects of the ultrasound occur through the mechanical vibration of the cells. Warming the sound gel in one of the available commercial warmers, may improve the comfort to the patient when the gel is applied to the tissue. Because of the variety of sound heads available, most of the clinical applications using ultrasound can be done directly to the tissue-direct contact. A water immersion technique can be used if the treated area is smaller than the diameter of the sound head available or if the area is irregular with bony prominences. A bladder technique or commercially available gel pack can also be used for these areas if an appropriate size sound head is unavailable. The gel pack will transmit the ultrasound energy into the underlying tissue as effectively when a gel coupling agent is applied to both sides of the gel pack. If water immersion techniques are used for a thermal effect, the transducer should be moved parallel to the treated area and the intensity should be increased to ensure adequate heating of the tissue (Klucinec, Scheidler, & Denegar, 2000).

Because of the irregularity of the ultrasound beam and energy distribution, moving the sound head during the application of ultrasound is necessary to prevent focal "hot spots." As the sound head is moved throughout the treatment area the ultrasound beam is "averaged" out, providing a more balanced heat application. Moving the sound head will prevent the development and potentially damaging effect of standing waves and periosteal heating. The transducer should be moved in slowly, overlapping circular motions at 4 cm per second with the total treatment area approximately twice the size of the sound head (Kramer, 1984). If the sound head is moved too rapidly, or is not kept parallel to the surface area, the effects of the ultrasound will be lessened. Moving the transducer too rapidly will also decrease the overall absorption of the sound energy and may decrease the effects. The transducer should be kept in direct contact with the skin and tissue being treated, moved in slow, circular motions with an adequate amount of firm pressure applied that is comfortable to the patient and not excessive or too "light." As always, if the patient complains of pain or discomfort, the therapist should revise their application by either lowering the intensity or modifying the parameters, adding additional gel, or by moving the sound head more (Figure 7-9).

# Treatment Frequency and Documentation

Ultrasound is an effective, easy-to-apply technology. Most often, ultrasound is administered once a day or every other day. It can be safely used as long as there is continued improvement in the patient's condition. As with any treatment intervention, ongoing reassessment of the patient's condition, response to intervention, and attainment of goals and outcomes is necessary. There are no hard and fast answers with

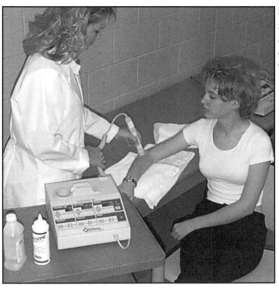

**Figure 7-9.** Ultrasound application—note the small sound head to localize the sound energy and the use of gel to ensure adequate contact during treatment. A 3 MHz frequency is used for superficial tissue.

regard to the number of treatment sessions using ultrasound. Clinically, many therapists have adhered to a course of 9 to 12 sessions as long as improvement is noted. The patient's condition is then monitored for approximately 2 weeks. If the condition worsens during that time, an additional series of treatments can be implemented or therapeutic parameters modified. Ultrasound treatment can continue as long as there is noted improvement in the patient's condition and functional abilities. Acute conditions may require more frequent treatments over a shorter time frame, while chronic conditions may require a longer period of treatment time, but fewer treatments (McDiamid & Burns, 1987). For chronic conditions, ultrasound can be applied on alternating days, continuing as long as improvement is noted.

Some clinical conditions, such as Dupuytren's contractures, may require an extended period of treatment. It should be noted that there are no controlled studies indicating that extended periods of treatment are detrimental, particularly if the patient continues to make progress. Treatment time is based on four primary factors: *area of tissue to be treated, intensity, frequency*, and *level of desired heating*. If the volume of the treated area is comparable to approximately three times the size of the sound head, the duration should be increased. Higher intensities also may decrease the treatment time. If vigorous heating is required, then higher intensities or longer durations at lower intensity should be applied. Though there is an inverse relationship between depth of penetration and frequency—3 MHz providing a more superficial effect and 1 MHz penetrating deeper—there is also more energy provided to the tissue when using higher frequency levels. The result will be faster heating of the structures being treated using thermal settings at a frequency of 3 MHz, so duration of the application should be decreased by approximately one-third. In determining duration of application, consideration of the treatment goal, therapeutic effect, and tissue type are important variables that must be taken into account. As a general rule, more vigorous levels of heat require either longer durations of application or higher intensity levels when using a frequency of 1 MHz. Review of clinical treatment parameters should be part of an on-going reasoning process based on both subjective and objective information gathered during the treatment sessions.

Clear and accurate documentation is necessary to assure continuity between therapists and third party intermediaries. When documenting ultrasound, therapists should note the patient's position, the area being treated, the technique being used (moving sound head, immersion), the frequency (1 MHz or 3 MHz), pulse ratio, intensity, sound head size, and the duration of the treatment. Clearly documenting the sequence of the treatment protocol and the activities and techniques involved, as well as the patient's response to the intervention, is also important. Any adverse reactions or subjective comments should also be reported.

## ULTRASOUND PRECAUTIONS AND CONTRAINDICATIONS

### Precautions

- Acute inflammation
- Fractures
- Breast implants
- Patients with cognitive, language, or sensory limitations

### Ultrasound Contraindications

- During pregnancy
- Over the reproductive organs
- Over the eyes
- Thrombophlebitis
- Plastic components
- Area of cardiac pacemaker
- Central nervous system tissue: stellate or cervical ganglia
- Over epiphyseal plates of children
- Malignancy or tumors
- Areas with active bleeding or infections

# Precautions and Contraindications

As with any treatment modality, careful observation of the effect of the intervention is important. Therapeutic ultrasound should never be applied over the eye, over the heart, over the pregnant uterus, or over reproductive organs. Due to the possibility of metastasis and increased tumor growth at therapeutic parameters, sonification to malignant tissue should be avoided. Care should also be used when applying ultrasound over areas with decreased circulation or over areas of thrombophlebitis, due to the possibility of clotting or dislodging a thrombus. Growth plates in children should be avoided if possible, particularly when using higher intensities (De Deyne & Kirsch-Volders, 1995; Sicard-Rosenbaum, Lord, & Danoff, 1995; Sicard-Rosenbaum & Danoff, 1993). Continuous ultrasound should be avoided in acute or postacute conditions due to the thermal effects of the ultrasound on the tissue.

Therapists should avoid using a stationary transducer technique due to an increased risk of "hot spots" in the sound field. Patients should not feel the ultrasound and should not experience discomfort during the session. If the patient complains of pain, it is usually an indication of periosteal heating. Decreasing the intensity or moving the transducer more quickly should prevent patient discomfort. Patients with surgical metal implants and those with prosthetic joint implants or replacements can safely receive therapeutic ultrasound if appropriate application techniques are followed. There is the possibility of a standing wave developing in metal implants, as the metal reflects approximately 90% of the ultrasound. Plastic is similar to bone in its response to ultrasound, and absorbs a large percentage of the ultrasound. Using the proper application techniques of moving the sound head over the area to be treated and setting the correct treatment parameters is necessary. In general, it is safe to apply ultrasound over implanted materials if proper techniques and precautions are followed (Kotenber & Ambrose/Mosher, 1986; Lehman, 1980; Skouba-Kristensen, 1982; Ter harr, 1987). Care must also be taken when applying ultrasound to areas around the heart and in those patients with cardiac pacemakers. Thermal ultrasound should also be applied carefully if the treatment area has decreased sensation or the patient has limitations due to language, cognitive, or sensory issues.

## Case Study

Jim is a 32-year-old male employed as a production worker on the midnight shift at a small injection molding factory. He lives in a rural town with his wife, a 10-year-old son practicing for the softball team, and two daughters, aged 5 and 7, who are involved in gymnastics and dance. Jim's wife works full time at a local agricultural plant. Jim is an active outdoors type who enjoys gardening, fishing, and bike riding. He is responsible for getting the kids off to school, taking care of the household, making dinner, and helping the kids with their homework when they return from school. Jim has experienced a major trauma in his life that will affect his role as a provider and have a negative impact on all of his occupational roles over the course of the next 12 to 16 weeks.

Jim was referred to occupational therapy by his orthopedic surgeon following an accident at work. Jim does not know exactly what caused the accident, but when he reached over to remove a small part wedged in the press, the press fired. The press came down squarely on the dorsal surface of his dominant right hand, crushing the dorsal aspect of the hand and lacerating the extensor tendons of his index, middle, and ring fingers.

Jim is still shaken when he talks about the accident and the subsequent surgery to repair his tendons. The physician immobilized the digits for almost 2 weeks secondary to a wound infection, and unfortunately Jim waited an additional week to schedule an occupational therapy appointment. Jim's hand is discolored, edematous, and painful, with limited functional or passive movement. Although he is thankful that he did not lose his fingers, Jim's life and roles have dramatically changed. Jim wants to know if he will ever be able to use his hand again or return to work; the Workers' Compensation coordinators, as well as the orthopedic surgeon, ask the same question.

How do we facilitate healing to expedite the return to occupational roles in so traumatic an injury? One approach is to incorporate therapeutic ultrasound into the traditional treatment. Jim's case is not unusual for many occupational therapists treating orthopedic injuries. The approach that we as occupational therapists use with these types of patients is unique, however. It is the occupational therapist's holistic focus and careful consideration of the media and methods used as part of the treatment process that places us in an excellent position to utilize physical technologies including therapeutic ultrasound as part of our treatment repertoire.

## Jim's Response to Ultrasound

Jim presented with a number of deficit areas, including decreased tendon gliding over the metacarpophalangeal joints, wound infection with decreased healing, and an inability to perform functional activities and occupations requiring bilateral manipulation or lifting. Circumferential measurements, ROM, grip and pinch strength, sensory testing, wound and scar evaluation, and assessment of functional activities were all component areas assessed and documented. His goals included increasing tendon gliding, increasing ROM, improving prehension patterns and functional use of the hand, improving functional abilities, and returning to competitive employment and rates of production.

Therapeutic ultrasound was selected as an adjunct to Jim's treatment due to the small area of injury and because of the tendency for the collagen rich tendon and joint capsules to selectively "absorb" the sound energy. Because the tissue area was superficial, the ultrasound frequency selected was 3 MHz/0.2 W/cm$^2$, pulsed at 20% duty cycle for 5 minutes. The smallest transducer (2 cm) was selected to localize the sound energy. A low intensity was chosen because of the subacute nature of the condition and for the nonthermal benefits to facilitate the wound healing process. Low intensity was also used because of the reflection at the tissue-bone interface, which could increase the intensity by a small amount. Therapeutic ultrasound preceded active motion incorporating flexion and limited excursion, active and full passive movement into extension in order to enhance tendon gliding and to facilitate the healing process.

As Jim improved and as the treatment sessions progressed, measurement of change was documented, and ultrasound parameters were revised to achieve a thermal effect to facilitate tissue elongation. The frequency continued to be 3 MHz, but intensity was increased to 1.0 W/cm$^2$ at 100% duty cycle. The lifting requirements and prehension patterns needed to safely and effectively perform his job requirements also were incorporated into Jim's treatment plan. Jim eventually returned to competitive employment; was able to play catch with his son again; and resumed his occupational roles as husband, father, provider, and caretaker of the children. Therapeutic ultrasound played an important and vital part of his overall treatment program.

## Clinical Reasoning Questions

1. When would you choose to use thermal ultrasound rather than nonthermal ultrasound?

2. How would you select the appropriate frequency for this condition?

3. What precautions and contraindications would you need to be aware of before using ultrasound in the treatment process?

4. What other physical agent modalities might be beneficial in this case?

5. What is happening physiologically to the tissue during the application of ultrasound?

6. How do you determine the appropriate length/time of ultrasound application?

# Summary

Therapeutic ultrasound can be an effective adjunct in the occupational therapist's treatment repertoire. The ability of ultrasound to increase tissue extensibility, decrease pain and muscle spasm, and facilitate tissue healing and repair make it a vital addition to the treatment program for selected patients and conditions. The occupational therapist using ultrasound as an adjunct to treatment should have a thorough understanding of the physics, biophysical effects, precautions, and contraindications involved in order to achieve the maximum benefit of the effects of ultrasound. Continued research related to dosage and treatment parameters will help to refine clinical applications.

# Evidence Based Research

1. Rosim, G., Barbieri, C., Lancas, F., & Mazzer, N. (2005). Diclofenac phonophoresis in human volunteers. *Ultrasound in Medicine and Biology, 31*(3), 337-343.

A quantitative study of sodium diclofenac (Voltaren Emulgel, Novartis, Cambridge, MA) phonophoresis was undertaken in humans. Fourteen healthy human volunteers were submitted to ultrasound irradiation on two 225-$cm^2$ areas on the dorsum (group A), followed by the application of the medication gel; and the plasma diclofenac mass was measured at 1, 2, and 3 hours later by high performance liquid chromatography. The same procedure was repeated 1 month later with the same volunteers but with the ultrasound equipment switched off for the control group (group B). The plasma diclofenac mass was significantly higher in group A than in group B at 1 h (0.0987 microg/mL as opposed to 0.0389 microg/mL; p=0.01) and 2 h (0.0724 microg/mL as opposed to 0.0529 microg/mL; p=0.01), but not at 3 h (0.0864 microg/mL as opposed to 0.0683 microg/mL; p=0.16). The authors conclude that previously applied therapeutic ultrasound irradiation enhances the percutaneous penetration of the topical diclofenac gel, although the mechanism remains unclear.

2. Byl, N. N. (1995). The use of ultrasound as an enhancer for transcutaneous drug delivery: Phonophoresis. *Physical Therapy, 75*, 539-553.

Phonophoresis is the use of ultrasound to enhance the delivery of topically applied drugs. The purposes of this article are 1) to review the basic principles of transcutaneous drug delivery, 2) to summarize the functional anatomy of the skin pertinent to phonophoresis, 3) to outline the physiological principles of ultrasound as an enhancer of topically applied drugs, 4) to review the literature on the efficacy of phonophoresis, 5) to discuss the relevance of ultrasound as an enhancer of topical drugs in the practice of physical therapy, and 6) to outline areas of needed research. Seventy-five percent of the studies reviewed reported positive effects of ultrasound on local subcutaneous drug diffusion, but some systemic effects were reported. This research review indicates that to maximize the clinical effectiveness of phonophoresis: 1) the topical drug (both the drug and the carrying agent) should transmit ultrasound; 2) the skin should be pretreated with ultrasound, heating, moistening, or shaving; 3) the patient needs to be positioned to maximize circulation during treatment; 4) a dressing that seals the area and prevents the escape of moisture should be applied after treatment; 5) an intensity of 1.5 $W/cm^2$ should be used to capture both the thermal and nonthermal effects of the ultrasound; and 6) low-intensity ultrasound (0.5 $W/cm^2$) should be used when treating open wounds or acute injuries. Research is needed to clarify what parameters of ultrasound will most efficiently facilitate topical drug diffusion, how often and for what duration ultrasound should be used to maximize local absorption of drugs, and which topical drugs can most effectively be used for phonophoresis.

3. Koeke, P. U., Parizotto, N. A., Carrinho, P. M., & Salate, A. C. (2005). Comparative study of the efficacy of the topical application of hydrocortisone, therapeutic ultrasound and phonophoresis on the tissue repair process in rat tendons. *Ultrasound in Medicine & Biology, 31,* 345-350.

The purpose of this study was to compare the treatment efficacy of topical application of hydrocortisone, therapeutic ultrasound, and phonophoresis on the rat's Achilles tendon (tendo calcaneus) repair process after tenotomy. The two treated groups with ultrasound were made in a pulsed mode. The irradiation of ultrasound was performed at a frequency of 1 MHz and an intensity of 0.5 W/cm$^2$ (SATA), for 5 minutes each session. The tendons were analyzed using the polarized light microscopy. The results showed that the treated group with the topical application of hydrocortisone has not been delivered transdermally and that the molecule of collagen responds to the ultrasonic stimulation. The treatment with phonophoresis was the more efficient method. These findings allow us to conclude that ultrasound stimulates the acceleration of tissue repair processes and induces the transdermal delivery of hydrocortisone in a therapeutic concentration on the tendon.

4. Batavia, M. (2004). Contraindications for superficial heat and therapeutic ultrasound: Do sources agree? *Archives of Physical Medicine and Rehabilitation, 85,* 1006-1012.

Objectives: To determine the amount of agreement among general rehabilitation sources for both superficial heating and therapeutic ultrasound contraindications. Data sources: English-language textbook and peer-reviewed journal sources, from January 1992 to July 2002. Searches of computerized databases (HealthSTAR, CINAHL, MEDLINE, Embase) as well as Library of Congress Online Catalogs, Books in Print, and AcqWeb's Directory of Publishers and Venders. Data selection: Sources were excluded if they 1) were published before 1992, 2) failed to address general rehabilitation audiences, or 3) were identified as a researcher's related publication with similar information on the topic. Data extraction: Type and number of contraindications, type of audience, year of publication, number of references, rationales, and alternative treatment strategies. Data synthesis: Eighteen superficial heat and 20 ultrasound sources identified anywhere from 5 to 22 and 9 to 36 contraindications/precautions, respectively. Agreement among sources was generally high but ranged from 11% to 95%, with lower agreement noted for pregnancy, metal implants, edema, skin integrity, and cognitive/communicative concerns. Seventy-two percent of superficial heat sources and 25% of ultrasound sources failed to reference at least 1 contraindication claim. Conclusions: Agreement among contraindication sources was generally good for both superficial heat and therapeutic ultrasound. Sources varied with regard to the number of contraindications, references, and rationales cited. Greater reliance on objective data and standardized classification systems may serve to develop more uniform guidelines for superficial heat and therapeutic ultrasound.

5. Chan, C. W., Qin, L., Lee, K. M., Cheung, W. H., Cheng, J. C., & Leung, K. S. (2006). Dose-dependent effect of low-intensity pulsed ultrasound on callus formation during rapid distraction osteogenesis. *Journal of Orthopaedic Research*, *24*, 2072-2079.

Distraction osteogenesis of bone or callotasis causes poor bone formation when the distraction rate is beyond the optimal rate. Low-intensity pulsed ultrasound was reported to enhance fracture healing, treatment of nonunion, and accelerate bone maturation and remodeling during consolidation stage of distraction osteogenesis. In this study, we evaluated the efficacy of different durations of LIPUS treatments during rapid bone lengthening. After a 7-day latent period, osteotomized New Zealand white rabbit tibiae were lengthened at the rate of 2 mm per day for 1 week. Two different LIPUS treatment durations of 20 minutes and 40 minutes were selected for treatment groups. Rabbits without treatment served as the control group. Plain X-ray, peripheral quantitative computed tomography (pQCT), and histology were performed to assess bone acquisition in the distraction callus. The results showed that LIPUS increased bone mineral content and volume of the mineralized tissue of distraction callus in a dose-dependent manner. The different regions of distraction callus exhibited various spatial response to LIPUS treatment. Moreover, LIPUS enhanced dose-dependant endochondral formation. Compared with 20-minute treatment, the 40-minute LIPUS treatment was a more favorable treatment duration for bone regeneration in the distraction callus. In conclusion, LIPUS was able to enhance bone regeneration under rapid distraction, and its effect was dose-dependent.

6. Giannini, S., Giombini, A., Moneta, M. R., Massazza, G., & Pigozzi, F. (2004). Low-intensity pulsed ultrasound in the treatment of traumatic hand fracture in an elite athlete. *American Journal of Physical Medicine & Rehabilitation*, *83*, 921-925.

We report a case of complex traumatic hand fracture successfully treated with low-intensity ultrasound in an elite soccer goalkeeper. A single 20-minute daily application of low-intensity pulsed ultrasound (frequency, 1.5 Mhz; intensity, 30 mW/cm$^2$) provided by Exogen's Sonic Accelerated Fracture Healing System (Memphis, TN) was administered for 24 days on end. Plain radiographs, ultrasonography, and computed tomographic scans were performed to diagnose and to follow-up the evolution of the fracture during the treatment. After 24 days, the athlete was allowed to recommence his specific sport activity with a modified soccer glove and functional taping. After 2 months, radiographs demonstrated the complete healing, with no displacement, of the fracture sites.

# References

Apfel, R. (1989). Acoustic cavitation: A possible consequence of biomedical uses of ultrasound. *British Journal of Cancer*, *45*, 140.

Arnheim, D. (Ed.). (1989). *Modern principles of athletic training.* St. Louis, MO: Mosby.

Artho, P. A., Thyne, J. G., Warring, B. P., Willis, C. D., Brismee, J. M., & Latman, N. S. (2002). A calibration study of therapeutic ultrasound units. *Physical Therapy*, *82*, 257-263.

Baba-Akbari Sari, A., Flemming, K., Cullum, N. A., & Wollina, U. (2006). Therapeutic ultrasound for pressure ulcers. *Cochrane Database of Systematic Reviews (Online)*, *3*, CD001275.

Balmaseda, M. T., Jr, Fatehi, M. T., Koozekanani, S. H., & Lee, A. L. (1986). Ultrasound therapy: A comparative study of different coupling media. *Archives of Physical Medicine and Rehabilitation*, *67*, 147-150.

Bandow, K., Nishikawa, Y., Ohnishi, T., Kakimoto, K., Soejima, K., & Iwabuchi, S. et al. (2007). Low-intensity pulsed ultrasound (LIPUS) induces RANKL, MCP-1, and MIP-1beta expression in osteoblasts through the angiotensin II type 1 receptor. *Journal of Cellular Physiology, 211*(2):392-8.

Batavia, M. (2004). Contraindications for superficial heat and therapeutic ultrasound: Do sources agree? *Archives of Physical Medicine and Rehabilitation, 85*, 1006-1012.

Binder, A., Hodge, G., Greenwood, A. M., Hazleman, B. L., & Page Thomas, D. P. (1985). Is therapeutic ultrasound effective in treating soft tissue lesions? *BMJ (Clinical Research Ed.), 290*, 512-514.

Buchtala, V. (1952). The present state of ultrasonic therapy. *British Journal of Physical Medicine, 15*, 3-6.

Busse, J. W., Bhandari, M., Kulkarni, A. V., & Tunks, E. (2002). The effect of low-intensity pulsed ultrasound therapy on time to fracture healing: A meta-analysis. *Canadian Medical Association Journal, 166*, 437-441.

Byl, N. N. (1995). The use of ultrasound as an enhancer for transcutaneous drug delivery: Phonophoresis. *Physical Therapy, 75*, 539-553.

Cameron, M. H., & Monroe, L. G. (1992). Relative transmission of ultrasound by media customarily used for phonophoresis. *Physical Therapy, 72*, 142-148.

Casarotto, R. A., Adamowski, J. C., Fallopa, F., & Bacanelli, F. (2004). Coupling agents in therapeutic ultrasound: Acoustic and thermal behavior. *Archives of Physical Medicine and Rehabilitation, 85*, 162-165.

Casimiro, L., Brosseau, L., Robinson, V., Milne, S., Judd, M., & Well, G., et al. (2002). Therapeutic ultrasound for the treatment of rheumatoid arthritis. *Cochrane Database of Systematic Reviews (Online), (3)*, CD003787.

Chan, C. W., Qin, L., Lee, K. M., Cheung, W. H., Cheng, J. C., & Leung, K. S. (2006). Dose-dependent effect of low-intensity pulsed ultrasound on callus formation during rapid distraction osteogenesis. *Journal of Orthopaedic Research, 24*, 2072-2079.

Citak-Karakaya, I., Akbayrak, T., Demirturk, F., Ekici, G., & Bakar, Y. (2006). Short and long-term results of connective tissue manipulation and combined ultrasound therapy in patients with fibromyalgia. *Journal of Manipulative and Physiological Therapeutics, 29*, 524-528.

Claes, L., Ruter, A., & Mayr, E. (2005). Low-intensity ultrasound enhances maturation of callus after segmental transport. *Clinical Orthopaedics and Related Research, 430*, 189-194.

Claes, L., & Willie, B. (2007). The enhancement of bone regeneration by ultrasound. *Progress in Biophysics and Molecular Biology, 93*, 384-398.

Cullum, N., Nelson, E. A., Flemming, K., & Sheldon, T. (2001). Systematic reviews of wound care management: (5) beds; (6) compression; (7) laser therapy, therapeutic ultrasound, electrotherapy and electromagnetic therapy. *Health Technology Assessment (Winchester, England), 5*, 1-221.

Daniel, D. M., & Rupert, R. L. (2003). Calibration and electrical safety status of therapeutic ultrasound used by chiropractic physicians. *Journal of Manipulative and Physiological Therapeutics, 26*, 171-175.

De Deyne, P., & Kirsch-Volders, M. (1995). In vitro effects of therapeutic ultrasound on nucleum of human fibroblasts. *Physical Therapy, 75*, 629-633.

Draper, D. (1998). Guidelines to enhance therapeutic ultrasound treatment outcomes. *Athletic Therapy Today, 6*, 7.

Draper, D., Castel, J., & Castel, D. (1995). Rate of temperature increase in human muscle during 1 MH z and 3 MHz continuous ultrasound. *Journal of Orthopaedics and Sports Physical Therapy, 22*, 142-150.

Draper, D., & Prentice, W. (2002). Therapeutic ultrasound. In W. Prentice (Ed.), *Therapeutic modalities for physical therapists* (pp. 290-292). Chicago, Ill: McGraw Hill.

Draper, D. O., & Ricard, M. D. (1995). Rate of temperature decay in human muscle following 3 MHz ultrasound: The stretching window revealed. *Journal of Athletic Training, 30*, 304-307.

Draper, D. O., Sunderland, S., Kirkendall, D. T., & Ricard, M. (1993). A comparison of temperature rise in human calf muscles following applications of underwater and topical gel ultrasound. *Journal of Orthopaedic and Sports Physical Therapy, 17*, 247-251.

Dudda, M., Pommer, A., Muhr, G., & Esenwein, S. A. (2005). Application of low intensity, pulsed ultrasound on distraction osteogenesis of the humerus. Case report. *Der Unfallchirurg, 108*, 69-74.

Dyson, M., & Suckling, J. (1978). Stimulation of tissue repair by ultrasound: A survey of the mechanisms involved. *Physiotherapy, 64*, 105-108.

Ebenbichler, G. R., Resch, K. L., Nicolakis, P., Wiesinger, G. F., Uhl, F., & Ghanem, A. H. et al. (1998). Ultrasound treatment for treating the carpal tunnel syndrome: Randomised "sham" controlled trial. *BMJ (Clinical Research Ed.), 316*, 731-735.

Ennis, W. J., Valdes, W., Gainer, M., & Meneses, P. (2006). Evaluation of clinical effectiveness of MIST ultrasound therapy for the healing of chronic wounds. *Advances in Skin & Wound Care, 19*, 437-446.

Fieldhouse, C. (1979). Ultrasound for relief of painful episiotomy scars. *Physiotherapy, 65*, 217.

Flemming, K., & Cullum, N. (2000). Therapeutic ultrasound for venous leg ulcers. *Cochrane Database of Systematic Reviews (Online), 4*, CD001180.

Fyfe, M. C., & Bullock, M. (1985). Therapeutic ultrasound: Some historical background and development in knowledge of its effects on healing. *Australian Journal of Physiotherapy, 31*, 220-224.

Fyfe, M. C., & Parnell, S. M. (1982). The importance of measurement of effective transducers radiating area in the testing and calibration of "therapeutic" ultrasonic instruments. *Health Physics, 43*, 377-381.

Giannini, S., Giombini, A., Moneta, M. R., Massazza, G., & Pigozzi, F. (2004). Low-intensity pulsed ultrasound in the treatment of traumatic hand fracture in an elite athlete. *American Journal of Physical Medicine & Rehabilitation, 83*, 921-925.

Green, S., Buchbinder, R., & Hetrick, S. (2003). Physiotherapy interventions for shoulder pain. *Cochrane Database of Systematic Reviews (Online), 2*, CD004258.

Heckman, J. D., Ryaby, J. P., McCabe, J., Frey, J. J., & Kilcoyne, R. F. (1994). Acceleration of tibial fracture-healing by non-invasive, low-intensity pulsed ultrasound. *Journal of Bone and Joint Surgery, 76*, 26-34.

Hekkenberg, R., Oosterbaan, W., & Van Beekum, W. (1986). Evaluation of ultrasound therapy devices. *Physiotherapy, 72*, 390-395.

Hill, G. E., Fenwick, S., Matthews, B. J., Chivers, R. A., & Southgate, J. (2005). The effect of low-intensity pulsed ultrasound on repair of epithelial cell monolayers in vitro. *Ultrasound in Medicine & Biology, 31*, 1701-1706.

Ito, M., Azuma, Y., Ohta, T., & Komoriya, K. (2000). Effects of ultrasound and 1,25-dihydroxyvitamin D3 on growth factor secretion in co-cultures of osteoblasts and endothelial cells. *Ultrasound in Medicine & Biology, 26*, 161-166.

Kennedy, J. E., Ter Haar, G. R., & Cranston, D. (2003). High intensity focused ultrasound: Surgery of the future? *British Journal of Radiology, 76*, 590-599.

Kimura, I. F., Gulick, D. T., Shelly, J., & Ziskin, M. C. (1998). Effects of two ultrasound devices and angles of application on the temperature of tissue phantom. *Journal of Orthopaedic and Sports Physical Therapy, 27*, 27-31.

Klucinec, B., Scheidler, M., & Denegar, C. (2000). Transmission of coupling agents used to deliver acoustic energy over irregular surfaces. *Journal of Orthopaedic and Sports Physical Therapy, 30*, 263-269.

Koeke, P. U., Parizotto, N. A., Carrinho, P. M., & Salate, A. C. (2005). Comparative study of the efficacy of the topical application of hydrocortisone, therapeutic ultrasound and phonophoresis on the tissue repair process in rat tendons. *Ultrasound in Medicine & Biology, 31*, 345-350.

Kollmann, C., Vacariu, G., Schuhfried, O., Fialka-Moser, V., & Bergmann, H. (2005). Variations in the output power and surface heating effects of transducers in therapeutic ultrasound. *Archives of Physical Medicine and Rehabilitation, 86*, 1318-1324.

Kotenber, R., & Ambrose, L./ Mosher, R. (1986). Therapeutic ultrasound effect on high density polyethylene and polymethyl methacrylate. *Archives of Physical Medicine and Rehabilitation, 67*, 618.

Kramer, J. F. (1984). Ultrasound: Evaluation of its mechanical and thermal effects. *Archives of Physical Medicine and Rehabilitation, 65*, 223-227.

Kuitert, J. H., & Harr, E. T. (1955). Introduction to clinical application of ultrasound. *Physical Therapy Review, 35*, 19-25.

Lehman J. (1980). Ultrasound: Considerations for use in the presence of prosthetic joints. *Archives of Physical Medicine and Rehabilitation, 61*, 502.

Lehman J., Warren, C., & Guy, A. (1978). *Ultrasound: Its applications in medicine and biology*. New York: Elsevier Scientific.

Lehmann, J. F., & Herrick, J. F. (1953). Biologic reactions to cavitation, a consideration for ultrasonic therapy. *Archives of Physical Medicine and Rehabilitation, 34*, 86-98.

Leung, K. S., Cheung, W. H., Zhang, C., Lee, K. M., & Lo, H. K. (2004). Low intensity pulsed ultrasound stimulates osteogenic activity of human periosteal cells. *Clinical Orthopaedics and Related Research, 418*, 253-259.

Leung, M. C., Ng, G. Y., & Yip, K. K. (2004). Effect of ultrasound on acute inflammation of transected medial collateral ligaments. *Archives of Physical Medicine and Rehabilitation, 85*, 963-966.

Malizos, K. N., Hantes, M. E., Protopappas, V., & Papachristos, A. (2006). Low-intensity pulsed ultrasound for bone healing: An overview. *Injury, 37(Suppl 1)*, S56-62.

Markert, C. D., Merrick, M. A., Kirby, T. E., & Devor, S. T. (2005). Nonthermal ultrasound and exercise in skeletal muscle regeneration. *Archives of Physical Medicine and Rehabilitation, 86*, 1304-1310.

Mayr, E., Wagner, S., Ecker, M., & Ruter, A. (1999). Ultrasound therapy for nonunions. Three case reports. *Der Unfallchirurg, 102*, 191-196.

McDiamid, T. (1985). Ultrasound and the treatment of pressure sores. *Physiotherapy, 71*, 66-70.

McDiamid, T., & Burns, P. (1987). Clinical applications of therapeutic ultrasound. *Physiotherapy, 73*, 155.

Merrick, M. A., Bernard, K. D., Devor, S. T., & Williams, M. J. (2003). Identical 3-MHz ultrasound treatments with different devices produce different intramuscular temperatures. *Journal of Orthopaedic and Sports Physical Therapy, 33*, 379-385.

Michlovitz, S. (1996). *Thermal agents in rehabilitation.* Philadelphia, PA: FA Davis.

Morrisette, D. C., Brown, D., & Saladin, M. E. (2004). Temperature change in lumbar periarticular tissue with continuous ultrasound. *Journal of Orthopaedic and Sports Physical Therapy, 34*, 754-760.

Mukai, S., Ito, H., Nakagawa, Y., Akiyama, H., Miyamoto, M., & Nakamura, T. (2005). Transforming growth factor-beta1 mediates the effects of low-intensity pulsed ultrasound in chondrocytes. *Ultrasound in Medicine & Biology, 31*, 1713-1721.

Myer, J. W., Measom, G., & Fellingham, G. (2000). Significant intramuscular temperature rise obtained when topical analgesics: nature's chemist and biofreeze, were used as coupling agents during ultrasound treatment, *Journal of Athletic Training, 35*, 48.

Naruse, K., Miyauchi, A., Itoman, M., & Mikuni-Takagaki, Y. (2003). Distinct anabolic response of osteoblast to low-intensity pulsed ultrasound. *Journal of Bone and Mineral Research, 18*, 360-369.

Ng, C., & Ng, G. (2003). Therapeutic ultrasound improves strength of achilles tendon repair in rats. *Ultrasound in Medicine and Biology, 29*, 151-156.

Oh, Y. S., Early, D. S., & Azar, R. R. (2005). Clinical applications of endoscopic ultrasound to oncology. *Oncology, 68*, 526-537.

Okaro, E., & Condous, G. (2005). Diagnostic and therapeutic capabilities of ultrasound in the management of pelvic pain. *Current Opinion in Obstetrics & Gynecology, 17*, 611-617.

Peschen, M., Weichenthal, M., Schopf, E., & Vanscheidt, W. (1997). Low-frequency ultrasound treatment of chronic venous leg ulcers in an outpatient therapy. *Acta Dermato-Venereologica, 77*, 311-314.

Piersol, G. M., Schwan, H. P., Pennell, R. B., & Carstensen, E. L. (1952). Mechanism of absorption of ultrasonic energy in blood. *Archives of Physical Medicine and Rehabilitation, 33*, 327-332.

Pilla, A. A., Mont, M. A., Nasser, P. R., Khan, S. A., Figueiredo, M., & Kaufman, J. J. et al. (1990). Non-invasive low-intensity pulsed ultrasound accelerates bone healing in the rabbit. *Journal of Orthopaedic Trauma, 4*, 246-253.

Reid, D., & Cummings, G. (1973). Factors in selecting the dosage of ultrasound with particular reference to the use of various coupling agents. *Physiotherapy Canada, 63*, 255.

Rivest, M., Quirion-de Girardi, C., Seaborne, D., & Lambert, J. (1987). Evaluation of therapeutic ultrasound devices: Performance stability over 44 weeks of clinical use. *Physiotherapy Canada, 39*, 77-86.

Robertson, V. J., & Baker, K. G. (2001). A review of therapeutic ultrasound: Effectiveness studies. *Physical Therapy, 81*, 1339-1350.

Rose, S., Draper, D. O., Schulthies, S. S., & Durrant, E. (1996). The stretching window part two: Rate of thermal decay in deep muscle following 1-MHz ultrasound. *Journal of Athletic Training, 31*, 139-143.

Rosim, G. C., Barbieri, C. H., Lancas, F. M., & Mazzer, N. (2005). Diclofenac phonophoresis in human volunteers. *Ultrasound in Medicine & Biology, 31*, 337-343.

Samosiuk, I. Z., Miasnikov, V. G., & Klimenko, I. V. (1999). The use of low-frequency ultrasound in the combined therapy of pulmonary tuberculosis patients. *Voprosy Kurortologii, Fizioterapii, i Lechebnoi Fizicheskoi Kultury, (2)*, 9-11.

Sicard-Rosenbaum, L., Lord, D., & Danoff, J. (1995). Effects of continuous therapeutic ultrasound on growth and metastasis of subcutaneous murine tumors. *Physical Therapy, 75*, 3-13.

Sicard-Rosenbaum, L., & Danoff, J. (1993). Cancer and ultrasound: A warning. *Physical Therapy, 73*, 404-406.

Skouba-Kristensen, E. (1982). Ultrasound influence on internal fixation with a rigid plate in dogs. *Archives of Physical Medicine and Rehabilitation, 61*, 502.

Snow, C. J. (1982). Ultrasound therapy units in manitoba and northwestern ontario: Performance evaluation. *Physiotherapy Canada, 34*, 185-189.

Stein, H., & Lerner, A. (2005). How does pulsed low-intensity ultrasound enhance fracture healing? *Orthopedics, 28*, 1161-1163.

Stewart, H. F., Abzug, J. L., & Harris, G. R. (1980). Considerations in ultrasound therapy and equipment performance. *Physical Therapy, 60*, 424-428.

Stewart, H. F., Harris, G. R., Herman, B. A., Robinson, R. A., Haran, M. E., & McCall, G. R., et al. (1974). Survey of use and performance of ultrasonic therapy equipment in Pinellas County, Florida. *Physical Therapy, 54*, 707-715.

Swist-Chmielewska, D., Franek, A., Brzezinska-Wcislo, L., Blaszczak, E., Polak, A., & Krol, P. (2002). Experimental selection of best physical and application parameters of ultrasound in the treatment of venous crural ulceration. *Polski Merkuriusz Lekarski: Organ Polskiego Towarzystwa Lekarskiego, 12*, 500-505.

ter Haar, G., Dyson, M., & Oakley, E. M. (1987). The use of ultrasound by physiotherapists in britain, 1985. *Ultrasound in Medicine & Biology, 13*, 659-663.

ter Haar, G. (1987). Recent advances and techniques in therapeutic ultrasound. In M. Rapacholi, & M. Grandolfo (Eds.), *Ultrasound: Medical applications, biological effects and hazard potential* (pp. 333). New York: Plenum Press.

Uhlemann, C. (1993). Pain modification in rheumatic diseases using different frequency applications of ultrasound. *Zeitschrift Fur Rheumatologie, 52*, 236-240.

Walmsley, A. D. (1988). Applications of ultrasound in dentistry. *Ultrasound in Medicine & Biology, 14*, 7-14.

Wells, P. (1977). Ultrasonics in medicine and biology. *Physics in Medicine and Biology, 22*, 629-669.

Wilkin, L. D., Merrick, M. A., Kirby, T. E., & Devor, S. T. (2004). Influence of therapeutic ultrasound on skeletal muscle regeneration following blunt contusion. *International Journal of Sports Medicine, 25*, 73-77.

Williams, A. (1983). *Ultrasound: Biological effects and potential hazards.* London: Academic Press.

Williams, R., McHales, I., & Bowditch, M. (1987). Effects of humans. *Ultrasound in Medicine & Biology, 13*, 249.

Young, S., & Dyson, M. (1990). The effect of therapeutic ultrasound on angiogenesis. *Ultrasound in Medicine & Biology, 16*, 261-269.

# PRINCIPLES OF ELECTROTHERAPY

*Alfred G. Bracciano, EdD, OTR/L, FAOTA*
*Kirk Peck, PT, PhD, CSCS*

## Learning Objectives

1. Describe foundational principles and concepts of electricity.
2. Identify the waveforms of electrical stimulation and their characteristics.
3. Describe the physiological effects of electrical stimulation on the body.
4. Explain the rationale for selecting various electrical stimulation parameters.
5. Discuss the types and selection of electrodes and their placement.

## Terminology

| | | |
|---|---|---|
| Action potential | Electrode | Phase duration |
| Alternating current (AC) | EMS | Polyphasic |
| Biphasic | ESTR | Propagation |
| Capacitance | FES | Pulsatile current |
| Conductance | Frequency | Pulse duration |
| Decay time | Impedance | Reactance |
| Depolarization | Modulation | Resistance |
| Direct current (DC) | Monophasic | Rise time |
| Duty cycle | NMES | Wave form |

## Background

The use of electric current to stimulate muscle contraction has a long and color-ful history dating as far back as 48 AD when a Roman physician named Scribonius Largus used torpedo fish in the treatment of chronic headache and gout. During the late 1700s, Luigi Galvani revealed through experimentation that a frog's legs jumped when stimulated by static electric charges from lightening conducted through copper downspouts and railings. Over the years, numerous claims of medical cures attributed to electricity have surfaced. Some were propagated by the "snake oil salesmen" of the time. Others have had a more thorough grounding in science and research leading to contemporary applications of electricity in medicine and rehabilitation. For example,

Kratzenstein reported the use of electrification to treat a paralyzed limb while Seiler reported treating scoliosis patients, and Deluc pioneered the concept of ion transfer through bodily tissues by experimenting on rabbits (Geddes, 1984; Hunter, Mackin, & Callahan, 1995; Licht, 1983).

Growth in the use of electrical stimulation has accelerated since 1965, in part due to research conducted by Melzack and Wall (1965) and application of their proposed Gate Control Theory of blocking pain, still advocated by experts today. Advances in technology have also contributed to an increased use of therapeutic electrical current in part due to manufacturers who continue to develop smaller, more portable units with greater options for the clinician and easier use for patients.

To better understand the application of electrotherapy, occupational therapists must possess a basic knowledge of commonly used terminology and principles of electricity. There are numerous methods of applying electrical stimuli on patients to accomplish a variety of therapeutic goals, and proper use of electrical terminology is essential. Common types of clinical electrical stimulation include: neuromuscular electrical stimulation (NMES) for muscle reeducation and strengthening, functional electrical stimulation (FES), electrical stimulation for tissue and wound repair (ESTR), transcutaneous electrical nerve stimulation (TENS) for pain control, and use of direct current (DC) to stimulate denervated muscle. Terms commonly used by clinicians include: NMES, TENS, FES, and High-voltage Pulsed Current (HVPC) (American Physical Therapy Association, 1990).

*NMES* is the use of pulsed alternating electrical current (AC) to stimulate a motor response by depolarizing intact peripheral nerves. FES and functional neuromuscular stimulation (FNS) are alternative methods of applying NMES, and serve the purpose of acting as a substitute modality for an orthotic to assist in functional activities such as grasping an object. NMES is clinically used to reduce muscle spasm, increase muscle strength, facilitate muscle reeducation, and to reduce edema by creating a "muscle pumping" action through intermittent delivery of current.

*TENS* is an acronym commonly recognized as being a synonymous term for the use of electrical stimulation to reduce pain, even though technically it encompasses all forms of electrical stimulation. The application of TENS requires use of electrodes applied to the surface of the skin to deliver electricity across the dermal layers. The goal of treatment is to reduce pain either by sensory analgesia or through the release of chemical endorphins depending on how the parameters of current are modulated.

*High-voltage galvanic stimulation* is electrical stimulation used commonly for tissue repair (ESTR) and pain control, and refers to a type of stimulator using an interrupted monophasic twin-peak wave form with an output greater than 150 volts. Electrical stimulation for tissue repair has been used in the treatment of chronic and acute edema, chronic and acute pain, wound healing, muscle spasm, delaying muscle atrophy, and increasing blood flow.

*Iontophoresis* is the induction of topically applied ions into bodily tissue by application of a low-voltage direct galvanic electrical current. Iontophoresis is typically used for treatment of inflammatory conditions such as tendinitis, bursitis, myositis, and scar tissue modification.

Determining the type and characteristics of therapeutic electrical current for patient treatment is dependent upon the pathology involved, the desired functional outcomes, and the primary goals of therapy. Common uses for electrotherapy in the clinical setting include muscle reeducation, strengthening, restoration or enhancement of functional motor use, pain control, tissue and wound repair, and to also stimulate denervated muscle following neurological injury.

## Basic Electrical Principles

Electrical current is the flow or movement of electrons or charged particles from one point to another with a purpose to reestablish balance between negative and positive charges. Electricity is a type of energy that is capable of producing magnetic, chemical, mechanical, and thermal effects. The flow of charged particles occurs when there is an imbalance in the number of electrons located at two different points. Electrical current always takes a path of least resistance, and characteristically flows from an area of high electron concentration (cathode) to an area with less concentration (anode), or positively charged pole. A variety of electrical waveforms (e.g., pulsatile, waveform shapes, modulated, and nonmodulated) are available for clinical use depending on the manufacturer. Choosing the correct pulsed waveform can be confusing since little research exists to support one type over another. Since patient response and tolerance to electrical stimulation is highly varied the selection of pulsed waveform should primarily be based upon patient comfort. Three primary types of electrical current output are typically used in the clinical setting: *direct current (DC)*, *alternating current (AC)*, and *pulsatile or pulsed current (PC)* (American Physical Therapy Association, 1990).

# Electrical Current Output

## Direct Current

DC is a unidirectional flow of electrons being either positively or negatively charged. DC is also referred to as "galvanic current" to describe the uninterrupted, unidirectional flow of charged particles. The direction of the current flow, from a negative electrode to a positive electrode or vice versa, can be selected depending on the options available on the electrical stimulation unit being used.

The polarity of electrical current selected for treatment remains unchanged unless it is altered either manually or automatically by the electrical device. The most common depiction of DC electrical current flow is a square wave and a straight horizontal line indicating that current is flowing in a continuous manner until the circuit is disconnected or the battery is turned off (Forester & Palastanga, 1981). Clinicians must use caution with DC since it has the potential to cause chemical reactions in body tissues, especially the dermal layers. An acidic reaction can occur at the anode due to oxidation of the anions, and an alkaline reaction can occur at the cathode. Although patients must be monitored for these potentially negative effects, they may actually be a desired treatment goal by the clinician in situations where scar tissue modification is a priority.

DC can also be used to directly stimulate denervated muscle with the goal of preventing or reducing muscle fiber atrophy, however, limited research exists to support this use of electrical current for this purpose (Binder, 1981). Finally, DC is clinically used to facilitate the movement of ionized medication through the skin by a process called iontophoresis, which will be covered more thoroughly in a later chapter.

## Alternating Current

AC is a type of current characterized by a continuous change in direction of electron flow, and is the current typically used to supply electricity for common household appliances. The flow of electrons is bidirectional (e.g., positive and negative) and can be interrupted or not interrupted depending on the device and goals of patient treatment. Due to the constant changing in direction of charged particles there is an absence of net charge in either positive or negative electrons at either pole. As a result AC is characterized as having the absence of a positive or negative pole since there is an equal balance between the two charges.

The terms *biphasic waveform* and *bidirectional current* have both been used to describe AC. Minimal chemical effects occur on body tissues as a result of using AC due to a lack of accumulation of either negative or positive electrons. Hertz (Hz) is a term used to measure the number of times electrical current reverses direction in a period of one second (e.g., cycles per second). A 1 megahertz (MHz) current means electron flow changes direction and polarity 1 million times per second.

## Pulsatile Current

Most electrical stimulators deliver current using one of three pulsatile waveforms: monophasic, biphasic, or polyphasic. The type of waveform being delivered by an electrical unit may be identified by reviewing the technical section of the manufacturer's owner's manual. It is important to remember that selecting the appropriate type of electrical current to use in the clinic is dependent upon desired treatment outcomes. For example, different electrical stimulation parameters are required to treat or modulate pain, reduce muscle spasm, facilitate muscle contractions, decrease edema, or to promote wound healing. A variety of electrical waveforms (e.g., pulsatile or waveform shapes) are available for clinical use depending on the manufacturer. The selection of pulsed waveform can be confusing to the clinician since little research exists to validate use of one form over another. Therefore, most clinicians choose one waveform or another based predominately on patient response to the sensation of the stimulation and their perceived comfort (Figure 8-1).

The term pulsatile or pulsed current is used to describe modulations made to electrical current whereby electron flow is periodically interrupted (see Figure 8-1). Pulsed current can flow in a unidirectional (monophasic) or bidirectional (biphasic) pattern. The current is interrupted for only brief periods of time (e.g., milliseconds [ms] or microseconds [μm]). With pulsed current, the flow of electrons is turned on and off in rapid fashion and can be visualized best if one imagines the flashing sensation of a strobe light. The current, in effect, is pulsed over time and the reaction on the tissue is dependent on whether the parameters are set for a unidirectional or bidirectional effect (Kloth & Cummings, 1990).

# Electrical Waveforms

The geometric or visual representation of an electrical current flow or stimulus is known as the waveform (Alon & De Domenico, 1987). The geometric shape of the wave characterizes the amplitude and the pulse duration of each stimulus. The basic properties of the electrical current flow are the amplitude (e.g., intensity) and the duration (or pulse length) of the current. The isoelectric point is the level which sets the baseline where the electrical potential between the two poles is considered equal, or zero, with no current flow. The amplitude is the level or distance that the impulse rises above or below (positive or negative respectively) the baseline. The pulse duration is the horizontal distance or length required to complete the shape of the electrical flow.

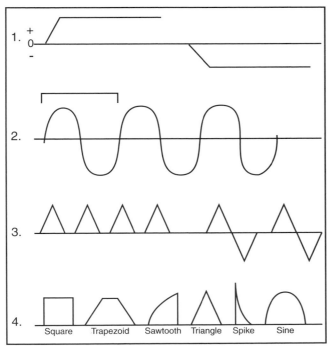

**Figure 8-1.** Types of current: 1) Direct current, 2) alternating current, 3) pulsatile current, and 4) classifiers of interrupted direct current, on phase of AC, or one phase of a pulse (Illustration by Kim Bartlett, used with permission).

Pulse width is a term used synonymously with pulse duration but standardization of electrical terminology now precludes its use. The total area within the waveform represents the volume of current being delivered to the tissue (Lake, 1992).

Most electrical stimulators deliver current using one of three pulsatile waveforms: *monophasic*, *biphasic*, or *polyphasic*. The type of waveform being delivered by an electrical unit may be identified by reviewing the technical section of the manufacturer's owner's manual. Selecting the appropriate electrical current to use in the clinic is dependent on the desired effects for patient treatment. For example, a therapist may use a biphasic waveform in treating a shoulder subluxation in a patient who has suffered a CVA. A patient who is being treated for epicondylitis and inflammation may require the use of a monophasic waveform in the delivery of medication to the area using iontophoresis (Figure 8-2).

## Monophasic

A monophasic waveform has one phase to a single pulse with a unidirectional flow of electrons. Current flows in only one direction, and is either negative or positive in polarity depending on the setting of the unit. Clinical uses for monophasic current typically include direct stimulation of denervated muscle and to deliver medication transdermally through iontophoresis.

## Biphasic

Biphasic current consists of two opposing electrical phases (positive and negative) constructing a single pulse. The pulse is bidirectional with the lead phase of the pulse above the baseline and the second phase below the baseline. A *symmetrical* biphasic pulse occurs when the two phases deviate from the baseline in an identical and equal

**Figure 8-2.** Pulsatile waveform classifications: monophasic, biphasic, and polyphasic. Biphasic waveforms can be symmetrical or asymmetrical, and balanced or unbalanced (Illustration by Kim Bartlett, used with permission).

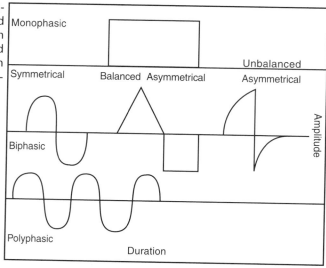

amount (e.g., one phase in a positive direction and one phase in the negative direction have equal area under the graph). The two phases of the pulse are equal in magnitude and duration and therefore produce a zero net charge (ZNC).

An electrical pulse is characterized as being *asymmetrical* biphasic when the positive and negative phases are not identical. In this case, a net electrical charge is created by the asymmetric waveform, and physiological effects on tissue are made possible due to a build up of positive and negative ions. This type of pulse is described as being an unbalanced asymmetrical biphasic waveform. Many commercial neuromuscular stimulation and TENS units are capable of producing both balanced and unbalanced asymmetrical biphasic waveforms, however, the symmetrical biphasic waveforms are generally found to be more comfortable for patient use. Assymetrical biphasic waveforms are used more often for stimulation of the small muscles of the forearm with the negative electrode being placed over the motor nerve as it is more active than the positive electrode. This application provides a better isolation of specific, small muscles. A symmetrical biphasic waveform is more efficient for stimulation of large muscles such as the quadriceps, hamstring, or muscles of the back or when combined muscle function is required (e.g., wrist and finger extension). Symmetrical waveforms tend to be more comfortable to the patient and are often easier and more efficient in treating multiple motor points or for large muscle contraction (see Figure 8-2).

## Polyphasic

Polyphasic waveforms consist of a burst of three or more electrical phases. A burst is characterized as being a series of pulses delivered as a single charge. Some experts claim that this type of current is clinically unique, but there are no documented physiologic advantages to using this type of current that is often perceived by humans as being a single pulse (Ward & Shkuratova, 2002).

Polyphasic pulses of current are used in electrical generators that also produce "medium frequency" currents such as *interferential stimulation* and *russian stimulation*. These electrical currents employ a train of pulses, separated by an interpulse interval, to deliver current to tissue in what is termed *burst frequency*. Each burst of polyphasic current technically consists of multiple pulses, but are considered to be a single burst unit for the purpose of describing the rate (frequency) of current. For example, an electrical device delivering current at 30 polyphasic burst-pulses per second would be equivalent to saying a current is delivering 30 single pulses per second for the purpose of describing the rate of electrical current. The difference between the two currents is that the pulses being delivered in burst format is actually comprised of multiple pulses (polyphasic) separated by an interburst interval; whereas the nonmedium frequency current would be delivering single pulses (e.g., not polyphasic) for its rate (Bennie, Petrofsky, Nisperos, Tsurudome, & Laymon, 2002).

# Medium Frequency Current

## Interferential

*Interferential* current utilizes alternating, low-frequency current that has been modified and uses two medium frequency currents: one which is preset by the equipment (the carrier frequency) and the other which is adjusted by the clinician. The primary clinical applications for the use of interferential frequency is for pain relief, decreasing edema, increasing blood flow and muscle stimulation. These two medium frequency currents are transmitted through the tissues almost simultaneously allowing the electrical current paths to cross and "interfere" with each other. This interference between the two currents creates a "beat" frequency which can vary between 1 to 150 Hz. The beat frequency is adjusted from the machine and is adjusted based on the clinical need. For example, a motor response or muscle contraction to tetany is between 20 to 50 pps, while 50 to 150 pps are used for pain management and 1 to 5 pps is often used for acupuncturelike pain relief. The electrical current is gradually increased until there is a sensory or motor response depending on the therapeutic parameters set. Treatment time is usually between 10 and 20 minutes long (Fourie & Bowerbank, 1997; Hou, Tsai, Cheng, Chung, & Hong, 2002; Hurley, Minder, McDonough, Walsh, Moore, & Baxter, 2001; Hurley, Minder, McDonough, Walsh, Moore, & Baxter, 2001; Minder et al., 2002). Interferential current uses four electrodes in a quadripolar configuration which allows for a centralization of the electrical current over the treatment or painful area.

## Russian Stimulation

*Russian* stimulation was initially developed for use by the Russian Olympic team as a method of improving athletic performance by increasing the muscle mass and force gains. Russian current used a stimulator which delivers a medium-frequency 2000 to 10,000 Hz, polyphasic alternating current waveform. The original therapeutic format using Russian current followed a pattern of 10 seconds of stimulation followed by 50 seconds rest, repeated for 10 minutes (Figure 8-3).

# Electrical Parameters

A variety of electrical stimulation units are available on the market today. Selecting the appropriate piece of equipment to use for patient treatment is based in part on the clinical goals, the equipment available, and the perceived comfort of the waveform. Though patient compliance and comfort will vary, the symmetrical biphasic waveform

**Figure 8-3.** Common waveforms used on electrotherapy equipment.

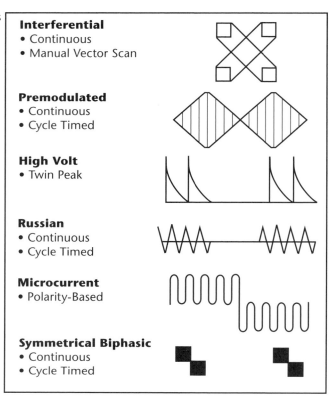

**Interferential**
• Continuous
• Manual Vector Scan

**Premodulated**
• Continuous
• Cycle Timed

**High Volt**
• Twin Peak

**Russian**
• Continuous
• Cycle Timed

**Microcurrent**
• Polarity-Based

**Symmetrical Biphasic**
• Continuous
• Cycle Timed

**Figure 8-4.** A) Peak amplitude and B) peak to peak amplitude (Illustration by Kim Bartlett, used with permission).

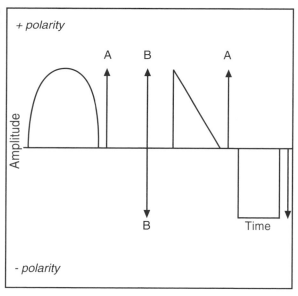

appears to provide the highest tolerance and comfort level (Baker, 1979; Karselis, 1973). Three parameters associated with the electrical waveform must be taken into consideration when selecting an appropriate electrotherapeutic unit for clinical use: amplitude, duration, and rate (Figure 8-4).

## Amplitude

The maximum amount of current or voltage delivered during a single phase of a pulse is known as the peak amplitude. Increasing the amplitude will also increase the total average current output of the unit. *Average current* is defined as the total current per unit of time and is determined by averaging the current amplitude over the duration or length of the waveform. Milliamps or microamps are the measurements used to describe the peak amplitude in current though some manufacturers use voltage (volts) as the preferred measure. The amplitude of electrical current is more commonly known as *pulse intensity*. The peak amplitude measures the magnitude of the stimulus during a monophasic pulse, and is characterized as being the amount of current flow from the point of zero output to a point of maximum output, either in the positive or negative direction. Peak to peak amplitude is measured from the point of maximal positive charge to an adjacent point of maximal positive charge when describing a biphasic (AC) waveform.

## Duration

*Pulse duration* is defined as being the amount of time that elapses between the onset of one phase in an electrical pulse to the end-point of the second phase in the same pulse, including the intrapulse interval. In a case where monophasic current is being delivered, the phase and pulse duration are synonymous and considered to be indefinite. In the case of biphasic current, the pulse duration is equal to the time it takes for both phases (e.g., negative and positive) to elapse, including the intrapulse interval if present.

The *phase duration* is a significant factor in determining the type of tissue to be stimulated, the depth of current penetration, and the perceived level of comfort induced by the electrical unit. As the phase duration increases, the depth of electrical current will also increase. There is also a direct effect to the degree of chemical changes occurring in the tissue. As phase duration is increased, the chemical effects on body tissues will also increase. A shorter pulse and short phase duration result in better conductivity of the current into the tissue with less impedance (Gracanin & Trnkoczy, 1975) (Figure 8-5).

## Rate/Frequency

*Rate* is defined as the number of pulse cycles being delivered to body tissues, and is generally expressed as pulses per second (pps) (Alon & De Domenico, 1987). The faster the rate of electrical current equates to a greater number of pulses per second being delivered to the tissue. Modulating the rate to be either fast or slow is dependent upon patient treatment goals and the desired physiological effects of electrical current. For example, a slow rate setting (e.g. 1 to 5 pps) may be used to create a muscle pumping effect with NMES or to simulate the release of endorphins with acupuncture-type TENS. Setting the rate at a fast pace will help facilitate the recruitment of more muscle fibers with NMES, and will be more comfortable to the patient when using TENS to control pain.

The frequency of electrical current output is also known as the *carrier* frequency. The carrier frequency is the base frequency of the AC sine wave and is described in hertz (Hz) or cycles per seconds (cps). The carrier frequency consists of three primary classifications: low-frequency currents (<1000 Hz), medium-frequency currents (1000-10000 Hz), and high-frequency currents (>10000 Hz). In general, most therapeutic electrical stimulation units deliver low-frequency currents.

**Figure 8-5.** Strength duration curve demonstrates the relationship between amplitude and duration. As phase duration increases, less amplitude is requred to achieve threshold (Illustration by Kim Bartlett, used with permission).

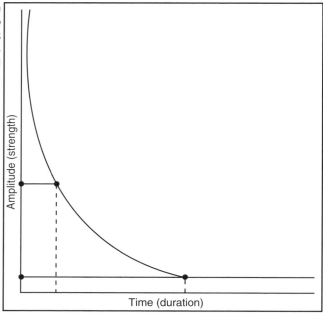

Some manufacturers have developed equipment that uses an AC carrier frequency which administers a medium-frequency current as an electrical burst. The burst rate is a series of cycles that results in depolarization of the sensory and motor nerves (DeVahl, 1992). On most electrical stimulators, the parameter of frequency is adjustable and often labeled on the unit as the pulse "rate." An inverse relationship exists between the pulse frequency of a current and the capacitive resistance of the tissue meaning that low-frequency currents encounter greater tissue resistance than medium- and high-frequency currents. As a result, the intensity (amplitude) of the electrical unit may need to be increased to accommodate greater resistance with low-frequency currents. Frequency settings in a range from 1 pps to 120 pps are effective for most therapeutic purposes (Charman, 1990; DeVahl, 1992).

## Characteristics of Electricity and Physiological Implications

The ability to store a charge in an electric field and oppose change in the flow of current is termed *capacitance*. Nerve and muscle membranes serve as *capacitors*, while the nerve-muscle complex functions as the conductors. Conversely, skin and adipose tissue function as *insulators*, and subsequently resist current flow. *Conductance* is the ease by which electrons flow and is largely dependent on the water content of bodily tissue. Tissues with low water content are less conductive to the flow of electrons. Nerve and muscle components possess higher water content and serve to facilitate electron flow even though the membrane surfaces of these tissues provide a high degree of reactance.

Skin is also a factor to the flow of electrons since the amount of moisture within the skin will affect the flow of current, particularly if the skin is dry. Skin provides the greatest resistive element to the flow of electrical current since it contains very little fluid. Increasing the moisture of the skin through heat, which also increases the surface salt content, facilitates conductivity of the current (Forster & Palastange, 1981; Wadsworth & Chanmugam, 1983).

## Impedance

*Impedance* is the opposition to the flow of electrons in tissue and is characterized as being the "resistance" to the current. Impedance consists of the properties of resistance and reactance. Reactance is also termed capacitive resistance and is the result of counter-voltage, which occurs due to electrolytic polarization when current is conducted through the tissues. Ions accumulate at the tissue interface and cell membrane, creating a charge that is opposite of the voltage being applied at the electrode. This counter-voltage is called reactance or capacitive resistance.

## Resistance

*Resistance* is the property of a substance that opposes or resists the flow of current. Units of resistance are measured in ohms, and the amount of resistance of a given material is determined by Ohm's law. The greater the resistance or "impedance" in an electrical circuit, the lower the rate of electrical flow. The flow of electrical current is directly proportional to amount of applied voltage. If there is an increase in voltage combined with constant resistance, the flow of current increases. Current flow is also inversely related to resistance. If there is an increase in resistance combined with constant voltage, the flow of current will decrease. Ohm's law accounts for the relationship between amperage, voltage, and resistance, and can be shown by the following equations:

$$I = V/R \text{ or } V = I*R$$

I is the current intensity in amperes; V is the potential difference in volts; and R is the resistance in Ohms. The voltage (V) must be sufficient to overcome the resistance for the current (I) to exist. Clinically, this concept is important since high skin impedance necessitates a high voltage to allow the current to penetrate into deeper tissues (Forster & Palastange, 1981; Wadsworth & Chanmugam, 1983). The ability of a material to conduct a current rather than resist the current is known as conductance and is considered the inverse of resistance.

## Depth of Penetration

Commercial electrical stimulation units are typically classified as being either high- or low-voltage devices. A unit using high-voltage output has the potential to also produce high peak amplitude. Low-voltage units are those in the range of one to 100 volts. High-voltage units typically have an output of 500 volts. A relationship exists between peak amplitude and the depth of the electrical current penetration. If the biological tissue to be stimulated is similar, the higher the voltage applied will equate to a greater amount of current penetrating the tissue. Low-voltage stimulation, on the other hand, delivers less current through the tissue. The conductivity of the tissue being stimulated will determine the depth of penetration (Mehreteab, 1994). Tissue such as bone, fat, or adipose are poor conductors of electricity (e.g., high impedance) and, subsequently, have a decreased depth of electron penetration.

**Figure 8-6.** A) Peak amplitude, B) rise time, C) decay time, and D) intrapulse interval (Illustration by Kim Bartlett, used with permission).

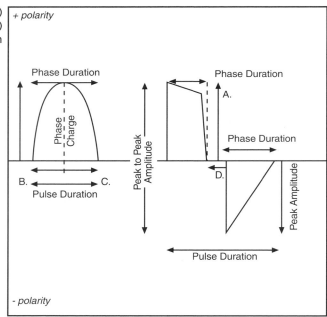

## Rise Time and Decay Time

Rise and decay values are associated with the amount of time needed for the amplitude (e.g., intensity) to increase from zero to a peak voltage level and then back to zero. A short rate of rise time will cause a more rapid nerve depolarization as compared to longer rates of rise. If the rate of rise is too slow, the nerve membrane has a greater chance to accommodate or adjust to the electrical stimulation, and may limit the effectiveness of the stimulating current. The rate of rise time for electrical stimulation is measured in nanoseconds (Ns) (one-billionth) of a second, up to several hundred ms (thousandth of a second) or longer. The amount of time it takes for the amplitude of current to decrease from its peak level back to 0 volts is known as the decay time, and is expressed also in Ns or ms (Figure 8-6).

## Duty Cycle

The duty cycle refers to a ratio of the amount of time electrical stimulation is turned on, and the amount of time that current is not being delivered. Other terms commonly used to describe this concept include the on/off cycle, or reciprocate. The on-time consists of the length of time that current is actually being delivered to body tissues. The off-time is the period of time when the current has been interrupted, or stopped.

The duty cycle is often expressed as a percentage, or ratio. For example, a current which is on for 5 seconds and off for 20 seconds would have a ratio of 1:4. To express the duty cycle as a percentage, one divides the time the current is on by the total cycle time (e.g. the time the current is on plus the off-time). Using the previous example, an on-time of 5 seconds and off time of 20 seconds would equate to the following:

On-Time (5 seconds) x 100
On-Time (5 seconds) + Off-Time (20 seconds) = 5 seconds (On-Time) x 100
25 seconds (Total Cycle Time) = 0.2 x 100 = 20% duty cycle

The duty cycle is a critical factor when calculating the total stimulation time and is important in determining the amount of potential muscle fatigue. Fatigue is related to the duty cycle and the ratio selected for electrical stimulation. A duty cycle with a short off-time (e.g. 10 seconds) will cause muscle to fatigue at a faster rate as compared to a duty cycle with a longer off-time (e.g., 40 seconds) (Leo, 1984) (see Figure 8-6). Conversely, an on-time of 15 seconds will cause a faster rate of muscle fatigue as compared to an on-time of 5-seconds. Deciding the length and ratio of the total stimulation time are critical decisions as they will affect the extent of potential muscle fatigue. When the off-time is longer than the on-time, less muscle fatigue will occur; however, as the patient's condition improves, the duty cycle can be gradually increased. Determining the proper amount of on- and off-times for electrical current requires a clinical reasoning based on patient treatment goals, and desired physiological effects.

## Current Modulation

Modulating electrical current occurs when there is a random alteration in any parameter of electrical output including amplitude, pulse duration, or rate/frequency. Depending on the unit, electrical parameters can be modified individually or in combination. Modulating the parameters of electrical current may be accomplished manually by the clinician or automatically by the electrical device depending on the manufacturer. The most common therapeutic purpose for intentionally modulating electrical current is to increase comfort and to prevent physiological accommodation to prolonged stimulation. One form of modulation is the ramping of the current to change the pulse intensity or duration (Karnes, Mendel, & Fish, 1992).

## Ramp Time

Ramp time refers to the amount of change in pulse intensity or duration from zero current to a point of peak intensity. Adjusting current intensity from a starting point of zero to a point of maximum tolerance or electrical output is termed ramping up. When current is decreased from a predetermined maximum toleration or electrical output, it is termed ramping down (Figure 8-7). The intensity of electrical current may be adjusted to gradually increase over a predetermined period of time, most often between 1 and 8 seconds. Ramp down refers to the gradual decrease of intensity at the end of the on-time, or the length of time it takes electrical current to move from its peak amplitude back to zero.

The ramp time describes the change in amplitude of the current over a specific time period of the current flow and is different from the rise time which describes the amplitude of a single pulse (Bassett, 1989; Karnes, Mendel, & Fish, 1992; Xuan, Hu, & Li, 2006). Therapeutic electrical stimulation devices generally allow therapists to adjust the ramp time, but in some cases this parameter is preset within the unit and cannot be modulated.

Clinically, the purpose of modifying the ramp time for electrical stimulation is to offer a degree of patient comfort during initial stimulation and to reproduce a normal muscle contraction when using current for neuromuscular education or strengthening. In general, a 2-second ramp time is usually sufficient for this purpose. If a muscle contracts too rapidly or the stimulation is too painful to the patient, a longer ramp time should be used. In addition, when calculating the total time for electrical stimulation during the on-time, the ramp up time must be included in the calculation.

**Figure 8-7.** Current increased by increasing: 1) peak amplitude, 2) pulse frequency, and 3) phase duration (Illustration by Kim Bartlett, used with permission).

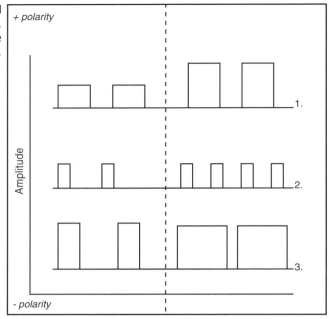

# Physiological Basis of Nerve and Muscle Excitation

When electrical current is delivered in sufficient quantity to body tissues, alterations in the physiological process of the tissue will occur at a localized or cellular level. Electrical current can modify the physiologic response and chemical effects of the tissue. Tissues possess unique properties and are considered either excitable or non-excitable. Nerve and muscles are considered *excitable tissues* and their ability to initiate and propagate an action potential is the basis for electrotherapeutic interventions. The sudden alteration of the membrane's potential is known as an *action potential*. Excitable tissues such as nerves or muscles have the ability to initiate and propagate an action potential if the stimulation parameters are of sufficient intensity. In essence, an action potential will occur if any electrical, mechanical, chemical, thermal, or hormonal stimulus of sufficient magnitude changes the cell's permeability and causes depolarization. A general review and understanding of the fundamental neurophysiology of nerve and muscle excitation are necessary to properly apply the principles of electrical stimulation in the clinical setting.

Nerve and muscle cells are considered to be excitable tissues and have the ability to maintain an electrical potential across the cell membrane as well as to respond with an alteration in the electrical potential. The resting membrane potential for a nerve and muscle cells is between -60 and -90 millivolts (mV). The cell interior is negative in relation to the external tissues and consists of larger amounts of potassium ions with lower levels of sodium ions. At rest, there is an unequal ionic distribution across the membrane due to the increased permeability of the membrane and an active sodium pump. Action potentials occur when a stimulus excites the nerve cell causing membrane depolarization and may be caused by thermal, mechanical, chemical, or electrical stimuli.

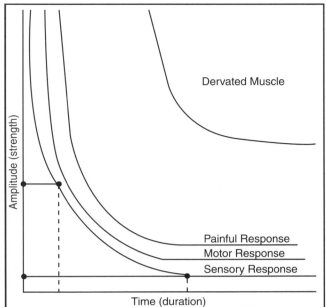

**Figure 8-8.** Strength-Duration curve. Relationship between Strength-Duration curves for nerve fibers and denervated skeletal muscles. Less amplitude is needed to reach threshold as time/duration increases (Illustration by Kim Bartlett, used with permission).

When an action potential occurs, the result is an increase in cell permeability to sodium ions. The sudden influx of positively charged sodium ions into the cell causes further depolarization of the membrane and facilitates an increased opening of the sodium/potassium channels. As sodium ions flow into the cell, potassium ions are permitted to exit resulting in an imbalanced concentration gradient. When an equilibrium potential for sodium is reached the sodium ion flow decreases and the membrane channels close. The original diffusion gradient with selective potassium permeability returns and results in a potassium dominated potential once again (e.g., negatively charged on the inside of the cell and positively charged on the outside of the cell).

Cellular depolarization and stimulation of an action potential occurs in approximately 1 to 2 ms. Action potentials are an all-or-none occurrence; when the threshold of stimulation is reached, the action potential occurs and the cell depolarizes. For the action potential to occur, the stimulus must be of sufficient intensity and duration to cause the ions to move across the membrane. Excitable tissues will respond to an electrical stimulus in the same fashion regardless of the intensity of stimulus. For example, once an action potential is reached, the potential cannot be graded by changing the intensity or duration of the electrical stimulus. Following excitation of the tissue, there is a brief period during which the tissue is not excitable to a second stimulus and therefore cannot be depolarized. This phase is known as the absolute refractory period, and during this brief period, a second action potential cannot occur. The action potential threshold of tissues varies between muscle and nerve fibers with variations occurring among nerve fibers (Figure 8-8).

## Propagation of Electrical Current

When electrical current is applied the to body, it will cause physiological and physiochemical changes due to the body's ability to conduct electrical current through

## Table 8-1

### TISSUE IMPEDANCE

| Type of Tissue | Approximate Water Content | Electrical Impedance | Electrical Conduction |
|---|---|---|---|
| Bone | 5% | Highest | Poorest |
| Epidermis | 10% | Higher | Poorer |
| Fat | 15% | High | Poor |
| Muscle | 75% | Low | Good |
| Nerve | 80% | Lower | Better |
| Blood | 90% | Lowest | Best |

the water in the tissues. Tissues composed of higher levels of water content are good transmitters of electricity. In contrast, tissues composed of low water content transmit electrical current poorly. For example, bone, tendon, fascia, and adipose tissue are composed of approximately 5% to 15% water content and are, therefore, poor conductors of electricity. In contrast, muscle, nerve, and blood are composed of 70% to 90% water making them good conductors of electricity. As noted previously, the outer layer of skin is also a poor conductor of electricity due to its low water content (Table 8-1).

When an action potential is reached, the excitable membrane may also cause an action potential to occur in adjoining tissues. In a nerve or muscle fiber, the action potential can be propagated across the entire membrane following the path of least resistance. Continuous electrical stimulation can generate continuous action potentials in the tissue.

The rate at which an action potential is propagated is dependent on the diameter of the nerve fiber and the degree of myelination. Conduction occurs at a faster rate in myelinated fibers than in unmyelinated fibers. Larger diameter fibers also have lower resistance to the conduction current which is generated by the action potential. The number of nerve fibers recruited increases as the amplitude and the pulse duration increase. Following an action potential, there is a period of recovery which limits the frequency of the number of action potentials.

The effect of the electrical current on muscle is dependent on a number of factors including the number of fibers in the motor unit and the amount of stimulation provided by the device. The size of motor units varies and is dependent upon its specific function. For example, motor units in the hand are composed of only a small number of muscle fibers per unit which allows for fine muscle control. Larger numbers of fibers, 200 or more (up to thousands), are found in large motor units and produce gross motor movement, such as in the muscles making up the quadriceps. When a cell membrane or tissue receives an unchanging stimulus over a period of time, the cell membrane will begin to adapt to the stimulus and require higher levels of stimulation to trigger an action potential. This is called *accommodation*. Also, following stimulation and an onset of an action potential in a nerve cell membrane, there will be a short recovery period so the membrane can recoup from its excitability. This recovery time is known as the absolute refractory period.

The effect of electrical current on muscle tissue is determined by the output of stimulation provided and temperature of the tissue. The amplitude and pulse duration determine the threshold for stimulation of the muscle and the quality of the sensation. The frequency determines the degree of tetany and the rate of fatigue. The duty cycle also influences the amount of fatigue, while the rise time affects the rate of accommodation to the electrical stimulus, as well as influencing the action of the muscle-spindle stretch reflex. In addition, electrical conduction may also increase when the temperature of body tissues is increased.

## Voluntary Verses Electrical Stimulation of Muscle

Normal voluntary stimulation of an efferent motor fiber causes depolarization of the motor unit at the neuromuscular junction. The process of depolarization serves as the impetus for an action potential resulting in a muscle contraction. During normal voluntary contractions, the nerve fibers that innervate muscle tissue fire asynchronously with small motor units being recruited first and large motor units recruited only when the muscle is required to produce an increased force output. This sequence of motor unit recruitment results in a smooth controlled muscle contraction during normal voluntary movements.

In muscle fibers stimulated by use of an electrical device, fiber size recruitment occurs in reverse sequence as compared to normal voluntary contractions (e.g., large motor fibers are recruited first in a synchronous pattern, followed by smaller muscle fibers). Motor fiber recruitment using electrical stimulation is a result of the anatomic position of large motor fibers being more superficially located to the skin surface as compared to small motor fibers. Large motor fibers are more easily stimulated by electrical stimulation using surface electrodes. When the skin surface is stimulated, the sensory receptors will be activated before the signal is propagated to the motor or pain nerves. A primary factor that determines response to electrical stimulation and nerve recruitment is the location of the nerve fibers and their relationship to the electrode placement. In essence, the closer the nerve fiber is to the electrode, the more likely it will be stimulated. Since small-diameter fibers frequently lie closer to the surface of the skin, it is common for superficial touch or pressure receptors to be stimulated first in which the electrical current will cause "pins and needles" or a tingling sensation in the area where the electrode is placed. Furthermore, when the intensity of the stimulus is increased, the stimulation will initially spread to the deeper lying tissues to recruit motor fibers and then spread to the fibers which will subsequently convey a pain signal. If the stimulus frequency is sufficient enough, a muscle twitch contraction will also become fused in synchronous rapid succession and the contraction will become tetanic. By stimulating the motor nerve in clinical applications, a muscular contraction can be produced. In innervated muscle tissue with electrical current sufficient for muscle membrane depolarization, a muscle contraction will occur. This stimulation is considered an all-or-none response (Benton, Baker, & Towman, 1980; Nelson, Hayes, & Currier, 1987). Yet, when the electrodes are placed in an area with no skeletal muscle fibers or motor nerve fibers, a painful response will not occur until the electrical stimulation intensity is increased.

Muscle fatigue is another factor that must be respected by the clinician when using electrical stimulation devices for motor fiber recruitment. The recruitment bias of large muscle fibers with electrical stimulation tends to cause fatigue of large muscle fibers more rapidly than normally occurs during voluntary contractions. Modulating the parameters of pulse amplitude, rate, and duration will all affect the speed at which muscle fibers fatigue. In addition, electrical stimulation of large muscle fibers produces

**Figure 8-9.** Common electrodes which act as an interface between the body and the electrical stimulator. There is an inverse relationship to electrode size and current density (Courtesy of Chattanooga Group Inc).

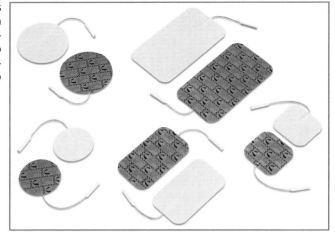

contractions that lack the finely controlled quality of normal voluntary movement that occurs when small muscle fibers are recruited first. As a result, experts are mixed on the question of how functional the use of electrical stimulation is on facilitating muscle contractions for rehabilitation (Baker, Bowman, & McNeal, 1988; Byl et al., 1994; Gregory, Williams, Vandenborne, & Dudley, 2005; Kantor, Alon, & Ho, 1994; Quevedo, Patla, & Cliquet, 1997).

# Electrodes and Skin Care

Clinical electrodes act as an interface between the skin surface and the electrical stimulator. In addition, they serve to facilitate the penetration of electrical current through the skin. A wide range and variety of clinical electrodes are commercially available to the clinician. Electrodes are designed in varying shapes, sizes, and flexibility depending on the manufacturer and based on clinical use. The electrode is composed of an electrically conductive material surrounded by a nonconductive material. The size, type, and placement of the electrodes help determine the effectiveness and ease of treatment (Figure 8-9).

Electrodes are made out of a variety of materials including metal, carbon-impregnated silicone rubber, or metallic meshed cloth. An interface, or medium, between the electrode and the skin is often needed to decrease skin-electrode resistance. Moistened sponges are frequently used with metal electrodes to decrease the skin-electrode impedance. Carbon-rubber electrodes often use a conducting gel, but sponges and gauze saturated with water often suffice. Conducting gel should be applied liberally to the entire conducting surface area of the carbon-rubber or metal electrodes to decrease the skin-electrode resistance and to improve patient comfort (De Domenico, 1988; Karnes, Mendel, & Fish, 1992).

Electrodes may be self-adhesive, but with nonadhesive electrodes adhesive patches or tape are used. Care must be used to ensure enough gel is used to completely cover the electrode surface to facilitate full contact between the electrode and the skin. Carbon-impregnated rubber electrodes degrade over time and with prolonged use and should, therefore, be replaced often to prevent the development of hot spots on the electrode. The hot spot in carbon-rubber electrodes may cause skin irritation and

## Table 8-2

### FACTORS AFFECTING ELECTRODE CONDUCTION

Resistance from skin surface due to dirt, sweat, lotions

Areas of excessive adipose tissue

Dry skin, skin irritation, or breakdown

Perspiration residues

Hair (excessive hair can be cut short, and/or cropped close to the skin, avoid shaving the area)

Poor electrode contact with the skin

Electrode spacing (electrodes placed too closely together)

patient discomfort frequently described as a biting or stinging sensation. If the patient complains of discomfort during electrical stimulation, the safest remedy is to replace the electrodes.

Self-adhering electrodes may be reusable with a foil or metal mesh and a synthetic gel or conductive karaya covered with an adhesive surface. These electrodes do not require strapping or taping for adherence making them convenient to use and helps facilitate patient compliance when home units are prescribed for treatment.

Many electrodes used in patient care are safe if left on the skin for extended periods of time. However, instruction in proper skin care and hygiene is crucial to prevent skin irritation or skin breakdown with prolonged use. Carbon-rubber electrodes allow the greatest amount of current to be delivered with the least amount of skin impedance. As a result, carbon-rubber electrodes may be more comfortable for the patient. Large electrodes tend to have a lower resistance to electrical conductivity as compared to smaller electrodes.

Electrodes are attached to the stimulator through the use of leads or lead wires. Lead wires most often attach to two electrodes by a metal tip that inserts into the electrode. There are a number of different types of electrode-lead wire configurations available such as the pin, pigtail, or snap-to-pin. The tips are prone to corrosion and should be cleaned on a regular basis. Patients who have difficulty with fine motor control or who have poor vision may be more comfortable using the snap-to-pin configuration. In addition, a number of factors exist, including skin resistance, presence of adipose tissue, excessive hair, or poor electrode contact with the skin, which may interfere with electrical conduction and result in increase resistance to the current (Table 8-2).

## Electrode Size

Careful selection of electrode size is crucial to achieve clinical goals for the purpose of either pain relief or to stimulate muscle contractions. An inverse relationship exists between the density of the electrical current and the size of the electrode. In other words, as the size of the electrode decreases, the current density increases. With large electrodes, the total amount of current is distributed over a larger surface area as compared to a small electrode which effectively creates an electrode with less current density.

Increased current density (as with small electrodes) creates a subsequent increase in perception of the electrical current under the electrode and a greater potential for physiologic changes to occur on the skin directly under the electrode. If the current density is too high, it can lead to surface burns and potential tissue damage. Therefore, it is important to monitor the skin surface when using electrical stimulation units for treatment.

Selecting the appropriate electrode size to treat various muscle tissues is also clinically important. Large muscle tissue is better stimulated using large electrodes to disburse the current while smaller muscle tissue will respond effectively by using smaller electrodes. For example, a larger electrode should be used to facilitate a muscle contraction of the biceps brachii, as compared to facilitating a muscle contraction of the intrinsic muscles in the hand.

# Electrode Placement

Placement of electrodes for clinical use is also crucial to achieve patient treatment goals. Correct placement of the electrodes will improve the effectiveness of the electrical current and facilitate patient comfort. Electrodes that are placed too closely together will increase the electrical current density between the two electrodes and may cause patient discomfort. In contrast, electrodes placed further apart will result in greater patient comfort due to less centralized current density.

The distance between two treatment electrodes also affects the depth of penetration of the electrical current. In general, the more distance between two electrodes the deeper the penetration into the tissue. This is clinically important when the goal of treatment is to stimulate tissue located below superficial tissues.

The orientation of the electrodes also needs to be considered when the goal is to stimulate muscle tissue. Muscle fibers are more conductive when electrical current flows in the same direction as does the muscle fibers. Therefore, electrodes placed longitudinally to the target muscle fibers will generally result in a stronger force of contraction. Finally, electrodes may be configured to be *monopolar, bipolar,* or *quadrapolar.*

## Monopolar Placement

Monopolar techniques involve the use of an active electrode and dispersive electrode (McCulloch, Kloth, & Feedar, 1995). The active electrode is placed over the target area where the treatment effect will occur and is generally smaller in size than the dispersive electrode. The dispersive electrode is used to complete the circuit and is larger with placement at a distance from the target electrode. Because of the higher current density, the effect of the treatment is concentrated under the smaller or active electrode. Monopolar techniques are used most often for the stimulation of trigger points or during wound healing (Baker et al., 1988; Myklebust & Robinson, 1989).

## Bipolar Placement

Bipolar techniques require the use of two electrodes from one channel of equal or near-equal size. Bipolar techniques are most often used for stimulating large muscle tissues. The patient will perceive an equal amount of stimulation or response under each electrode if equal sized. If the electrodes are not of equal size, then the net effect will generally be greater under the smaller electrode where the current density is

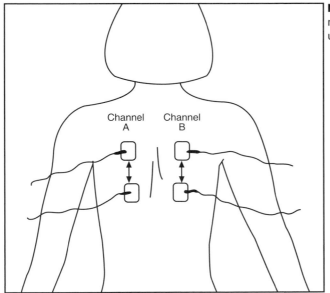

**Figure 8-10.** Bipolar electrode placement (Illustration by Kim Bartlett, used with permission).

greater. If a motor response is the goal, one electrode should be placed over the motor point, with the other electrode being placed at a different location on the muscle belly. If a larger area is targeted or a combination of movement is required, the leads can be bifurcated (Figure 8-10).

## Quadripolar Placement

Quadripolar techniques use two channels and two sets of electrodes. This arrangement requires four electrodes located within the treatment area. With a quadripolar arrangement, the electrical currents will cross each other thus causing an increased area of current density at the point of intersection. This may be beneficial when the goal of treatment is to target an area located at the point where both currents intersect. Quadripolar techniques are often used to stimulate large areas for pain management and for the purpose of stimulating antagonistic muscle groups to facilitate functional goals in rehabilitation (Figure 8-11).

# Stimulation of Muscle and Nerve Fibers

When using electrical current to stimulate healthy muscle tissue, it is not the muscle fiber being stimulated directly, but rather the nerve fibers that innervates the target muscle. Nerve fibers have lower electrical thresholds and are more excitable to action potentials as opposed to muscle fibers. As a result, nerve fibers react to electrical stimulation at lower electrical intensities and shorter pulse durations. Muscle fibers in contrast require longer pulse durations to achieve the same response. This is important when determining if electric stimulation is clinically indicated and when choosing the type of current to use.

Nerve fibers small in diameter (e.g., sensory and pain fibers) require greater electrical intensities with longer pulse durations to achieve a physiological response. Larger diameter nerve fibers on the other hand will respond to lower intensities and shorter

**Figure 8-11.** Quadrapolar electrode placements (Illustration by Kim Bartlett, used with permission).

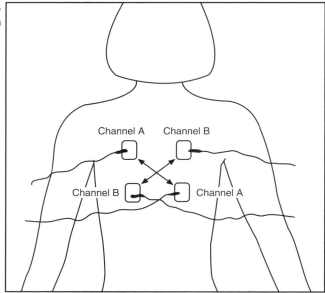

durations to achieve a response. When stimulating denervated muscle tissues, however, long pulse durations are required as it is necessary to stimulate the muscle fiber directly since the nerve fiber is no longer intact. Denervated muscle generally requires the use of galvanic or DC currents to be effective (Baker et al., 1988; Benton et al., 1980).

Research related to treating denervated muscle tissues is often contradictory and confusing. One school of thought adheres to the idea that denervated muscle needs to be stimulated during the early phases following injury to reduce atrophy of muscle fibers and inhibit the proliferation of fibrous connective tissues. To accomplish this, treatment must occur before this process begins. However, if the prognosis of recovery from denervation is good then stimulation may not be necessary as muscle atrophy and connective tissue formation will reverse naturally. If denervation is prolonged and atrophy occurs, stimulation of muscle tissue may be indicated. Denervated skeletal muscles lack contractile activity and subsequently lose mass and force generation. However, stimulated-denervated muscles maintained higher mass and force (Dow, Carlson, Hassett, Dennis, & Faulkner, 2006; Gallasch et al., 2005; Kern et al., 2004). FES training is effective in reverting long-term denervation atrophy and dystrophy. The recovery of muscle mass seems to be the result of both a size increase of the surviving fibers and the regeneration of new myofibers (Kern, Salmons, Mayr, Rossini, & Carraro, 2005; Russo et al., 2007). Other researchers have found that electrical stimulation can protect muscle histology, electrophysiology and enzymic histochemistry of denervated skeletal muscle from the degeneration (Modlin et al., 2005; Xu, Tu, & Gu, 2003).

There has been a great deal of research over the years advocating the use of electrical stimulation to enhance muscle strength and performance. NMES has been found to selectively stimulate large, fast twitch muscle fibers prior to slow twitch fibers. In contrast, traditional physical exercise to promote muscle strengthening selectively recruits smaller, slow twitch, type I fibers prior to stimulating type II fibers. Therefore, some experts claim that NMES is not an adequate substitute for voluntary exercise to strengthen muscle fibers since it does not functionally recruit muscle fibers in the same order as do voluntary contractions.

Table 8-3

| RECRUITMENT | | | | | |
|---|---|---|---|---|---|
| Recruitment Order | Fiber Type and Class | Diameter (μm) | Amplitude | Phase Duration | Pulse/Phase |
| 1st | A-Beta | 6 to 12 | Lowest | Shortest | Lowest |
| 2nd | A-Gamma | 2 to 8 | | | |
| 3rd | A-Delta | 1 to 6 | | | |
| 4th | C IV | <1 | Highest | Lowest | Highest |

Following injury and a period of immobilization, muscle atrophy first occurs in fast twitch, large fibers. To promote an increase in strength of fast twitch muscle fibers following injury, an individual would need to exercise at a high intensity level between 78% and 119% of maximal voluntary isometric muscle contraction (Delitto, Rose, et al., 1988; Delitto, McKowen, McCarthy, Shively, & Rose, 1988; Delitto & Snyder-Mackler, 1990; Lake, 1992). However, exercising at this level of intensity requires a significant increase in cardiac output primarily due to an increase in heart rate. If high intensity exercise is contraindicated for a patient, such as with the elderly and those suffering from cardiovascular disease, then selecting NMES as a substitute may be a better choice for therapeutic muscle strengthening. If an individual is able to safely perform volitional exercise at a high enough intensity to stimulate muscle strengthening then NMES may not be the best choice for therapy. Selecting NMES to augment strength is best indicated during the early phases of rehabilitation when the individual is unable to perform volitional exercise and activities at required levels of intensity (Bax, Staes, & Verhagen, 2005; Caggiano, Emrey, Shirley, & Craik, 1994; Cameron, Broton, Needham-Shropshire, & Klose, 1998; Chae, 2003; Currier & Mann, 1983; Delitto et al., 1988; Delitto & Snyder-Mackler, 1990). NMES over the pectoralis and abdominal muscles might improve cough capacity and pulmonary function in cervical spinal cord injury with tetraplegia (Cheng, Chen, Wang, & Chung, 2006) (Table 8-3).

# Physiologic Effects to Electrical Stimulation

Specific physiologic responses occur at the cellular level, tissue level, or segmentally within muscle fibers that are electrically stimulated. The intensity of stimulation is one factor which will determine if the effect enhances or suppresses a specific response. At the cellular level, electrical stimulation may modify the activity of fibroblasts and osteoblasts. In addition, electricity may facilitate increased microcirculation, and increase the metabolic rate of activity. Electrical current may also have an effect on smooth muscle contraction or relaxation secondary to its effect on circulation and influence tissue regeneration and remodeling.

Muscle contractions also affect lymphatic, arterial, and venous blood flow. Systemically, there may be a decrease in pain due to the stimulation effect on neurotransmitters and an increase in endogenous opiates (Ainsworth et al., 2006; Al-Smadi et al., 2003; Allais et al., 2003; Aydemir, Tezer, Borman, Bodur, & Unal, 2006; Benedetti, 2007).

General indications for the use of electrotherapy for innervated muscle tissue, or NMES, include:

1. Range of motion (ROM)
2. Inhibition of spasticity or muscle spasm
3. Muscle strengthening or disuse atrophy
4. Improving endurance
5. Muscle reeducation or neuromuscular facilitation
6. Orthotic substitution
7. Edema control in both acute and chronic conditions

In denervated muscle tissue, electrical stimulation can be used to maintain muscle integrity, strengthen adjacent muscle groups, or to teach compensatory movements, such as in the case of an incomplete spinal cord injury. Electrical stimulation may also be effective for stimulating tissue repair through improved circulation and/or edema control, promote wound healing, and facilitate the transcutaneous delivery of medications though the process of iontophoresis (Ciombor & Aaron, 2005; Evans, Foltz, & Foltz, 2001; Gardner, Frantz, & Schmidt, 1999).

# Summary

Electrotherapy is a dynamic and growing area of clinical practice and research. Recent advances in technology and the use of electrotherapy for a variety of clinical conditions and applications include stimulation for hemiparesis, tetraplegia, dysphagia, and cerebral palsy; to improve healing; and to decrease pain. These warrant careful consideration and review of this modality for the unique needs of each patient. Therapists are encouraged to continue to review the research in order to maintain current with the technological innovations in this area.

# References

Ainsworth, L., Budelier, K., Clinesmith, M., Fiedler, A., Landstrom, R., Leeper, B. J., et al. (2006). Transcutaneous electrical nerve stimulation (TENS) reduces chronic hyperalgesia induced by muscle inflammation. *Pain, 120*, 182-187.

Allais, G., De Lorenzo, C., Quirico, P. E., Lupi, G., Airola, G., Mana, O., et al. (2003). Non-pharmacological approaches to chronic headaches: Transcutaneous electrical nerve stimulation, laser therapy and acupuncture in transformed migraine treatment. *Neurological Sciences, 24 Suppl 2*, S138-42.

Alon, G., & De Domenico, F. (1987). *High-voltage stimulation: An integrated approach to clinical electrotherapy.* Chattanooga, TN: Chattanooga Group.

Al-Smadi, J., Warke, K., Wilson, I., Cramp, A. F., Noble, G., & Walsh, D. M., et al. (2003). A pilot investigation of the hypoalgesic effects of transcutaneous electrical nerve stimulation upon low back pain in people with multiple sclerosis. *Clinical Rehabilitation, 17*, 742-749.

American Physical Therapy Association. (1990). Electrotherapy standards committee of the section on clinical electrophysiology of the American Physical Therapy Association: Electrotherapeutic terminology in physical therapy. *Section on Clinical Electrophysiology and the American Physical Therapy Association.* Alexandria, VA: APTA.

Aydemir, G., Tezer, M. S., Borman, P., Bodur, H., & Unal, A. (2006). Treatment of tinnitus with transcutaneous electrical nerve stimulation improves patients' quality of life. *Journal of Laryngology and Otology, 120*, 442-445.

Baker, L. (1979). Effect of carrier frequency on comfort with medium frequency electrical stimulation. *Physical Therapy, 69*, 373.

Baker, L. L., Bowman, B. R., & McNeal, D. R. (1988). Effects of waveform on comfort during neuromuscular electrical stimulation. *Clinical Orthopaedics and Related Research, 233*, 75-85.

Bassett, C. A. (1989). Fundamental and practical aspects of therapeutic uses of pulsed electromagnetic fields (PEMFs). *Critical Reviews in Biomedical Engineering, 17*, 451-529.

Bax, L., Staes, F., & Verhagen, A. (2005). Does neuromuscular electrical stimulation strengthen the quadriceps femoris? A systematic review of randomised controlled trials. *Sports Medicine (Auckland, N.Z.), 35*, 191-212.

Benedetti, F. (2007). Placebo and endogenous mechanisms of analgesia. *Handbook of Experimental Pharmacology, 177*, 393-413.

Bennie, S. D., Petrofsky, J. S., Nisperos, J., Tsurudome, M., & Laymon, M. (2002). Toward the optimal waveform for electrical stimulation of human muscle. *European Journal of Applied Physiology, 88*, 13-19.

Benton, L., Baker, L., & Towman, B. (1980). *Functional electrical stimulation: A practical clinical guide.* Downey, CA: Rancho Los Amigos Rehabilitation Engineering Center.

Binder, S. (1981). Applications of low and high-voltage electrotherapeuticcurrents. In S. Wolf (Ed.), *Electrotherapy.* Edinburg, Scotland: Churchill Livingstone.

Byl, N. N., McKenzie, A. L., West, J. M., Whitney, J. D., Hunt, T. K., Hopf, H. W., et al. (1994). Pulsed microamperage stimulation: A controlled study of healing of surgically induced wounds in Yucatan pigs. *Physical Therapy, 74*, 201-13; discussion 213-8.

Caggiano, E., Emrey, T., Shirley, S., & Craik, R. L. (1994). Effects of electrical stimulation or voluntary contraction for strengthening the quadriceps femoris muscles in an aged male population. *Journal of Orthopaedic and Sports Physical Therapy, 20*, 22-28.

Cameron, T., Broton, J. G., Needham-Shropshire, B., & Klose, K. J. (1998). An upper body exercise system incorporating resistive exercise and neuromuscular electrical stimulation (NMS). *Journal of Spinal Cord Medicine, 21*, 1-6.

Chae, J. (2003). Neuromuscular electrical stimulation for motor relearning in hemiparesis. *Physical Medicine and Rehabilitation Clinics of North America, 14*, S93-109.

Charman, R. (1990). Cellular reception and emission of electromagnetic signals. *Physiotherapy, 76*, 509.

Cheng, P. T., Chen, C. L., Wang, C. M., & Chung, C. Y. (2006). Effect of neuromuscular electrical stimulation on cough capacity and pulmonary function in patients with acute cervical cord injury. *Journal of Rehabilitation Medicine, 38*, 32-36.

Ciombor, D. M., & Aaron, R. K. (2005). The role of electrical stimulation in bone repair. *Foot and Ankle Clinics, 10*, 579-93, vii.

Currier, D. P., & Mann, R. (1983). Muscular strength development by electrical stimulation in healthy individuals. *Physical Therapy, 63*, 915-921.

De Domenico, G. (1988). *Interferential stimulation.* Chattanooga, TN: Chattanooga Group.

Delitto, A., McKowen, J. M., McCarthy, J. A., Shively, R. A., & Rose, S. J. (1988). Electrically elicited co-contraction of thigh musculature after anterior cruciate ligament surgery. A description and single-case experiment. *Physical Therapy, 68*, 45-50.

Delitto, A., Rose, S. J., McKowen, J. M., Lehman, R. C., Thomas, J. A., & Shively, R. A. (1988). Electrical stimulation versus voluntary exercise in strengthening thigh musculature after anterior cruciate ligament surgery. *Physical Therapy, 68*, 660-663.

Delitto, A., & Snyder-Mackler, L. (1990). Two theories of muscle strength augmentation using percutaneous electrical stimulation. *Physical Therapy, 70*, 158-164.

DeVahl, J. (1992). *Neuromuscular electrical stimulation (NMES) in rehabilitation.* Philadelphia: FA Davis.

Dow, D. E., Carlson, B. M., Hassett, C. A., Dennis, R. G., & Faulkner, J. A. (2006). Electrical stimulation of denervated muscles of rats maintains mass and force, but not recovery following grafting. *Restorative Neurology and Neuroscience, 24*, 41-54.

Evans, R. D., Foltz, D., & Foltz, K. (2001). Electrical stimulation with bone and wound healing. *Clinics in Podiatric Medicine and Surgery, 18*, 79-95, vi.

Forester, A., & Palastanga or Palastange, N. (1981). *Clayton's electrotherapy: Theory and practice.* London: Tindall Books.

Fourie, J. A., & Bowerbank, P. (1997). Stimulation of bone healing in new fractures of the tibial shaft using interferential currents. *Physiotherapy Research International, 2*, 255-268.

Gallasch, E., Rafolt, D., Kinz, G., Fend, M., Kern, H., & Mayr, W. (2005). Evaluation of FES-induced knee joint moments in paraplegics with denervated muscles. *Artificial Organs, 29*, 207-211.

Gardner, S. E., Frantz, R. A., & Schmidt, F. L. (1999). Effect of electrical stimulation on chronic wound healing: A meta-analysis. *Wound Repair and Regeneration, 7*, 495-503.

Geddes, L. A. (1984). A short history of the electrical stimulation of excitable tissue. including electrotherapeutic applications. *The Physiologist, 27*, S1-47.

Gracanin, F., & Trnkoczy, A. (1975). Optimal stimulus parameters for minimum pain in the chronic stimulation of innervated muscle. *Archives of Physical Medicine and Rehabilitation, 56*, 243-249.

Gregory, C. M., Williams, R. H., Vandenborne, K., & Dudley, G. A. (2005). Metabolic and phenotypic characteristics of human skeletal muscle fibers as predictors of glycogen utilization during electrical stimulation. *European Journal of Applied Physiology, 95*, 276-282.

Hou, C. R., Tsai, L. C., Cheng, K. F., Chung, K. C., & Hong, C. Z. (2002). Immediate effects of various physical therapeutic modalities on cervical myofascial pain and trigger-point sensitivity. *Archives of Physical Medicine and Rehabilitation, 83*, 1406-1414.

Hunter, J., Mackin, E., & Callahan, A. (1995). Rehabilitation of the hand: Surgery and therapy (4th ed., pp. 1508-1519). St. Louis, MO: Mosby.

Hurley, D. A., Minder, P. M., McDonough, S. M., Walsh, D. M., Moore, A. P., & Baxter, D. G. (2001). Interferential therapy electrode placement technique in acute low back pain: A preliminary investigation. *Archives of Physical Medicine and Rehabilitation, 82*, 485-493.

Kantor, G., Alon, G., & Ho, H. S. (1994). The effects of selected stimulus waveforms on pulse and phase characteristics at sensory and motor thresholds. *Physical Therapy, 74*, 951-962.

Karnes, J. L., Mendel, F. C., & Fish, D. R. (1992). Effects of low-voltage pulsed current on edema formation in frog hind limbs following impact injury. *Physical Therapy, 72*, 273-278.

Karselis, T. (1973). *Descriptive medical electronics and instrumentation.* Thorofare, NJ: SLACK Incorporated.

Kern, H., Boncompagni, S., Rossini, K., Mayr, W., Fano, G., & Zanin, M. E., et al. (2004). Long-term denervation in humans causes degeneration of both contractile and excitation-contraction coupling apparatus, which is reversible by functional electrical stimulation (FES): A role for myofiber regeneration? *Journal of Neuropathology and Experimental Neurology, 63*, 919-931.

Kern, H., Salmons, S., Mayr, W., Rossini, K., & Carraro, U. (2005). Recovery of long-term denervated human muscles induced by electrical stimulation. *Muscle & Nerve, 31*, 98-101.

Kloth, L., & Cummings, J. (1990). *Electrotherapeutic Terminology in Physical Therapy.* Alexandria, VA: Section on Clinical Electrophysiology and the American Physical Therapy Association.

Lake, D. A. (1992). Neuromuscular electrical stimulation. An overview and its application in the treatment of sports injuries. *Sports Medicine (Auckland, N.Z.), 13*, 320-336.

Leo, K. (1984). Perceived comfort levels of modulated versus conventional TENS current. *Physical Therapy, 64*, 745.

Licht, S. (1983). History of electrotherapy. In G. Stillwell (Ed.), *Therapeutic electricity and ultraviolet radiation* (3rd ed.). Baltimore, MD: Williams & Wilkins.

McCulloch, J., Kloth, L., & Feedar, J. (1995). Wound healing: Alternatives in management (2nd ed., p. 64). Philadelphia, Pa: F.A. Davis.

Mehreteab, T. (1994). Therapeutic electricity. In B. Hecox (Ed.), *Physical agents: A comprehensive text for physical therapists* (pp. 225-283). Norwalk, CT: Appleton & Lange.

Melzack, R., Wall, P. D. (1965). Pain mechanisms: A new theory. *Science, 150*, 971.

Minder, P. M., Noble, J. G., Alves-Guerreiro, J., Hill, I. D., Lowe, A. S., & Walsh, D. M., et al. (2002). Interferential therapy: Lack of effect upon experimentally induced delayed onset muscle soreness. *Clinical Physiology and Functional Imaging, 22*, 339-347.

Modlin, M., Forstner, C., Hofer, C., Mayr, W., Richter, W., & Carraro, U., et al. (2005). Electrical stimulation of denervated muscles: First results of a clinical study. *Artificial Organs, 29*, 203-206.

Myklebust, B., & Robinson, A. (1989). Instrumentation. *Clinical Electrophysiology, Electrotherapy and Electrophysiologic Testing,* 31-32-40-41.

Nelson, R., Hayes K. W., & Currier, D. (1987). *Clinical electrotherapy.* Tamford CT: Appleton & Lange.

Quevedo, A. A., Patla, A. E., & Cliquet, A., Jr. (1997). A methodology for definition of neuromuscular electrical stimulation sequences: An application toward overcoming small obstacles. *IEEE Transactions on Rehabilitation Engineering, 5*, 30-39.

Russo, T. L., Peviani, S. M., Freria, C. M., Gigo-Benato, D., Geuna, S., & Salvini, T. F. (2007). Electrical stimulation based on chronaxie reduces atrogin-1 and myoD gene expressions in denervated rat muscle. *Muscle & Nerve, 35*, 87-97.

Wadsworth, J., & Chanmugam, A. (1983). *Electrophysical agents in physiotherapy: Therapeutic and diagnostic use*. Marrickville, NSW: Science Press.

Ward, A. R., & Shkuratova, N. (2002). Russian electrical stimulation: The early experiments. *Physical Therapy, 82*, 1019-1030.

Xu, J. G., Tu, Y. Q., & Gu, Y. D. (2003). Effect of electric stimulation on denervated skeletal muscle atrophy. *Chinese Journal of Reparative and Reconstructive Surgery, 17*, 396-399.

Xuan, X., Hu, G., & Li, D. (2006). Joule heating effects on separation efficiency in capillary zone electrophoresis with an initial voltage ramp. *Electrophoresis, 27*, 3171-3180.

# NEUROMUSCULAR ELECTRICAL STIMULATION

## APPLICATIONS AND INDICATIONS

## Learning Objectives

1. Describe the clinical application of electrical stimulation in rehabilitation.
2. Outline and discuss the clinical reasoning process used to determine selection of electrotherapy and appropriate application parameters.
3. Discuss the issues and factors which impact on neuromuscular electrical stimulation (NMES) efficacy.
4. Discuss indications and contraindications for NMES use.
5. Identify appropriate electrode placement for treatment protocols.

## Terminology

| | |
|---|---|
| Accommodation | Glenohumeral subluxation |
| Current density | NMES |
| Electrotherapeutic agents | Sensory electrical stimulation |
| Functional electrical stimulation | SOAP documentation |

## Background

The field of electrotherapy has grown dramatically in the course of the past 5 years due in part to advances in technology, instrumentation, and demand. To ensure that therapists are speaking the same language, it is important to have a concise definition of what constitutes an electrotherapeutic agent. *Electrotherapeutic agents* are those procedures or interventions that are systematically applied to modify specific client factors which may be limiting occupational performance; and which use electricity and the electromagnetic spectrum to facilitate tissue healing, improve muscle strength and endurance, decrease edema, modulate pain, decrease the inflammatory process and modify the healing process; and which are used as an adjunctive or preparatory method to engagement in occupation. Many of the recent advances and clinical applications use electrotherapeutic agents to facilitate functional movement in the performance of occupational tasks. In fact, use of electrotherapeutic agents in this fashion strengthens and reinforces the patterns of movement and function and facilitates independence (Chae, 2003; Cheng, Chen, Wang, & Chung, 2006; Crevenna, Marosi, Schmidinger, & Fialka-Moser, 2006; de Carvalho, Martins, Cardoso, & Cliquet, 2006; Han et al., 2003).

Clinically, NMES is used to selectively evoke muscle contraction through stimulation of the intact or partially intact peripheral nervous system. Though there is an increasing body of research and practical clinical applications supporting its use with a variety of clinical conditions, NMES use is rarely considered as an adjunctive method to facilitate occupational performance by most therapists. As research and clinical applications continue to evolve supporting the use of NMES, clinicians should consider its use and application as an additional tool in their therapeutic repertoire, particularly with those patients impacted with central nervous system (CNS) injuries. NMES can be used to strengthen or prevent disuse atrophy during or following immobilization or inactivity, maintain or improve range of motion (ROM), facilitate voluntary motor control, decrease edema through its muscle pumping action, decrease spasticity and muscle spasm, and act as a substitute for orthotic devices allowing for engagement in functional movements and activities. The goal and consideration for the occupational therapist is to clinically determine how electrical stimulation can effectively be incorporated into the therapeutic process and to strengthen research related to its use (Alon, 2003; Aoyagi & Tsubahara, 2004; Dromerick, Lum, & Hidler, 2006).

## Stimulating to Maintain Muscle Mass

Research over the years has shown that the electrical stimulation of healthy, innervated tissue showed little difference from muscle tissue put through traditional exercise and maximum isometric contraction. However, when faced with a patient demonstrating submaximal effort, such as a patient who is holding back due to anticipated pain, electrical stimulation may be a viable intervention until maximum effort can be achieved through traditional activity and exercise. Strength gains occur through the overload principle. Overload occurs during exercise programs consisting of a small number of high intensity contractions (e.g., a minimum of 70% of maximal contraction for 10 repetitions). Patients with orthopedic and traumatic injuries appear to demonstrate greater strength gains with NMES than with straight exercise alone.

Combining NMES with occupational activity can further enhance gains. Electrical stimulation should not replace voluntary muscle contraction but is most effective when used as an adjunct to exercise and activity (Caggiano, Emrey, Shirley, & Craik, 1994; Cameron, Broton, Needham-Shropshire, & Klose, 1998; Delitto & Snyder-Mackler, 1990; Selkowitz, 1985).

## Stimulation to Maintain or Gain Range of Motion

Electrical stimulation may be employed on patients who demonstrate moderate to high levels of spasticity. This may occur more frequently in patients with neurological impairments or with orthopedic patients. In neurologically impaired patients, increased spasticity may affect movement and ROM, which may impact skin integrity and engagement in occupational performance. Patients with mild levels of spasticity may respond to passive range of motion activities better than patients with moderate or severe spasticity. Traditional ROM techniques in home exercise programs, particularly when spasticity is moderate or severe, may become ineffective over time. NMES can be used as an adjunct to passive range of motion and in conjunction with serial casting or splinting. NMES can be applied to either the spastic muscle or the antagonist. With appropriate parameters, this results in a muscle contraction sufficient to move the joint through its complete range of motion. In applying electrical stimulation to an individual with severe spasticity, care should be taken to use a long ramp up time. Lengthening the ramp up time will decrease the likelihood of stimulating the spastic response and will result in a more balanced muscle contraction. As with all uses of electrical stimulation, the practitioner should be fully versed in the treatment protocol necessary with clear goals outlined (Kamper, Yasukawa, Barrett & Gaebler-Spira, 2006; Ozer, Chesher, & Scheker, 2006; Gorgey, Mahoney, Kendall, & Dudley, 2006).

## Electrical Stimulation to Facilitate Voluntary Motor Control

There have been multiple studies that evaluated the effectiveness of electrical stimulation in the treatment of healthy individuals and with orthopedic or neurological patients. Several studies have shown the improvement of functional performance following electrical stimulation. NMES can facilitate improvement of performance and efficiency of muscle recruitment (Kim, Schmit, & Youm, 2006; Schmidt, Sorowka, Hesse, & Bernhardt, 2003; Teasell, Bhogal, Foley, & Speechley, 2003; van der Salm et al., 2005).

Electrical stimulation as a muscle facilitation technique works best when it is part of a highly structured program with active patient participation. It has been postulated that one reason for electrical stimulation's effectiveness may be due to the increase in sensory information to the CNS. This increased sensory feedback may result in the individual's increased ability to activate specific muscle groups (Bowman, Baker, & Waters, 1979; Chen, Chang, Chen, Sheu, & Chen, 2003; Durfee, Mariano, & Zahradnik, 1991; Hara, Ogawa, & Muraoka, 2006; Kim et al., 2006; Mauritz, 2004; Phillips, Koubek, & Hendershot, 1991). A voluntary contraction that is enhanced and augmented by NMES can be used to facilitate and strengthen a weak response of the muscle group (Baker, Yeh, Wilson, & Waters, 1979; Carpinella, Mazzoleni, Rabuffetti, Thorsen, & Ferrarin, 2006). Incorporation of the NMES and stimulation at the appropriate time within an occupational task strengthens the results and outcomes. Utilizing NMES during functional activity, such as grasp and release, or for upper extremity positioning to recruit weak muscle groups will be rewarding to the patient and reinforce the re-education of the motor pattern.

## Electrical Stimulation for the Management of Spasticity

Research into the use of electrical stimulation for the control of spasticity has demonstrated only short-term control in neurologically impaired patients due to the underlying CNS abnormality. Long-term muscle control is usually not achieved through the use of NMES. NMES treatment protocols for spasticity interrupt the abnormal cycle that stimulates the motor neuron through muscle fatigue using high-frequency stimulation. ROM may improve due to a break in the pain-spasm cycle of spasticity. Numerous studies performed on both agonist and antagonist spastic muscles indicate that stimulation of the antagonist muscles causes an inhibition of the agonist. Even with stimulation of the agonist, however, minimal long-term improvement may affect functional outcomes due to the underlying pathology with use of NMES as a part of treatment. Other studies have indicated improvement in patient abilities and outcomes. Severe hand impairment was reduced after a short duration of NMES therapy for individuals with chronic stroke. NMES-assisted grasping trended towards greater functional benefit than traditional NMES-activation of wrist flexors/extensors (Santos, Zahner, McKiernan, Mahnken, & Quaney, 2006). Though the underlying cause and muscle tone may vary, NMES has been used in upper limb rehabilitation towards restoring motor hand function and should be a consideration as part of the treatment process (de Castro & Cliquet, Jr., 2000).

NMES should also be considered as an additional therapeutic tool in the treatment of cerebral palsy. Research has found that use of NMES as an adjunct to treatment in children with cerebral palsy can improve hand function and independence but may require additional splinting to maintain functional positioning (Carmick, 1995; Carmick, 1997). The use of NMES and bracing for improved functional use of the hand and upper extremity may, however, require continuous application to maintain the positive effects (Ozer, Chesher, & Scheker, 2006). NMES was also found to be an effective therapeutic technique to improve strength and motor function of a child with spastic diplegic cerebral palsy (Daichman, Johnston, Evans, & Tecklin, 2003). In improving wrist and hand control and movement, an NMES treatment protocol affected wrist extension by improving the strength of the wrist extensor muscles, possibly through decreased flexor coactivation (Scheker, Chesher, & Ramirez, 1999; Scheker & Ozer, 2003).

## Electrical Stimulation Used as an Orthotic Substitute

Electrical stimulation has been used effectively in place of orthotics and in conjunction with bracing to increase patient motor control and to facilitate occupational performance. Many manufacturers are developing electrically stimulated orthotic devices that position the extremity in a functional position and stimulate specific muscle groups to increase, for example, grasp and release patterns in the hand (Figure 9-1). Because the use of electrical stimulation is to gain control of function of targeted muscle groups, it is often referred to as functional electrical stimulation (FES).

Electrical stimulation can be an effective substitute for orthotics when activating innervated but paretic muscles. NMES has been used in upper limb rehabilitation with the goal of restoring motor hand function or paralyzed muscles. FES has been used to facilitate standing and ambulation in spinal cord injured patients, for idiopathic scoliosis, and as dorsiflexion assistance with patients with CVA (Baker, 1982; Phillips, 1989). An intervention that is often used clinically incorporates electrical stimulation as a substitute for orthotics in the treatment of CVA. Training weakened or paretic musculature using electric stimulation in a hemiplegic shoulder may reduce shoulder subluxation. A number of studies suggested that the use of electrical stimulation for reducing shoulder subluxation or improving the function of wrist and finger extensors is effective during or shortly after the daily treatment period and should be initiated as soon as possible following a stroke to prevent loss of integrity of the joint capsule (Aoyagi & Tsubahara, 2004; Baker & Parker, 1986; Chae et al., 2005).

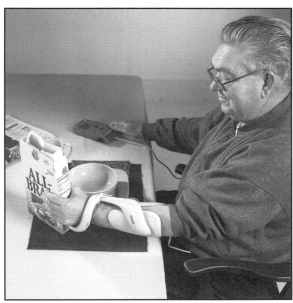

**Figure 9-1.** Bioness Inc, NESS H 200 functional electrical stimulation system. The platform or static wrist orthosis provides stability to the wrist allowing stimulation of the muscles for contraction of the digits for grasp and release activities (Reprinted with permission from Bioness, Santa Clarita, California).

# Factors Affecting Neuromuscular Electrical Stimulation

There is a wide variety of electrical equipment available for clinical use. Researchers are exploring the effectiveness of both surface and percutaneous electrodes on the CNS and muscular function (Chae, Yu, & Walker, 2001; Daly, 2006). It has been found that electrical stimulation also has long-term beneficial therapeutic effects on motor control and function, and that NMES training-induced neural adaptations were maintained after discontinuation of treatment (Gondin, Duclay, & Martin, 2006a). Though the research and technology indicate improved outcomes in a variety of clinical conditions, therapists are often hesitant to use NMES as an adjunctive tool. Because of the diversity of equipment available and variations in clinical and research parameters, clinicians are often cautious to use NMES—citing methodological "flaws" in the research, including timing of NMES initiation, NMES training dose, isolation of the NMES training from the training of specific tasks or functions, and confinement of stimulation to only one to two muscle groups (Alon, 2003). Because of these variations, clinicians should familiarize themselves with the type and parameters of the equipment available in their department before using electrical stimulation as part of a treatment program. Additionally, a thorough understanding and review of anatomical landmarks and kinesiology is crucial to determine appropriate electrode placement and muscle movement (Figure 9-2).

Each electrotherapeutic device may have unique characteristics and parameters which must be adjusted to achieve appropriate outcomes. It is critical to remember that use of electrical stimulation does not take precedence over engagement of the patient in appropriate activities and occupations, but is most effective when used in conjunction with occupation or activity (Baker, Parker, & Sanderson, 1983; Carmick, 1993). Clinicians should be familiar with the operation of the equipment available to them and thoroughly review the operating manual of their respective equipment. Incorporating NMES into functional movements and activities will reinforce the pat-

**Figure 9-2.** Electrode placement for wrist extension. Note wrist extension without radial or ulnar deviation, full extension of the digits. Electrode placement, frequency, amplitude, and pulse duration affect the strength of the muscle contraction. Intensity may need to be increased after 5 to 10 minutes of stimulation due to accomodation.

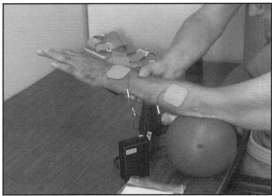

terns and improve the effectiveness and outcomes of the stimulation promoting occupational performance.

Some basic considerations and parameters need to be taken into account prior to using neuromuscular stimulation as part of a treatment protocol. The amplitude, pulse duration, resistance/impedance, electrode size and placement, and frequency will all affect the quantity or the amount of current required to stimulate motor nerves causing depolarization. The frequency and duty cycle affect the quality of the muscle contraction, the strength of the contraction and the rate of fatigue. The amplitude will provide the subjective comfort level and determine the magnitude of the sensory or motor response. The strength or force of the muscle contraction can also be manipulated by adjusting the intensity which will affect motor unit recruitment. Higher levels of intensity and contraction will increase muscle fatigue. Using a low frequency and high intensity will decrease fatigue in the muscle (Binder-Macleod & Snyder-Mackler, 1993). Pulse duration will affect the subjective comfort level of the stimulation and will also affect both the current density and release of endorphins. During electrical stimulation, the length of the pulse duration leads to greater penetration and the release of endorphins. Rise times that are set for a gradual onset facilitate patient comfort by avoiding a sudden onset of the stimulation which may startle the patient (Butterfield, Draper, Ricard, Myrer, Schulthies, & Durrant, 1997; Ralston, 1985). Longer rise times, between 6 to 8 seconds, should be used with more spastic muscles to avoid stimulating a spastic response.

The amount of time that the current stimulates and contracts the muscles, or the "on" time, will be a factor in affecting the strength and endurance of the muscle. The duty cycle (on-time/off-time) should be adjusted based on the condition of the patient. Historically, a 1:5 ratio is recommended for strengthening, but a 1:3 ratio may be used for a debilitated patient; a 1:2 ratio for an individual with average musculature; 1:1 ratio for athletic or conditioned individuals; and a 1:1 ratio can also be used to fatigue muscles since the "rest" time or "off" period is much shorter not allowing the muscles to recover. To produce a conditioning or strengthening effect, the longer the on-time, the greater the exercise that occurs. An objective method of documenting improvement in a patient is through documenting a decrease in the on-time/off-time. The force of the electrically stimulated contraction is related to the patient's perception of pain and may limit the outcomes and goals if the patient is hesitant and apprehensive towards use of electrical stimulation. Therapists should be aware of the impact of adaptations to a specific amplitude, pulse duration, and frequency to ensure effectiveness and patient compliance (Gorgey, Mahoney, Kendall, & Dudley, 2006). Other factors that influence the effectiveness and action of electrical stimulation on the target tissue include:

1. *Current Density*: The amount passing into the skin from an electrode is affected by the size of the electrode. There is an inverse relationship to electrical current and electrode size; the smaller the electrode the higher the current density per square inch. When the same amount of current is used, the larger the electrode, the lower the current is per square inch. Electrodes should be selected based on the area of muscle which is to be stimulated. Larger electrodes will be more comfortable, but will also cause recruitment of surrounding muscle which may not be intended. As a general rule of thumb, smaller electrodes are used for the upper extremity and larger electrodes should be used to stimulate the muscles of the lower extremity. Electrodes can be cut down to smaller sizes to stimulate or isolate smaller muscles of the forearm and hand.

2. *Accommodation*: This is the automatic rise in the threshold of excitation resulting from a gradually increasing stimulus applied to excitable tissue. As the tissue is stimulated it will accommodate to the stimulus, resulting in increasing stimulus being necessary to achieve the desired result or a decreased response to the same amount of stimulus. The intensity of the stimulation should be slowly increased after approximately five to ten minutes to prevent accommodation from occurring. Longer-lasting stimulation programs may also require the therapist to slowly increase the intensity to a higher level in order to achieve the same degree of muscle contraction.

3. *Electrode Placement*: In stimulating healthy innervated muscle tissue one can use either monopolar or bipolar techniques. Monopolar stimulation uses a small active electrode over the motor point of the muscle. A dispersive pad is used on the same side of the body. The dispersive pad is usually larger to decrease the current density. This allows a higher current density under the active electrode, thus stimulating the motor point with greater comfort. Bipolar stimulation utilizes two electrodes of approximately the same size and is the most commonly used form of stimulation for muscle re-education. The electrodes are placed over a single muscle group or group of muscles at each end of the muscle belly. The current is then passed through the muscle belly and results in contraction of the muscle. Additional research is being undertaken looking at the effectiveness of in-dwelling or percutaneous NEMS (P-NEMS) in which the electrodes are surgically implanted below the skin (Renzenbrink & Ijzerman, 2004; Van Til, Renzenbrink, Groothuis, & Ijzerman, 2006).

   Improper electrode preparation and placement may result in higher current density in some areas and a burn may occur under that area of the electrode. The skin should always be cleaned with a gentle soap and water prior to electrode application. Use of rubbing alcohol has a tendency to dry the skin and may affect conduction of the electrical current. The electrodes should be placed directly on the skin and should not be pulling up in the corners or lift off the tissue during a muscle contraction.

4. *Tolerance of Muscle Tissue to Electric Stimulation*: Following repeated stimulation to achieve muscle contraction, fatigue of the muscle will result. This is usually noted by tremors in the muscle during contraction and a decrease in overall strength of the contraction and movement desired. To continue stimulation at the intended strength, it may be necessary to increase the intensity to achieve the desired degree of contraction. Care must be used however, as continually increasing the intensity during a treatment session results in little benefit and possible damage to the muscles.

# Contraindications for Neuromuscular Electrical Stimulation

NMES can be a safe and effective treatment with minimal contraindications in its use. When using NMES it should be noted that there are some specific conditions for which stimulation is contraindicated or which have precautions against the use of stimulation. Precautions and contraindications should always be a consideration during the evaluation when goals, objectives, and treatment interventions are being considered. One common adverse reaction to the electrical stimulation is transient skin irritation. This irritation appears as a reddened area under the electrode and may be due to the misapplication of the electrode with uneven contact, skin composition, poor cleansing of the skin prior to the treatment, or removing the self-adherent electrodes too forcefully following treatment. It is possible for the patient to develop electrical burns if the intensity is too high or the electrode is placed unevenly. Responding to a patient's subjective report or comment is crucial. The therapists should always remember to monitor a patient's skin condition and electrode placement prior to application and following the treatment.

As with any electrical device, application of electrical stimulation to patients with implantable cardioverter defibrillators (ICDs) is contraindicated. Though there is some research that has indicated that long-term *NMES* of thigh muscles appears to be safe in patients with ICDs, this would require that the individual be screened from a cardiac standpoint and be excluded prior to the application if there were any inconsistencies in the cardiac screening (Crevenna et al., 2004). Other research has found that electromagnetic interference (EMI) may occur with electrical stimulation use in patients with ICDs, particularly if used in the neck and shoulder area. NMES should not be used unless it is tested with each particular patient who has an ICD with bipolar sensing, and physician consent should be obtained prior to application. One study of NMES treatment of thigh muscles using a combined NMES protocol to enhance strength and endurance capacity concluded that NMES appeared to be safe in patients with heart failure and implanted pacemakers with bipolar sensing, but therapists are cautioned that further research is needed to document patient safety with these devices (Crevenna et al., 2003).

# Neuromuscular Electrical Stimulation Applications

Neuromuscular electrical stimulation is often underutilized as a treatment option even though there are a wide variety of therapeutic applications for its use. As with any physical agent modality, the therapist should complete a thorough evaluation of the patient prior to NMES use to determine objective measurements and function which will assist in identifying appropriate goals and interventions. Patients suffering from CNS damage are often "deprived" of NMES and the therapeutic interventions as part of their neurorehabilitation process (Alon, 2003). Because of design flaws and variability, NMES use is typically not a primary consideration as part of the therapeutic approach to rehabilitation of these patients. Research, however, indicates that consideration and application of NMES as an adjunctive method and technique should be considered immediately after the CNS insult. In a number of studies, NMES use 48 hours post-stroke did not impede spontaneous recovery or have a negative complicating effect on the patient (Alon, 2003). NMES has been shown to be effective in facilitating movement in the upper extremity in "chronic" stroke

## CONTRAINDICATIONS AND PRECAUTIONS FOR THE USE OF ELECTRICAL STIMULATION

- Over the thoracic region as it may interfere with heart activity
- Patients with demand-type pacemakers
- Areas of phrenic nerve or bladder stimulators
- Over the carotid sinus as this may cause cardiac arrhythmias
- With hypertensive or hypotensive patients
- Peripheral vascular disorders such as venous thrombosis or thrombophlebitis
- Patients with cancer, infection, tuberculosis, or active hemorrhage
- Pregnant women, over a pregnant uterus during the first trimester
- Near diathermy devices
- Obese patients with excessive adipose tissue (may require higher levels of electrical current which may cause skin irritation or burning)
- Patients unable to provide clear feedback regarding the level of stimulation such as infants or young children, patients with dementia or cognitive disorders, or individuals with mental disorders
- Over areas with pathology of the cell body (e.g., polio)
- Over areas with pathology of the myelin sheath (i.e., diabetic neuropathy, MS, peripheral neuropathy)
- Over areas with pathology of the synapse points between muscle and nerve (e.g., myasthenia gravis)
- Over areas with pathology within the muscle (i.e., muscular dystrophy)
- Caution should be used in areas of absent or diminished sensation
- Patients with skin conditions such as eczema, psoriasis, acne, dermatitis
- Over or near superficial metal pins, plates, or hardware
- Over areas where movement is contraindicated or to be avoided

Adapted from Hunter, Mackin, & Callahan, 1995; Robinson & Snyder-Mackler, 1995.

patients, even 5 years post-stroke (Chae, Fang, Walker, & Pourmehdi, 2001; Sullivan & Hedman, 2004).

With the advances in electronics and equipment over the past decade, it is unfortunate that occupational therapists are not pursuing more aggressively the use of NMES as part of their treatment protocol with CVA patients. Electrical stimulation is particularly valuable when incorporated with functional movement and activities enhancing and strengthening the therapeutic outcomes which can be intrinsically rewarding to the patient and family as independence and movement increases. NMES use to facilitate movement in the upper extremity of CVA patients may also decrease pain, shoulder subluxation, and can be highly motivating to patients. Often, when occupational therapists are evaluating patients who have suffered a CVA, the patient will describe the affected side, particularly the arm, as being "dead." When NMES is used to facilitate movement in the extremity, patients can see their arm or hand move due to the stimulation, often leading to increased motivation and engagement to participate in treatment.

NMES is most effective when there is an intact or partially intact peripheral nerve pathway. Therapists should be aware of the contraindications and precautions of electrical stimulation, along with being well acquainted with the equipment that is available to them in their clinic prior to application. Because of the continuing advances in technology, equipment can be as small as a cigarette box or as large as a table top model. As there is a wide range of equipment available, the therapist should be familiar with the particular features of the selected equipment and thoroughly review the equipment manual. Informing the patient and family as to the goals and objectives, as well as the possible subjective feelings which the patient may experience when applying electrical stimulation, will help to allay the patient's fears.

In patients with severe neurological involvement, the sensory feedback loop may become distorted or impaired and subsequently alter the movement and tone. In patients with orthopedic issues, particularly those who have been immobilized, proprioception may become altered which can affect movement and tone. NMES can be utilized to effectively incorporate stimulation for voluntary muscle contractions, functional movement or activities, and to provide sensory feedback. NMES provides both a motor response as well as a sensory response, which can be beneficial. P-NMES has been found to potentially decrease shoulder pain in chronic hemiplegia. Electrical stimulation has both a motor effect as well as sensory effect (sensory electrical stimulation), which has been evaluated in research combined with motor level stimulation and may also be a component in the effectiveness of electrical stimulation with CNS injuries (Renzenbrink & Ijzerman, 2004; Sullivan & Hedman, 2004; Van Til et al., 2006). Electrical stimulation can also be used to increase strength through the overload principle and specificity with similar outcomes in muscle strength occurring if the same amount of force is produced (Hainaut, 1992; Wolf et al., 1986).

Though there are a number of potential applications for NMES, we will discuss those most frequently used by occupational therapists. It should be noted that there are a variety of applications and possible protocols for specific muscle groups, and the clinician is encouraged to explore other treatment approaches and electrode placements. Electrical stimulation can be used as an adjunctive treatment in managing many disorders including neuromuscular, musculoskeletal, vascular, and soft-tissue injuries. Clinical application of electrical stimulation can include muscle re-education and facilitation, decreasing spasticity or spasm, decreasing edema and pain, and to facilitate tissue repair and wound healing. It is important to stress again that, as with any physical agent, electrical stimulation should be used as an adjunctive method to occupational therapy treatment and when possible should be paired to active movement or engagement in occupational tasks and activities.

The following protocols provide recommended settings for wave form, intensity, pulse duration, frequency, on-/off-time, treatment time, and engagement in possible functional activities. These settings may vary with patients, medical diagnoses, and equipment, and are intended to guide the therapist's clinical reasoning.

# Maintaining or Increasing
# Active Range of Motion and Strength

Utilizing electrical stimulation in patients affected by stroke or damage to the CNS such as traumatic brain injury (TBI), and in patients with orthopedic conditions, can be effective to maintain or increase ROM, increase muscle strength, facilitate muscle re-education and movement, or decrease pain. Electrical stimulation provides muscle contraction that may be highly motivating to the patient, but also provides proprioceptive, kinesthetic, and sensory input to the CNS (Baldwin, Klakowicz, & Collins, 2006; Becker, Hayashi, Lee, & White, 1987; Dromerick et al., 2006; Gondin, Duclay, & Martin et al., 2006b; Liu, You, & Sun, 2005). A strengthening protocol can also be used when there is muscle weakness or atrophy which occurs secondary to immobilization or disuse from surgery, pain, or casting. NMES may also be beneficial in those patients with limited traumatic or orthopedic injuries who are demonstrating submaximal effort or hold back during therapy secondary to anticipated pain. A strengthening protocol may be used as it can be graded to the patient's limits and gradually increased until the patient achieves maximum voluntary effort through traditional activity or exercise. During immobilization or with decreased movement or casting, larger fast twitch muscle fibers are affected, first causing weakness and atrophy and affecting an individual's performance skills and their ability to perform occupational tasks and activities. Electrical stimulation recruits large, fast twitch nerve fibers first with the smaller muscle fibers recruited later (Trimble & Enoka, 1991). Electrical stimulation of the motor nerve results in stronger contractions with greater torque (Baldwin et al., 2006). Because electrically stimulated contractions are different than self-initiated or physiological contractions, the muscles fatigue more rapidly and fine motor control and smooth, coordinated movements are limited and asynchronous. Due to the increased fatigability of the muscles, longer rest periods are required between stimulation on-times and will require close monitoring by the clinician (Shields, Dudley-Javoroski, & Littmann, 2006; Stackhouse, Binder-Macleod, & Lee, 2005).

Maintaining or increasing AROM and strength can be accomplished using either asymmetrical or symmetrical biphasic waveforms. Most often, electrical stimulation of the upper extremity uses an asymmetrical waveform which will cause the motor nerve to depolarize under the negative (black) electrode, particularly when stimulating smaller muscles. Therapists should have a good understanding of the anatomy of muscles and their innervations in order to stimulate the muscles effectively. Smaller muscles of the upper extremity will require a smaller electrode to isolate the specific movements required or the electrode may be reduced in size. It is important to remember, however, that by decreasing the electrode size, the current density will increase— along with potential discomfort to the patient. A patient's perception of comfort during electrical stimulation appears to be affected by the physical and psychological results of the tingling sensation and the sensory response that occurs during contraction or by the force of the contraction itself. Therefore, the therapist should encourage the patient to relax the antagonists during the application of electrical stimulation when it is used for muscle strengthening. Whenever possible, the therapist should always superimpose active movement over electrically stimulated muscles to strengthen the response and training effect (Lyons, Leane, Clarke-Moloney, O'Brien, & Grace, 2004; Rooney, Currier, & Nitz, 1992).

Muscle stimulation provides a method of actively exercising the muscle in those patients unable to voluntarily contract the muscle. Stimulation of the muscle in patients with hemiplegia prevents or can reverse atrophy which may occur due to disuse or immobility, and facilitates peripheral circulation preventing fibrosis. In those patients who are displaying beginning return or motor control, NMES can also strengthen a weak response, improve muscle recruitment and strength, and assist occupational performance (Wolf et al., 1986). The success of NMES in a highly structured program that includes active patient involvement may be due in part to the increased sensory information to the CNS. Electrical stimulation facilitates modulatory effects on the central nervous system and can be used as an adjunct to conventional facilitory techniques in those patients with motor dysfunction caused by neurological injury (Field-Fote, 2004). Electrical stimulation provides the patient with proprioceptive and visual feedback which can be motivating to those patients with limited movement. The intent of facilitation and re-education is to flood the CNS with sensory and kinesthetic information that will link it with an anticipated motor response (Smith, Alon, Roys, & Gullapalli, 2003).

Electrical stimulation provides an external source for muscle contraction that can facilitate movement into functional, occupational movement patterns and activities. The duration of the treatment will depend on the selected goal and outcome desired, and on ensuring variation of functional activities which will result in carryover and integration of the pattern. Utilizing NMES during a functional activity such as grasp and release, object manipulation, or upper extremity positioning to recruit weak muscle groups can be intrinsically rewarding to the patient and reinforce the re-education of the motor pattern. Determining appropriate movements and electrode placement also requires creativity on the part of the therapist to ensure that the activity is intrinsically rewarding and meaningful.

# Treatment Parameters

The therapist should select the muscle or muscle group to be stimulated. Pulse duration is usually set at 200 to 300 microseconds (µs), with the frequency between 25 and 35 pulses per second (pps). Frequencies should be chosen which achieve the desired outcome, yet are comfortable to the patient. The intensity is increased to achieve tetany, which allows for a fair + muscle grade in the desired muscle. The on-/off-ratio should be 1:3 or higher to allow muscles a chance to recover between contractions. Treatment time is usually 30 minutes BID to TID for 5 sessions per week. Treatment should continue for 3 to 4 weeks with re-evaluation occurring to determine treatment effectiveness. To facilitate effectiveness of the intervention and carry-over, neuromuscular stimulators may often be used as part of a home exercise program. Proper patient and family training is a necessity to ensure that the patient and caregiver are familiar and comfortable with electrode placement, skin care, and the stimulating parameters of the equipment. Specific electrode placement for muscle groups will be discussed later.

NMES may be used when reinnervation has occurred and the patient is unable to achieve voluntary contraction without electric stimulation. The waveform can be asymmetrical or symmetrical biphasic, again depending on the muscle group targeted. The pulse duration is 300 µm with a frequency between 25 to 35 pps. The intensity should be gradually increased to the maximum tolerated contraction with an on-/off-time of 1:1 or 1:2. The recommended treatment is 10 to 20 repetitive contractions, 3 to

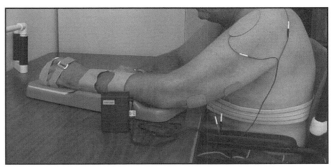

**Figure 9-3.** NMES can be used to stimulate paretic muscles following a CVA. NMES assists in maintaining approximation of the humeral head in the GH joint and can be paired with active movement to facilitate outcomes. Note electrode placement.

5 times per week. Treatment is usually continued until the patient can achieve maximal contraction of the target muscle without electric stimulation. Pairing the response to a functional movement or activity will increase the carryover effect and facilitate strengthening of the musculature.

## Neuromuscular Electrical Stimulation in the Treatment of the Hemiplegic Shoulder and for Muscle Re-Education

The use of electrical stimulation as a substitute for an orthotic device is known as "functional" electrical stimulation (FES). Many therapists erroneously refer to all forms of electrical stimulation as "functional", though this term should refer to specific use of electrical stimulation as an orthotic substitute to allow functional movement or activity engagement. FES is commonly used as an orthotic substitute to facilitate positional stability and mobility for a particular muscle function and movement. FES is an effective adjunct to treatment in that it can stimulate a muscle to contract volitionally during an active or functional movement. For example, the stimulation of innervated paretic or paralyzed muscles can decrease the dependence on slings, splints or orthotics through the development of increased strength and endurance of the paretic musculature. Electrical stimulation has also been used to facilitate motor learning in ankle dorsiflexion and wrist extension (Kimberley & Carey, 2002).

FES can be used when the peripheral nerve to the muscle is intact but not functioning appropriately such as with glenohumoral subluxation (GHS) secondary to hemiparesis after a cerebral vascular accident (CVA). Use of electrical stimulation for shoulder subluxation or flaccid paralysis following a CVA assists in maintaining approximation of the humeral head in the glenohumoral joint. FES can be effective for patients with hemiparesis who display shoulder subluxation during the flaccid phase of recovery (Figure 9-3). When muscle tone and voluntary control develop at the shoulder, normal glenohumoral alignment may not occur if the shoulder capsule becomes stressed by gravity causing stretching of the ligamentous capsule and soft-tissue structures. Other complicating conditions which can be associated with glenohumoral subluxation include an increased incidence of sympathetic reflex dystrophy of the upper limb and adhesive capsulitis (Dursun, Dursun, Ural, & Cakci, 2000; Gokkaya, Aras, Yesiltepe, & Koseoglu, 2006; Griffin, 1986a; Lo et al., 2003; Pinedo & de la Villa, 2001), rotator cuff injury (Chino, 1981; Paci, Nannetti, & Rinaldi, 2005), overstretching of ligaments and muscles (supraspinatus and deltoid), adhesive capsulitis (Culham, Noce, & Bagg, 1995; Daviet et al., 2002; Griffin, 1986b), tendonitis, adhesions of the bicipital tendons, and rupture of ligaments.

**Figure 9-4.** Neuromuscular electrical stimulation using a two channel, four electrode configuration for facilitating grasp and release patterns in the hand. Always pair electrical stimulation with a functional activity or movement to strengthen the response.

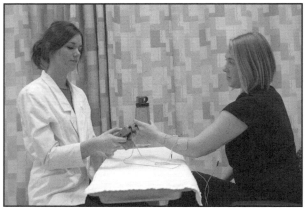

Although slings may be helpful to establish glenohumeral alignment, stimulation of the posterior deltoid and supraspinatus muscles may be more effective to improve the normal shoulder integrity and facilitate grasp-and-release activities. Incorporating electrical stimulation as part of an integrated approach including a home program may also facilitate return and function in the upper extremity (Sullivan & Hedman, 2004). As with any home program, it is crucial to properly educate clients and caregivers about the home program to ensure there will be continuity and carryover. Marking the electrode placements on the patient, clearly outlining family instructions, and having family demonstrate appropriate placement in the clinical setting will also foster confidence and carryover for the program (Aoyagi & Tsubahara, 2004; Liu et al., 2005).

Electrical stimulation is an effective intervention and is used to increase or maintain tone in the affected shoulder following a CVA. The electrical stimulator acts as a substitute to the traditional arm sling which many patients wear due to shoulder subluxation and flaccid paralysis of the affected extremity. Stimulation of the deltoid reapproximates the humeral head in the glenohumoral joint, decreasing subluxation of the shoulder. Treatment parameters are the same as those used for muscle strengthening and facilitation. Electrode placement is over the stimulated muscles' motor points. The easiest way to determine the electrode placement is to locate the "bulk" of the muscle, the muscle belly. An additional way to determine the motor point of a muscle is to use a probe electrode or to move the electrodes along the intended muscle during stimulation to observe the strength of the contraction (Figure 9-4).

There are multiple electrode placements for the treatment of shoulder subluxation and the therapist should determine the most appropriate placement based on the goals and subsequent muscle contraction (Chae et al., 2005). Bipolar electrode placement can be over the supraspinatus and posterior deltoid muscles. Additional electrode placements include bipolar electrode placement over the supraspinatus/upper trapezius and middle fibers of the deltoid which stimulates abduction of the shoulder; supraspinatus/upper trapezius and anterior fibers of the deltoid which stimulates shoulder flexion; supraspinatus/upper trapezius and posterior fibers of the deltoid which stimulates hyperextension of the shoulder; and anterior deltoid and posterior deltoid which results in reapproximation of the humeral head. Electrode placement selection is dependent on the goals and movements for the patient. A quadripolar pattern can also be used with electrode placement on the motor points of the deltoid and the three rotator cuff muscles: the supraspinatus, infraspinatus, and teres minor.

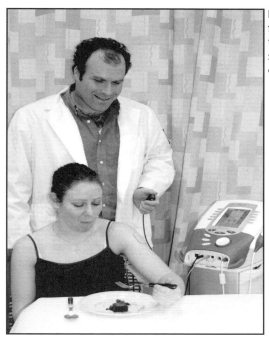

**Figure 9-5.** Neuromuscular electrical stimulation for shoulder subluxation. The stimulator can be triggered by the hand-held switch to decrease shoulder subluxation, strengthen shoulder muscles, and improve occupational performance.

The on-/off-ratio for a power program is 0.1 to 1 second for a power program, or 1.5 to 5 seconds for a strengthening program. NMES is effective in reducing shoulder subluxation, but is less effective in decreasing shoulder pain associated with the hemiplegic shoulder and further research is needed to document therapeutic parameters (Aoyagi & Tsubahara, 2004; Yu, 2004) (Figure 9-5).

A dual channel (four electrodes) pattern can also be used to stimulate a mass extensor or flexor pattern or to alternate between selected movements such as wrist flexion and extension. During two-channel stimulation, the electrical current can be adjusted to turn on concurrently (at the same time) or alternating (asynchronously). Dual channel protocols are frequently used when multiple muscle groups are targeted or the movement requires movement at two joints or in a mass pattern. The strength of the muscular contraction is varied by adjusting the intensity of the electrical stimulation which effectively recruits more, or less, motor units and muscle fibers. It is important to remember, however, that greater intensities with concurrent stronger muscle contractions can be perceived as painful by the patient and should be monitored.

Use of electrical stimulation for muscle re-education may be effective following neurologic injury or orthopedic surgery such as tendon transfers. The therapist should determine if the patient displays limitation of movement due to immobilization or disuse atrophy, weakness, or pain. Stimulation can be used to facilitate weak movement or to provide stability to a targeted muscle group. The therapist should identify the target muscle or muscle group. The waveform can be either asymmetrical or symmetrical biphasic pulse depending on the location. The pulse duration is set between 200 to 300 μs, with a frequency between 25 to 50 pps. The on-/off-ratio should be 1:3 dependent on identified goals. The intensity should be increased to achieve a tetanic contraction of appropriate size. As always, electrode placement is of great importance. The stimulator should be turned off and the electrodes relocated if the contraction is incorrect or the selected muscle group is not responding. During stimulation, the patient should attempt to actively move the targeted muscle group in conjunction with the stimulation. As greater voluntary control develops, the intensity can be gradually reduced to a sensory level and the patient instructed to actively contract the muscle with each "on" cycle. Treatment sessions are usually 30 minutes, 1 to 2 times per day, and can extend over 3 to 5 days per week.

## Facilitation of Tendon Excursion and Decreasing Edema

Orthopedic or neurological conditions which limit tendon excursion can be approached using either asymmetrical or symmetrical biphasic pulse waveforms. A thorough understanding of the patient's condition, particularly if surgical intervention has occurred, as well as the stage of wound healing is crucial before using electrical stimulation. A complete evaluation and review of the patient's history is required to assist in correctly identifying appropriate goals and interventions. Electrical stimulation should not be used if there is a question of a bony block, or if movement is contraindicated due to the surgery. It is always best to check with the patient's physician prior to using electrical stimulation with tendon repairs. Another factor that may influence the use of electrical stimulation is 3+ grade strength of muscle contraction if the intensity is set to tetany; higher intensity levels have subsequent higher muscle grades. If this amount of strength and movement is contraindicated for the patient's repair or condition, damage to the tendon or repaired structures may occur. The material properties of the tendon may also be degraded following paralysis such as spinal cord injury (SCI) and care must be taken to monitor the patient's response during treatment using electrical stimulation (Maganaris et al., 2006).

Surgery and trauma to the upper extremity may also cause edema to pool in the extremities within the interstitial spaces further limiting movement and function. Decreased venous and lymphatic return may also contribute to edema in these patients, causing pitting edema. Volitional muscle contractions cause a vascular pumping action that facilitates venous and lymphatic return. In some postsurgical and trauma patients, or those patients who are deconditioned due to immobility, pain, or musculoskeletal conditions, electrical stimulation of targeted muscles may prove beneficial. Electrical stimulation may also be effective as a mechanism to reduce swelling in individuals who do not fully activate the musculo-venous pump. Stimulation of the weakened muscles may improve circulation, increase venous return, and decrease edema through the pumping action of the muscular contractions (Figure 9-6). Electrical stimulation may decrease volume in the distal extremities by increasing venous return, reducing venous stasis and increasing lymph flow as well as interstitial hydrostatic pressure, thereby reducing capillary filtration and assisting in fluid reabsorption (Lake, 1992; Man, Morrissey, & Cywinski, 2007; Man, Lepar, Morrissey, & Cywinski, 2003). Electrical stimulation may also facilitate the healing process of the tendons and affected collagen structures (Michlovitz, 2005; Shi, 2005; Snyder, Wilensky, & Fortin, 2002).

To facilitate tendon excursion for innervated muscles, the pulse duration is set between 200 to 300 µm, with a frequency of 25 to 50 pps. Intensity is increased to achieve maximal contraction of the muscle so that a comfortable tendon excursion is noted. Intensity should never be set above the tolerable level of the patient. Lower intensity levels can be used at the start of treatment and increased as tolerance improves. On/off duration should be a 1:3 ratio. The recommended treatment time is 30 minute sessions 2 to 3 times daily, over a period of 3 to 5 days per week. Electrical stimulation may not be indicated once the patient can achieve a maximal contraction

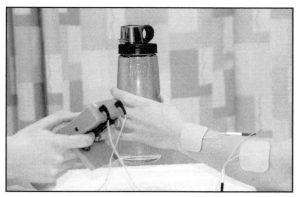

**Figure 9-6.** Amplitude, pulse duration, resistance/impedance, electrode size and placement, and frequency affect the amount of current needed to stimulate motor nerves causing depolarization and contraction.

of the target muscle voluntarily and re-evaluation of treatment goals and interventions should occur.

# Neuromuscular Electrical Stimulation for Relaxation of Muscle Spasm and Spasticity

As discussed earlier, NMES can be used to decrease the pain and tension accompanied by muscle spasm or spasticity. Often this pain and spasm is exacerbated by anxiety and leads to a cyclic pain-spasm-pain pattern causing further protective guarding and muscle spasm. The effectiveness of this technique with the neurologically involved patient is usually of short benefit due to the underlying pathology. However, NMES can be used with success in those orthopedic patients who are having muscle spasm due to injury. Electrical stimulation of the involved muscles facilitates muscle relaxation and increases circulation to the area. This increased circulation and stimulation of the affected muscles, may help to break the pain-spasm-pain cycle. NMES is typically used to fatigue a muscle, thus relaxing the spasm. Its most notable use is in the muscles of the shoulder which may be limiting functional movement due to pain and spasm. The waveform can be either asymmetrical or symmetrical biphasic pulse. The pulse duration is 300 µm with a frequency between 30 to 60 pps. The intensity is increased to patient tolerance and to achieve a gentle contraction. To achieve fatigue of the muscle group, the on-/off-ratio should be 1:1. The electrodes should be placed over the motor point with stimulation continuing until muscle fatigue is noted.

Inhibition of spasticity is dependent on the underlying pathology and degree of spasticity in the patient. If the PNS is intact, electrical stimulation can provide muscle contractions in those individuals who may be lacking volitional movement caused by CVA, cerebral palsy (CP), or TBI (Baker, Parker, & Sanderson, 1983; Patel, 2005; Pease, 1998). Though a relaxation response in the musculature can occur in the neurologically involved individual, the underlying cause of the spasticity may limit the overall effectiveness of the intervention. A thorough evaluation of the patient and the underlying cause should be completed to identify those areas that may respond better to the stimulation and have a prolonged effect.

Spasticity is associated with hypertonia, hyperactive deep tendon reflexes, and clonus; it is difficult to manage. NMES for decreasing spasticity in the neurologically involved patient can be used as an adjunct method to cooling, vibration, serial casting or splinting, and with medication or injections such as botulinum toxin (Detrembleur, Lejeune, Renders, & Van Den Bergh, 2002; Hesse, Brandi-Hesse, Bardeleben, Werner, & Funk, 2001). Reductions in muscle tone following stimulation can last for a minimum of 30 minutes to a maximum of 6 hours or longer if combined with other medications or techniques. Stimulating the spastic muscles may cause a decrease in muscle tone and the common posturing of flexor spasticity. Stimulation of the antagonist muscles in spastic patients may cause inhibition in the spastic agonist muscle. Alternating or reciprocal electrical stimulation between spastic and the weaker antagonist muscle may also decrease spasticity. Because of the increased risk for these patients to develop soft-tissue contractures, muscle shortening, and decreased movement, it is important that the therapist incorporate additional treatment interventions such as splinting, positioning, and home programs to maintain any gains that occur (Baker, Parker, & Sanderson, 1983b; Billian & Gorman, 1992; Daly et al., 1996; Scheker, Chesher, & Ramirez, 1999a; Scheker & Ozer, 2003).

## THREE PRIMARY METHODS OF APPROACHING THE PROBLEM OF SPASTICITY

1. Stimulation of the antagonist muscle to the spastic muscle. The treatment protocol is the same as described in increasing ROM. Stimulation is carried out three times daily for 30 minutes with expected results of 10 minutes to 2 hours of relief from spasticity.

2. Stimulation of the spastic muscle directly in order to achieve an overall muscle fatigue. This protocol is the same as stimulating the antagonist, only stimulation is to the spastic muscle directly.

3. Stimulating the antagonist and spastic muscle alternately. This protocol is the same as that used to increase AROM. The stimulator is set to alternately stimulate agonist and antagonist muscles. An additional application which may prove to be effective is stimulation of the acupuncture points, though the neurophysiological basis for its effectiveness is not clearly understood.

Joint contractures also present a challenging problem for the clinician. A complete evaluation to determine the cause of the contracture as well as the total active or passive movement available is necessary to aid in determining the appropriate approach. The end-feel is also of importance, as a bony block or hard end-feel may limit a positive outcome. As always, a thorough review of the patient's history, surgical intervention, and underlying pathology will help guide treatment goals. For orthopedic patients, it is valuable to review the x-rays and x-ray report if available. The treatment protocol used in treating a joint contracture is essentially the same protocol utilized for increasing AROM. Stimulation parameters are also similar with the addition of serial casting which can be modified with openings over the electrode sites. Use of electrical stimulation in conjunction serial casting or dynamic splinting can be reapplied in greater degrees of motion as progress is made (Scheker & Ozer, 2003).

# Electrical Stimulation for Wound Healing

Electrical stimulation can also be used to effectively facilitate tissue healing. It is well documented that electrical stimulation will stimulate bone growth and can enhance callus development and mineralization, with consequent improvement in the biomechanical properties of the bone (Park & Silva, 2004). In some individuals, the three phases of healing become delayed for a variety of reasons, including diabetes, ischemia in patients with and without diabetes, and by pressure, such as in "bedsores" (Kloth, 2005).

Direct current and high-voltage, pulsed current can have beneficial effects in the healing process since electrical stimulation can be used to transfer energy from the electrical current to a wound because of the current's polarity. Although the mechanism behind the efficacy of electrical stimulation to accelerate wound healing has not been fully identified, research has demonstrated that electrical stimulation can affect both the process of healing as well as the histochemical and circulatory effects on the targeted tissue (Petrofsky et al., 2005; Sun, Wise, & Cho, 2004). Electrical stimulation has beneficial effects during the inflammatory, proliferation, and maturation phases of a wound and can be used successfully in treatment of decubitis ulcers and chronic wounds, in combination with conventional therapies such as daily care and debridement of wounds (Demir, Balay, & Kirnap, 2004).

Direct electrical current occurs naturally in the body to control the healing process. When there is an injury to the tissue that disrupts the body's natural electrical field, a change is triggered in the current at the injured site that influences the histochemical substrates associated with the healing process. The wound will possess a positive electrical potential relative to the uninjured tissue and the body's bioelectric system will attract cells that will facilitate cellular secretion through the cell membranes, orient cell structures, and repair the skin defect. However, the healing will be arrested or incomplete if the current no longer flows while the wound is open. Treatment of chronic ulcers is based on "moist" wound healing, and the underlying pathology and local treatment must be taken into consideration. Local treatment of the wound is necessary and includes cleaning, debridement, the control of any infection, and the application of different topical agents, both medication and dressings (Moreno-Gimenez, Galan-Gutierrez, & Jimenez-Puya, 2005).

Electrical stimulation involving high-voltage, pulsed current can be effective for a variety of conditions. Clinicians, though, should be aware of the healing phase and the anticipated goals of the intervention since the use of electrical stimulation is not pathology dependent. The types of wounds in which the use of high-voltage, pulsed current are indicated include pressure ulcers (stage I through IV), diabetic ulcers (due to pressure, insensitivity, and dysvascularity), venous ulcers, traumatic wounds, surgical wounds, ischemic ulcers, vasculitic ulcers, donor sites, wound flaps, and burn wounds. The application of electrical stimulation during the proliferative phase of wound healing can affect biophysiological changes that will stimulate fibroblast and epithelial cells, generate DNA and protein synthesis, increase adenosine triphosphate (ATP) generation, improve cell membrane permeability and transport, produce better collagen matrix organization, and stimulate wound contraction (Evans, Foltz, & Foltz, 2001; Houghton et al., 2003).

During the remodeling phase of wound healing, electrical stimulation will stimulate epidermal cell reproduction and migration that will produce smooth and thin scarring. However, the wound must be kept moist with normal saline to maintain an optimal bioelectric charge, and dressings such as amorphous hydrogels and occlusive dressings should be utilized to promote the current in the injury. Since electrical stimulation with negative current can solubilize clotted blood, negative polarity can be used to treat wounds that have necrotic tissue. Therefore, a hematoma or hemorrhaging at the wound margin or on the granulating tissue will dissolve and become reabsorbed when a high-voltage, pulsed current with a negative pole is applied (Thawer & Houghton, 2001). Absorption of the hemorrhagic material should occur within 48 hours when negative polarity is used during the inflammatory phase of healing.

The protocols used for wound healing should be modified when the healing phase changes and in response to changes in the wound. Therefore, clinicians need to identify the wound healing phase when performing the assessment and diagnosis as this will influence which treatment protocols should be selected. It should be noted, though, that the pathogenesis of the wound will not affect the protocols or parameters. Before applying electrical stimulation to an open wound, the wound dressing should be removed so that the area can be cleaned of any slough, exudate, and petrolatum products, and sharp debridement of the necrotic tissue can be completed. The wound should then be gently packed with saline-soaked gauze (using saline-based amorphous hydrogels) to permit conduction of electrical current. When the gauze is attached to the lead of the stimulator with an alligator clip, it will act as the active treatment electrode. Aluminum foil can also be placed in or over the gauze to increase conductivity. The dispersive electrodes should be placed proximal to the wound, but care should be taken to avoid bony prominences. When the separation or distance between the active and dispersive electrode is increased, the current path will become deeper.

The waveforms that are commonly used for wound healing are direct current and low-voltage or high-voltage, multipulsed current. The outcomes during the inflammatory phase include necrosis free, erythema free, edema free, exudate free, and red granulation, and the expected outcomes during the proliferative phase include undermining and tunneling of the wound, and decreased wound size, open area, and depth. During the inflammatory and proliferation phases, the amplitude should be adjusted to the patient's tolerance level, but below the motor-level threshold. The polarity should be negative with a pulse rate of 30 pps. The treatment period should be 60 minutes daily for a frequency of 5 to 7 times per week, though these parameter settings may vary depending what type of equipment is utilized. Furthermore, when there is a great deal of blood exudate while using direct current, the amplitude should be decreased; conversely, when there is copious, serous drainage without any bleeding while using direct current, the amplitude should be increased. Although electrical stimulation produces a substantial improvement in the healing of chronic wounds, further research is needed to identify which electrical stimulation devices and which therapeutic parameters are the most effective (Baker, Chambers, DeMuth, & Villar, 1997; Bayat et al., 2006; Bogie, Reger, Levine, & Sahgal, 2000; Gardner, Frantz, & Schmidt, 1999; Nalty & Sabbahi, 2001).

# Electrode Placement

Electrode placement for NMES will vary depending on what muscle group is being stimulated and the goal of the program. A thorough understanding of the kinesiology, muscle insertion, and innervation of the targeted muscle as well as the underlying pathology is necessary to ensure appropriate response of the tissue. There is a wide variety of potential applications and electrode placements for NMES depending upon the identified goals and objectives. It is recommended that the clinician be familiar

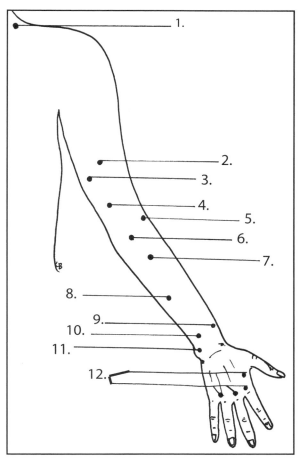

**Figure 9-7.** Neuromuscular electrical stimulation electrode placements—posterior view for stimulation of upper extremity extensor muscles (Illustration by Kim Bartlett, used with permission).

with the parameters of the equipment that they will be using and should familiarize themselves with electrode placements before applying electrical stimulation to patients.

The following electrode placements provide a sampling of possible electrode placements for use with NMES and are intended to serve as a general guide for some of the more common programs used in occupational therapy.

## Electrode Placements and General Parameters

➤ 1 to 12 are located on the posterior arm and are used in stimulating extensor muscles (Figure 9-7).

1. Over the supraspinatus muscle
2. Over the triceps muscle belly
3. Over the long head of the triceps muscles
4. Over the triceps tendon at the musculotendonous junction
5. Between the motor points of the ECU, ECRB, and ECRL muscles
6. Over the lateral epicondyle
7. Motor point of the ECRL

**Figure 9-8.** Neuromuscular electrical stimulation electrode placement for stimulation of upper extremity flexor muscle groups (Illustration by Kim Bartlett, used with permission).

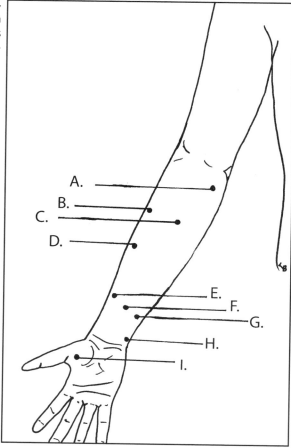

8. Between motor points of EDC and EIP muscles
9. Radial dorsal wrist
10. Dorsal wrist
11. Ulnar dorsal wrist
12. Motor points of posterior interossei muscles

➤ A to H are located on the anterior side and are used in stimulating the flexor muscle groups (Figure 9-8).

A. Between motor points of FCR and FCU
B. Motor point of brachioradialis
C. Between motor points of FDS and FDP
D. Motor point of FPL
E. Radial volar wrist
F. Volar wrist
G. Ulnar volar wrist
H. Ulnar nerve at Guyons Canal
I. Motor point of FPB

# Neuromuscular Electrical Stimulation Treatment Guide

The following protocols are recommended guidelines for the use of NMES. There are a variety of protocols and electrode placements which can be uniquely configured for each patient to meet their specific needs. It is the responsibility of the clinician to determine the appropriate application and use of NMES based on formal evaluation and patient need. For ease and clarity of application, the electrodes are labeled positive and negative. Because the protocols are using a biphasic waveform, the pulse is bidirectional. Either the negative or positive electrode could be placed on either motor point of the protocols unless the muscles are smaller (e.g., in the upper extremity and are more difficult to localize). In these cases, an assymetrical waveform should be used with the active electrode placed over the motor point. Some electrode leads use the colors of black and red, or brown and white. The clinician should review the manufacturer's information on the equipment being used and apply the guidelines based on their equipment (Table 9-1).

## Incorporating Functional Activities with Electrical Stimulation

As with any physical agent, NMES is most effectively used as an adjunct to the occupational therapy plan. NMES will be more effective when combined with voluntary movement facilitating an individual's occupational performance and should always be a consideration. NMES has an extrinsic value to the treatment process, but incorporating active, functional activities, and interventions adds intrinsic value and motivation to the treatment protocol for the patient. Many of the uses of NMES in occupational therapy are based on using the stimulation for functional electrical stimulation and engagement in a specific activity or movement pattern. NMES can be used to facilitate movement and muscular contractions in patients with minimal activity, as well as be used to strengthen or augment weak voluntary movement. Used functionally, NMES can be incorporated to strengthen a particular motor response, such as grasp and release activities of the finger flexors and extensors. NMES is also frequently used as a substitute for shoulder slings, with electrode placement used to strengthen shoulder flexion and abduction.

Treatment protocols for the shoulder may also provide some measure of pain relief to those patients with shoulder/hand syndrome. Patients who display essentially flaccid musculature of the shoulder due to hemiplegia may benefit from stimulation to the posterior deltoid and supraspinatus muscle to increase tone and decrease subluxation.

With any of the upper extremity protocols for strengthening or facilitation, incorporating a hand switch to trigger the stimulation can be an effective method for table activities and for producing functional grasp and release activities. There are some systems such as that offered by the Bioness Company (Santa Clarita, CA) use a static wrist support with surface electrodes and can be triggered automatically or by the therapist to stimulate a specific group of muscles or movements in the forearm (see Figure 9-1).

The Chattanooga Group (Chattanooga, TN) offers an integrated system, the Vectra Genysis, which utilizes both sEMG biofeedback and sEMG activated electrical stimulation. With this system, the patient and therapist can monitor the amount of motor activity and volitionally control the muscle activity and movement using the sEMG biofeedback. This feedback is then paired to the motor response with electrical stimulation. Once a set threshold is reached beyond the point where the patient can not

**Table 9-1**

## RECOMMENDED ELECTRODE PLACEMENTS FOR NMES
## OF THE UPPER EXTREMITY

| Treatment Protocol | Waveform | – Pad Location (motor point=mp) | + Pad Location (dispersive) |
|---|---|---|---|
| Wrist flexion | Asymmetrical biphasic | Small electrode over (A) mp of FCR, FCU | (F) Volar aspect of the wrist |
| Power grasp | Symmetrical biphasic | Small active eletrode over (c) mp between FCS and FDP | (H) ulnar nerve |
| Thumb IP flexion | Asymmetrical biphasic | Small electrode over (D) mp of the FPL | Larger inactive electrode over (F) volar wrist |
| Composite thumb flexion | Symmetrical biphasic | Small electrode over (D) mp of the FPL | (F) volar wrist |
| Lumbricals 3 & 4 | Asymmetrical biphasic | Small electrode over (C) mp btw FDS & FDP | Inactive electrode over (F) volar wrist |
| Combination with power grasp and extrinsic flexion w/ lumbrical 3 & 4 | Asymmetrical biphasic | Small active electrode over (C) btw mp of FDS & FDP and (H) ulnar nerve | Dispersive electrode over (E) and (G) ulnar & radial aspect of volar wrist |
| Wrist extension | Asymmetrical biphasic | Small electrode (5) btw motor points of ECRL, ECRB, and ECU | Large electrode at (1) dorsal wrist |
| Wrist extension with associated EDC facilitation | Asymmetrical biphasic | Small electrode over (5) mp btw ECRB, ECRL, & ECU muscles | Large electrode over (6) lateral epicondyle |
| Digital extension | Asymmetrical biphasic | Small electrode over (8) mp btw EDC & EIP | Large electrode over (10) dorsal wrist |
| Elbow extension | Symmetrical biphasic | Small electrode over (3) mp of the medial head of the triceps | Same size electrode over (4) between the mp of the long head and lateral head of the triceps |

*continued*

**Table 9-1, continued** _____

### RECOMMENDED ELECTRODE PLACEMENTS FOR NMES OF THE UPPER EXTREMITY

| Treatment Protocol | Waveform | − Pad Location (motor point=mp) | + Pad Location (dispersive) |
| --- | --- | --- | --- |
| 1st dorsal interossei | Asymmetrical biphasic | Small electrode placed at (12) the first intrinsic muscle; placement can be modified for the 2nd, 3rd, 4th interossi by moving the smaller electrode over appropriate muscle | Large electrode at (10) dorsal wrist |
| Composite digital and wrist extension | Symmetrical biphasic | Small electrode over (7) mp btw ECRL, ECRB, & ECU | Electrode placed at (8) btw mp of EDC & EIP |
| Wrist extension with grasp (two channels & four leads). Use alternate channel. | Asymmetrical biphasic | Pad placement for wrist extensors and extrinsic digital flexors | Pad placement for wrist extensors and extrinsic digital flexors |

functionally move, the NMES portion of the machine stimulates the targeted muscle completing the movement and strengthening the muscles; thereby, reinforcing the patterns and movements. This biofeedback paired with NMES is particularly effective in those patients who become "stuck" in flexor synergies and which have a tendency to override developing upper extremity extension patterns. With a conventional electrical stimulator, the therapist can use bifurcated leads, effectively targeting up to four muscle groups and facilitating a wide ROM and activities. Creativity and analysis of the movement patterns and activities desired are a necessary component of the evaluation and formative assessment (Figure 9-9).

As the spectrum of conditions and applications for NMES use in the treatment process will vary, the occupational therapist must be creative and adept at analyzing the activity and movement that is being facilitated by the stimulation to determine appropriate interventions. Though the activity and technique may be different for each client, the underlying benefit of greater effectiveness of NMES when combined with functional, active movement will be consistent with nearly all interventions and applications. Patient compliance and engagement in the treatment process and in setting appropriate and achievable goals is vital to success.

## Documentation

As with any other intervention, clear and concise documentation is important to ensure that there is a complete chronological record of the client's condition and

**Figure 9-9.** Chattanooga Group Vectra Genisys 4 Channel electrotherapy system and cart (Photo courtesy of Chattanooga Group).

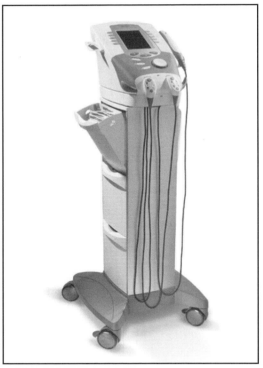

course of intervention. Appropriate documentation aids in facilitating communication with other team members and provides an objective means of determining the appropriateness and effectiveness of the intervention.

Documentation can include a narrative format or more commonly, a SOAP (S=subjective; O=objective; A=assessment; P=plan) format. When documenting the treatment parameters for NMES, the subjective information that is documented should include any subjective information or comments related to the therapist by the patient.

Objectively, the therapist should document the target area being treated and the location of the electrodes; the overall treatment time for the stimulation; the treatment goal or goals with the identified electrode placement; and all of the treatment parameters including the type of device used, on-/off-time, ramp time, and intensity. Specific treatment results or characteristics of the stimulation should also be identified and documented during an activity—volitional contraction or static resistance. Recording the patient's subjective comments and noting any objective

## DOCUMENTATION

- Treatment goal
- Electrode placement
- Treatment time
- On-/off-time
- Ramp time
- Intensity
- Subjective patient comments
- Objective observations related to movement
- Patient response to treatment

changes is also important. As with any therapeutic intervention, the documentation should present an external reader with a clear and concise record of what was done and how the patient responded to the intervention. Making sure that the documentation clearly demonstrates the relationship between the use of NMES and occupational performance areas will also assist in identifying the need and appropriateness of the intervention to external auditors such as third-party payers.

# Summary

NMES can be an effective adjunct in the treatment of a variety of conditions. Unfortunately, it is frequently overlooked by therapists as an adjunctive method to achieve patient goals and to facilitate functional outcomes. Combining sEMG biofeedback and electrical stimulation can strengthen appropriate motor patterns and movements which can improve occupational performance and independence. NMES can facilitate muscle contraction, improve or enhance the development of strength, re-educate muscles, and assist in the training of new muscle function. With less muscle atrophy, the patient displays better ability to voluntarily contract their muscles, leading to better clinical function and facilitating occupational performance.

Indirect benefits of NMES include increased blood flow, improved venous and lymphatic drainage, and the prevention of or loosening of adhesion formation. NMES can be effective in decreasing disuse atrophy, increasing ROM, facilitating functional use of muscles, decreasing tone in spastic musculature, and facilitating muscular contraction. Through evaluation and assessment, the therapist must identify the need and goal of NMES as part of the overall treatment process. NMES should be incorporated into the occupational therapy intervention with regard to the significance and importance of volitional movement and occupation. There are a number of electrical stimulators available on the market, and it is the clinician's responsibility to fully evaluate and understand the equipment that will be used with the client. The clinician also must be aware of the indications and contraindications to the use of NMES to safely and effectively incorporate electrical stimulation into treatment. NMES can be a useful technology and adjunct to occupational therapy, enhancing occupational performance, facilitating independence, and improving patient outcomes.

# Case Study

Mr. P is a 72-year-old male with a right middle cerebral artery thrombosis 5 weeks prior to his initial evaluation. Mr. P was an active individual before the stroke, continuing to farm, garden, and maintain an active lifestyle such as traveling and involvement with his church. Mr. P is married, his wife is in good health, and he has friends and family who live near him and assist him as needed. Mr. P has had good functional return since the initial onset; he is able to ambulate using a quad cane and ankle-foot orthosis (AFO). Assessment reveals active movement in the left upper extremity with better control distally. He has weak finger flexion and extension with weak grasp. Movement at the biceps and triceps is nearly full. Mr. P's primary difficulty is the lack of strength and endurance in the left shoulder. He displays approximately 65 degrees of active shoulder flexion and 70 degrees of abduction. He displays a one finger left shoulder subluxation and has been complaining of pain. A friend told him that he should be wearing a sling to "take the pressure off the shoulder," but he is concerned that his arm will "stiffen" if it is immobilized. He has been working on arm/hand placement activities with moderate success, but decreased endurance in the shoulder has limited his ability. After further assessment of the shoulder integrity, strength, sensation, skin condition, and obtaining a medical history from the patient and his family, treatment using NMES for functional electrical stimulation of the shoulder was implemented.

Therapeutic goals were to decrease the pain in the shoulder, facilitate active shoulder movement, and decrease subluxation and possible dependence on a sling. Sling use should be avoided in this type of patient, because posturally the use of a sling will cause internal rotation and adduction of the arm. FES consisted of active electrode placement over the posterior deltoid on the proximal one-third of the arm. The indifferent electrode was cut and placed to fit over the supraspinous fosa, above the scapula and over the supraspinatus. Intensity was increased to achieve tetany and a strengthening protocol was used. The electrical stimulation facilitated a more normal alignment of the humerus with the glenoid fossa, while allowing free functional use and movement of the forearm and hand. As the strength continued to return in the shoulder, electrode placements to stimulate shoulder flexion and abduction were implemented paired with reaching and grasping activities to reinforce the patterns and gains. For shoulder flexion and abduction, both electrodes were placed on the proximal third of the anterior arm, below the acromium. A space of a minimum of 1 inch was maintained between the electrodes, and intensity was increased to achieve a contraction with a strengthening protocol used. As Mr. P became more independent and functional, he was given a NMES unit for home use and instructed in electrode placement and strengthening protocols. Mr. P was eventually able to actively grasp and reach for objects in a controlled and fluid movement. He gained functional shoulder flexion and abduction to 100 degrees and used the stimulator as needed. With his new-found function, Mr. P was able to brush his teeth again, wash his hair using "both" hands, and began to work in the garden once again.

## Clinical Reasoning Questions

1. What other therapeutic techniques might be beneficial for this patient?
2. What precautions and contraindications would you need to be aware of prior to using NMES?
3. What signs does this patient display that would indicate that he might be a good candidate for use of NMES?
4. What muscle groups and motor patterns would be targeted to facilitate independence and why were these selected?
5. What instructions and training would you provide the patient and family for a home exercise program using electrical stimulation?

# Manufacturers of Electrical Stimulation Devices

The following manufacturers have assisted in the preparation of the chapters on electrotherapy and neuromuscular electrical stimulation through their contribution of materials and information. Many of the manufacturers have information, manuals, and treatment protocols specific to their equipment which is available to the clinician. Therapists are recommended to contact the companies directly or to contact their regional sales representative.

➤ Bioness, Inc.
25134 Rye Canyon Loop, Suite 300
Santa Clarita, California 91355
www.bionessinc.com

➤ Chatanooga Group, Inc.
4717 Adams Road, P.O. Box 489
Hixson, Tennessee 37343-0489
www.chattgroup.com

➤ Dynatronics
7030 Park Centre Drive
Salt Lake City, Utah 84121
www.dynatronics.com

➤ Electro-Med Health Industries
11601 Biscayne Boulevard
Suite 200-A
North Miami, Florida 33181-3151
www.egs-emhi.com

➤ EMPI, Inc.
1275 Grey Fox Road
St. Paul, Minnesota 55112-6989
www.empi.com

➤ Mettler Electronics Corp.
1333 South Claudina Street
Anaheim, California 92805
www.mettlerelectronics.com

➤ Rich-Mar Corp.
P.O. Box 879
Inola, Oklahoma 74036
www.richmarcorp.com

# References

Alon, G. (2003). Use of neuromuscular electrical stimulation in neureorehabilitation: A challenge to all. *Journal of Rehabilitation Research and Development, 40*, ix-xii.

Aoyagi, Y., & Tsubahara, A. (2004). Therapeutic orthosis and electrical stimulation for upper extremity hemiplegia after stroke: A review of effectiveness based on evidence. *Topics in Stroke Rehabilatation, 11*, 9-15.

Baker, L. (1982). Neuromuscular electrical stimulation in the restoration of purposeful limb movements. In S. Wolf (Ed.), *Clinics in physical therapy—electrotherapy* (pp. 25). New York, NY: Churchill Livingstone.

Baker, L. L., Chambers, R., DeMuth, S. K., & Villar, F. (1997). Effects of electrical stimulation on wound healing in patients with diabetic ulcers. *Diabetes Care, 20*, 405-412.

Baker, L. L., & Parker, K. (1986). Neuromuscular electrical stimulation of the muscles surrounding the shoulder. *Physical Therapy, 66*, 1930-1937.

Baker, L. L., Parker, K., & Sanderson, D. (1983). Neuromuscular electrical stimulation for the head-injured patient. *Physical Therapy, 63*, 1967-1974.

Baker, L. L., Yeh, C., Wilson, D., & Waters, R. L. (1979). Electrical stimulation of wrist and fingers for hemiplegic patients. *Physical Therapy, 59*, 1495-1499.

Baldwin, E. R., Klakowicz, P. M., & Collins, D. F. (2006). Wide-pulse-width, high-frequency neuromuscular stimulation: Implications for functional electrical stimulation. *Journal of Applied Physiology, 101*, 228-240.

Bayat, M., Asgari-Moghadam, Z., Maroufi, M., Rezaie, F. S., Bayat, M., & Rakhshan, M. (2006). Experimental wound healing using microamperage electrical stimulation in rabbits. *Journal of Rehabilitation Research and Development, 43*, 219-226.

Becker, W. J., Hayashi, R., Lee, R. G., & White, D. (1987). Modulation of reflex and voluntary EMG activity in wrist flexors by stimulation of digital nerves in hemiplegic humans. *Electroencephalography and Clinical Neurophysiology, 67*, 452-462.

Billian, C., & Gorman, P. H. (1992). Upper extremity applications of functional neuromuscular stimulation. *Assistive Technology, 4*, 31-39.

Binder-Macleod, S. A., & Snyder-Mackler, L. (1993). Muscle fatigue: Clinical implications for fatigue assessment and neuromuscular electrical stimulation. *Physical Therapy, 73*, 902-910.

Bogie, K. M., Reger, S. I., Levine, S. P., & Sahgal, V. (2000). Electrical stimulation for pressure sore prevention and wound healing. *Assistive Technology, 12*, 50-66.

Bowman, B. R., Baker, L. L., & Waters, R. L. (1979). Positional feedback and electrical stimulation: An automated treatment for the hemiplegic wrist. *Archives of Physical Medicine and Rehabilitation, 60*, 497-502.

Butterfield, D. L., Draper, D. O., Ricard, M. D., Myrer, J. W., Schulthies, S. S., & Durrant, E. (1997a). The effects of high-volt pulsed current electrical stimulation on delayed-onset muscle soreness. *Journal of Athletic Training, 32,* 15-20.

Caggiano, E., Emrey, T., Shirley, S., & Craik, R. L. (1994). Effects of electrical stimulation or voluntary contraction for strengthening the quadriceps femoris muscles in an aged male population. *Journal of Orthopaedic and Sports Physical Therapy, 20,* 22-28.

Cameron, T., Broton, J. G., Needham-Shropshire, B., & Klose, K. J. (1998). An upper body exercise system incorporating resistive exercise and neuromuscular electrical stimulation (NMS). *Journal of Spinal Cord Medicine, 21,* 1-6.

Carmick, J. (1997). Use of neuromuscular electrical stimulation and [corrected] dorsal wrist splint to improve the hand function of a child with spastic hemiparesis. *Physical Therapy, 77,* 661-671.

Carmick, J. (1995). Managing equinus in children with cerebral palsy: Electrical stimulation to strengthen the triceps surae muscle. *Developmental Medicine and Child Neurology, 37,* 965-975.

Carmick, J. (1993). Clinical use of neuromuscular electrical stimulation for children with cerebral palsy, part 2: Upper extremity. *Physical Therapy, 73,* 514-22; discussion 523-7.

Carpinella, I., Mazzoleni, P., Rabuffetti, M., Thorsen, R., & Ferrarin, M. (2006). Experimental protocol for the kinematic analysis of the hand: Definition and repeatability. *Gait & Posture, 23,* 445-454.

Chae, J. (2003). Neuromuscular electrical stimulation for motor relearning in hemiparesis. *Physical Medicine and Rehabilitation Clinics of North America, 14,* S93-109.

Chae, J., Fang, Z. P., Walker, M., & Pourmehdi, S. (2001). Intramuscular electromyographically controlled neuromuscular electrical stimulation for upper limb recovery in chronic hemiplegia. *American Journal of Physical Medicine & Rehabilitation, 80,* 935-941.

Chae, J., Yu, D., & Walker, M. (2001). Percutaneous, intramuscular neuromuscular electrical stimulation for the treatment of shoulder subluxation and pain in chronic hemiplegia: A case report. *American Journal of Physical Medicine & Rehabilitation, 80,* 296-301.

Chae, J., Yu, D. T., Walker, M. E., Kirsteins, A., Elovic, E. P., & Flanagan, S. R., et al. (2005). Intramuscular electrical stimulation for hemiplegic shoulder pain: A 12-month follow-up of a multiple-center, randomized clinical trial. *American Journal of Physical Medicine & Rehabilitation, 84,* 832-842.

Chen, Y. L., Chang, W. H., Chen, S. C., Sheu, P. F., & Chen, W. L. (2003). The development of a knee locker with closed-loop functional electrical stimulation (FES) for hemiplegia in gait training. *Disability and Rehabilitation, 25,* 916-921.

Cheng, P. T., Chen, C. L., Wang, C. M., & Chung, C. Y. (2006). Effect of neuromuscular electrical stimulation on cough capacity and pulmonary function in patients with acute cervical cord injury. *Journal of Rehabilitation Medicine, 38,* 32-36.

Chino, N. (1981). Electrophysiological investigation on shoulder subluxation in hemiplegics. *Scandinavian Journal of Rehabilitation Medicine, 13,* 17-21.

Crevenna, R., Marosi, C., Schmidinger, M., & Fialka-Moser, V. (2006). Neuromuscular electrical stimulation for a patient with metastatic lung cancer-a case report. *Supportive Care in Cancer, 14,* 970-973.

Crevenna, R., Stix, G., Pleiner, J., Pezawas, T., Schmidinger, H., & Quittan, M., et al. (2003). Electromagnetic interference by transcutaneous neuromuscular electrical stimulation in patients with bipolar sensing implantable cardioverter defibrillators: A pilot safety study. *Pacing and Clinical Electrophysiology, 26,* 626-629.

Crevenna, R., Wolzt, M., Fialka-Moser, V., Keilani, M., Nuhr, M., & Paternostro-Sluga, T. et al. (2004). Long-term transcutaneous neuromuscular electrical stimulation in patients with bipolar sensing implantable cardioverter defibrillators: A pilot safety study. *Artificial Organs, 28,* 99-102.

Culham, E. G., Noce, R. R., & Bagg, S. D. (1995). Shoulder complex position and glenohumeral subluxation in hemiplegia. *Archives of Physical Medicine and Rehabilitation, 76,* 857-864.

Daichman, J., Johnston, T. E., Evans, K., & Tecklin, J. S. (2003). The effects of a neuromuscular electrical stimulation home program on impairments and functional skills of a child with spastic diplegic cerebral palsy: A case report. *Pediatric Physical Therapy, 15,* 153-158.

Daly, J. J. (2006). Response of gait deficits to neuromuscular electrical stimulation for stroke survivors. *Expert Review of Neurotherapeutics, 6,* 1511-1522.

Daly, J. J., Marsolais, E. B., Mendell, L. M., Rymer, W. Z., Stefanovska, A., Wolpaw, J. R., et al. (1996). Therapeutic neural effects of electrical stimulation. *IEEE Transactions on Rehabilitation Engineering : A Publication of the IEEE Engineering in Medicine and Biology Society, 4,* 218-230.

Daviet, J. C., Salle, J. Y., Borie, M. J., Munoz, M., Rebeyrotte, I., & Dudognon, P. (2002). Clinical factors associate with shoulder subluxation in stroke patients. *Annales De Readaptation Et De Medecine Physique, 45,* 505-509.

de Carvalho, D. C., Martins, C. L., Cardoso, S. D., & Cliquet, A. (2006). Improvement of metabolic and cardiorespiratory responses through treadmill gait training with neuromuscular electrical stimulation in quadriplegic subjects. *Artificial Organs, 30,* 56-63.

de Castro, M. C., & Cliquet, Jr., A. (2000). An artificial grasping evaluation system for the paralysed hand. *Medical & Biological Engineering & Computing, 38,* 275-280.

Delitto, A., & Snyder-Mackler, L. (1990). Two theories of muscle strength augmentation using percutaneous electrical stimulation. *Physical Therapy, 70,* 158-164.

Demir, H., Balay, H., & Kirnap, M. (2004). A comparative study of the effects of electrical stimulation and laser treatment on experimental wound healing in rats. *Journal of Rehabilitation Research and Development, 41,* 147-154.

Detrembleur, C., Lejeune, T. M., Renders, A., & Van Den Bergh, P. Y. (2002). Botulinum toxin and short-term electrical stimulation in the treatment of equinus in cerebral palsy. Movement Disorders, 17, 162-169.

Dromerick, A. W., Lum, P. S., & Hidler, J. (2006). Activity-based therapies. *NeuroRx : Journal of the American Society for Experimental NeuroTherapeutics, 3,* 428-438.

Durfee, W. K., Mariano, T. R., & Zahradnik, J. L. (1991). Simulator for evaluating shoulder motion as a command source for FES grasp restoration systems. *Archives of Physical Medicine and Rehabilitation, 72,* 1088-1094.

Dursun, E., Dursun, N., Ural, C. E., & Cakci, A. (2000). Glenohumeral joint subluxation and reflex sympathetic dystrophy in hemiplegic patients. *Archives of Physical Medicine and Rehabilitation, 81,* 944-946.

Evans, R. D., Foltz, D., & Foltz, K. (2001). Electrical stimulation with bone and wound healing. *Clinics in Podiatric Medicine and Surgery, 18,* 79-95, vi.

Field-Fote, E. C. (2004). Electrical stimulation modifies spinal and cortical neural circuitry. *Exercise and Sport Sciences Reviews, 32,* 155-160.

Gardner, S. E., Frantz, R. A., & Schmidt, F. L. (1999). Effect of electrical stimulation on chronic wound healing: A meta-analysis. *Wound Repair and Regeneration, 7,* 495-503.

Gokkaya, N. K., Aras, M., Yesiltepe, E., & Koseoglu, F. (2006). Reflex sympathetic dystrophy in hemiplegia. *International Journal of Rehabilitation Research, 29,* 275-279.

Gondin, J., Duclay, J., & Martin, A. (2006a). Neural drive preservation after detraining following neuromuscular electrical stimulation training. *Neuroscience Letters, 409,* 210-214.

Gondin, J., Duclay, J., & Martin, A. (2006b). Soleus- and gastrocnemii-evoked V-wave responses increase after neuromuscular electrical stimulation training. *Journal of Neurophysiology, 95,* 3328-3335.

Gorgey, A. S., Mahoney, E., Kendall, T., & Dudley, G. A. (2006). Effects of neuromuscular electrical stimulation parameters on specific tension. *European Journal of Applied Physiology, 97,* 737-744.

Griffin, J. W. (1986). Hemiplegic shoulder pain. *Physical Therapy, 66,* 1884-1893.

Hainaut. (1992).

Han, B. S., Jang, S. H., Chang, Y., Byun, W. M., Lim, S. K., & Kang, D. S. (2003). Functional magnetic resonance image finding of cortical activation by neuromuscular electrical stimulation on wrist extensor muscles. *American Journal of Physical Medicine & Rehabilitation, 82,* 17-20.

Hara, Y., Ogawa, S., & Muraoka, Y. (2006). Hybrid power-assisted functional electrical stimulation to improve hemiparetic upper-extremity function. *American Journal of Physical Medicine & Rehabilitation, 85,* 977-985.

Hesse, S., Brandi-Hesse, B., Bardeleben, A., Werner, C., & Funk, M. (2001). Botulinum toxin A treatment of adult upper and lower limb spasticity. *Drugs & Aging, 18,* 255-262.

Houghton, P. E., Kincaid, C. B., Lovell, M., Campbell, K. E., Keast, D. H., Woodbury, M. G., et al. (2003). Effect of electrical stimulation on chronic leg ulcer size and appearance. *Physical Therapy, 83,* 17-28.

Hunter, J., Mackin, E., & Callahan, A. (1995). *Rehabilitation of the hand: Surgery and therapy* (4th ed., pp. 1508-1519). St. Louis, MO: Mosby.

Kamper, D. G., Yasukawa, A. M., Barrett, K. M., & Gaebler-Spira, D. J. (2006). Effects of neuromuscular electrical stimulation treatment of cerebral palsy on potential impairment mechanisms: A pilot study. *Pediatric Physical Therapy, 18,* 31-38.

Kim, Y., Schmit, B. D., & Youm, Y. (2006). Stimulation parameter optimization for functional electrical stimulation assisted gait in human spinal cord injury using response surface methodology. *Clinical Biomechanics (Bristol, Avon), 21,* 485-494.

Kimberley, T. J., & Carey, J. R. (2002). Neuromuscular electrical stimulation in stroke rehabilitation. *Minnesota Medicine, 85,* 34-37.

Kloth, L. C. (2005). Electrical stimulation for wound healing: A review of evidence from in vitro studies, animal experiments, and clinical trials. *International Journal of Lower Extremity Wounds, 4,* 23-44.

Lake, D. A. (1992). Neuromuscular electrical stimulation. an overview and its application in the treatment of sports injuries. *Sports Medicine (Auckland, N.Z.), 13,* 320-336.

Liu, J., You, W. X., & Sun, D. (2005). Effects of functional electric stimulation on shoulder subluxation and upper limb motor function recovery of patients with hemiplegia resulting from stroke. *Di Yi Jun Yi Da Xue Xue Bao, 25,* 1054-1055.

Lo, S. F., Chen, S. Y., Lin, H. C., Jim, Y. F., Meng, N. H., & Kao, M. J. (2003). Arthrographic and clinical findings in patients with hemiplegic shoulder pain. *Archives of Physical Medicine and Rehabilitation, 84,* 1786-1791.

Lyons, G. M., Leane, G. E., Clarke-Moloney, M., O'Brien, J. V., & Grace, P. A. (2004). An investigation of the effect of electrode size and electrode location on comfort during stimulation of the gastrocnemius muscle. *Medical Engineering & Physics, 26,* 873-878.

Maganaris, C. N., Reeves, N. D., Rittweger, J., Sargeant, A. J., Jones, D. A., & Gerrits, K., et al. (2006). Adaptive response of human tendon to paralysis. *Muscle & Nerve, 33,* 85-92.

Man, I. O., Lepar, G. S., Morrissey, M. C., & Cywinski, J. K. (2003). Effect of neuromuscular electrical stimulation on foot/ankle volume during standing. *Medicine and Science in Sports and Exercise, 35,* 630-634.

Man, I. O., Morrissey, M. C., & Cywinski, J. K. (2007). Effect of neuromuscular electrical stimulation on ankle swelling in the early period after ankle sprain. *Physical Therapy, 87,* 53-65.

Mauritz, K. H. (2004). Gait training in hemiparetic stroke patients. Europa Medicophysica, 40, 165-178.

Michlovitz, S. L. (2005). Is there a role for ultrasound and electrical stimulation following injury to tendon and nerve? *Journal of Hand Therapy, 18,* 292-296.

Moreno-Gimenez, J. C., Galan-Gutierrez, M., & Jimenez-Puya, R. (2005). Treatment of chronic ulcers. *Actas Dermo-Sifilograficas, 96,* 133-146.

Nalty, T., & Sabbahi, M. (2001). Electrical stimulation to promote wound healing. In T. Nalty, & M. Sabbahi (Eds.), *Electrotherapy: Clinical procedures manual* (pp. 105-129). New York: McGraw-Hill.

Ozer, K., Chesher, S. P., & Scheker, L. R. (2006). Neuromuscular electrical stimulation and dynamic bracing for the management of upper-extremity spasticity in children with cerebral palsy. *Developmental Medicine and Child Neurology, 48,* 559-563.

Paci, M., Nannetti, L., & Rinaldi, L. A. (2005). Glenohumeral subluxation in hemiplegia: An overview. J*ournal of Rehabilitation Research and Development, 42,* 557-568.

Park, S. H., & Silva, M. (2004). Neuromuscular electrical stimulation enhances fracture healing: Results of an animal model. *Journal of Orthopaedic Research, 22,* 382-387.

Patel, D. R. (2005). Therapeutic interventions in cerebral palsy. *Indian Journal of Pediatrics, 72,* 979-983.

Pease, W. S. (1998). Therapeutic electrical stimulation for spasticity: Quantitative gait analysis. *American Journal of Physical Medicine & Rehabilitation, 77,* 351-355.

Petrofsky, J., Schwab, E., Lo, T., Cuneo, M., George, J., Kim, J., et al. (2005). Effects of electrical stimulation on skin blood flow in controls and in and around stage III and IV wounds in hairy and non hairy skin. *Medical Science Monitor, 11,* CR309-16.

Phillips, C. A. (1989). Functional electrical stimulation and lower extremity bracing for ambulation exercise of the spinal cord injured individual: A medically prescribed system. *Physical Therapy, 69,* 842-849.

Phillips, C. A., Koubek, R. J., & Hendershot, D. M. (1991). Walking while using a sensory tactile feedback system: Potential use with a functional electrical stimulation orthosis. *Journal of Biomedical Engineering, 13,* 91-96.

Pinedo, S., & de la Villa, F. M. (2001). Complications in the hemiplegic patient in the first year after the stroke. *Revista De Neurologia, 32,* 206-209.

Ralston, D. (1985). High voltage galvanic stimulation: Can there be a "state of the art"? *Athletic Training, 20,* 291.

Renzenbrink, G. J., & Ijzerman, M. J. (2004). Percutaneous neuromuscular electrical stimulation (P-NMES) for treating shoulder pain in chronic hemiplegia. effects on shoulder pain and quality of life. *Clinical Rehabilitation, 18,* 359-365.

Robinson, A., & Snyder-Mackler, L. (1995). *Clinical electrophysiology: Electrtherapy and electrophysiologic testing.* Baltimore, MD: Williams & Wilkins.

Rooney, J. G., Currier, D. P., & Nitz, A. J. (1992). Effect of variation in the burst and carrier frequency modes of neuromuscular electrical stimulation on pain perception of healthy subjects. *Physical Therapy, 72,* 800-6; discussion 807-9.

Santos, M., Zahner, L. H., McKiernan, B. J., Mahnken, J. D., & Quaney, B. (2006). Neuromuscular electrical stimulation improves severe hand dysfunction for individuals with chronic stroke: A pilot study. *Journal of Neurologic Physical Therapy, 30,* 175-183.

Scheker, L. R., Chesher, S. P., & Ramirez, S. (1999). Neuromuscular electrical stimulation and dynamic bracing as a treatment for upper-extremity spasticity in children with cerebral palsy. *Journal of Hand Surgery (Edinburgh, Lothian), 24*, 226-232.

Scheker, L. R., & Ozer, K. (2003). Electrical stimulation in the management of spastic deformity. *Hand Clinics, 19*, 601-6, vi.

Schmidt, H., Sorowka, D., Hesse, S., & Bernhardt, R. (2003). Development of a robotic walking simulator for gait rehabilitation. *Biomedizinische Technik.Biomedical Engineering, 4*8, 281-286.

Selkowitz, D. M. (1985). Improvement in isometric strength of the quadriceps femoris muscle after training with electrical stimulation. *Physical Therapy, 65*, 186-196.

Shi, J. (2005). The research progress of accelerating tendon healing and preventing tendon adhesion. *Chinese Journal of Reparative and Reconstructive Surgery, 19*, 400-403.

Shields, R. K., Dudley-Javoroski, S., & Littmann, A. E. (2006). Postfatigue potentiation of the paralyzed soleus muscle: Evidence for adaptation with long-term electrical stimulation training. *Journal of Applied Physiology, 101*, 556-565.

Smith, G. V., Alon, G., Roys, S. R., & Gullapalli, R. P. (2003). Functional MRI determination of a dose-response relationship to lower extremity neuromuscular electrical stimulation in healthy subjects. *Experimental Brain Research, 150*, 33-39.

Snyder, M. J., Wilensky, J. A., & Fortin, J. D. (2002). Current applications of electrotherapeutics in collagen healing. *Pain Physician, 5*, 172-181.

Stackhouse, S. K., Binder-Macleod, S. A., & Lee, S. C. (2005). Voluntary muscle activation, contractile properties, and fatigability in children with and without cerebral palsy. *Muscle & Nerve, 31*, 594-601.

Sullivan, J. E., & Hedman, L. D. (2004). A home program of sensory and neuromuscular electrical stimulation with upper-limb task practice in a patient 5 years after a stroke. *Physical Therapy, 84*, 1045-1054.

Sun, S., Wise, J., & Cho, M. (2004). Human fibroblast migration in three-dimensional collagen gel in response to noninvasive electrical stimulus. I. characterization of induced three-dimensional cell movement. *Tissue Engineering, 10*, 1548-1557.

Teasell, R. W., Bhogal, S. K., Foley, N. C., & Speechley, M. R. (2003). Gait retraining post stroke. *Topics in Stroke Rehabilitation, 10*, 34-65.

Thawer, H. A., & Houghton, P. E. (2001). Effects of electrical stimulation on the histological properties of wounds in diabetic mice. *Wound Repair and Regeneration, 9*, 107-115.

Trimble, M. H., & Enoka, R. M. (1991). Mechanisms underlying the training effects associated with neuromuscular electrical stimulation. *Physical Therapy, 71*, 273-80; discussion 280-2.

van der Salm, A., Nene, A. V., Maxwell, D. J., Veltink, P. H., Hermens, H. J., & Ijzerman, M. J. (2005). Gait impairments in a group of patients with incomplete spinal cord injury and their relevance regarding therapeutic approaches using functional electrical stimulation. *Artificial Organs, 29*, 8-14.

Van Til, J. A., Renzenbrink, G. J., Groothuis, K., & Ijzerman, M. J. (2006). A preliminary economic evaluation of percutaneous neuromuscular electrical stimulation in the treatment of hemiplegic shoulder pain. *Disability and Rehabilitation, 28*, 645-651.

Wolf, S. L., Ariel, G. B., Saar, D., Penny, M. A., & Railey, P. (1986). The effect of muscle stimulation during resistive training on performance parameters. *American Journal of Sports Medicine, 14*, 18-23.

Yu, D. (2004). Shoulder pain in hemiplegia. *Physical Medicine and Rehabilitation Clinics of North America, 15*, vi-vii, 683-97.

# TRANSCUTANEOUS ELECTRICAL NERVE STIMULATION

## Learning Objectives

1. Define transcutaneous electrical nerve stimulation (TENS).
2. Describe the gate control theory.
3. Discuss the endorphin theory.
4. Identify the types of stimulation programs available for use in TENS.
5. Describe the biophysiological action of TENS.
6. Demonstrate appropriate clinical reasoning in the application and indications for TENS use.

## Terminology

| | |
|---|---|
| Acupunture point | Gate control theory |
| Conventional TENS | Motor point |
| Cranial electrotherapy stimulation (CES) | Subsensory TENS |
| Electroacupuncture | TENS |
| Electrode endogenous opiates | Trigger point |

## Transcutaneous Electrical Nerve Stimulation Theory

TENS is the application of electrical stimulation for pain control. TENS is a generic term used to describe a classification of electrotherapy that applies low-voltage electrical pulses to the nervous system using surface electrodes. There is a great deal of research which indicates that electrical stimulation can modify pain. TENS was developed as a noninvasive technique of afferent stimulation to control and modulate pain. There are a number of theories that have been postulated to explain how pain is transmitted. Many credit the work of Melzack and Wall (1968) for facilitating the development of TENS and pain theory with their Gate Control Theory in the mid-1960s. The two primary theories that postulate the modulation of pain associated with TENS are the *gate theory* and the *endorphin theory (aka opiate-mediated theory)*. Pain is a multidimensional issue and pain management involves controlling the perception and sensation of pain. Use of TENS as a component of pain management provides the therapist with a technology to provide an analgesic (absence of pain) effect that facilitates occupational performance and function.

## Gate Theory

In the mid-1960s, Melzack and Wall (1968) described their gate theory of pain, which further stimulated the interest, development, and manufacture of electrotherapeutic and TENS equipment, and facilitated further research into pain and pain perception. Melzack and Wall hypothesized that stimulation of non-nociceptors or their axons would interfere with the transmission of sensation from nociceptors to the higher cortical areas where pain is perceived. Small-diameter, slow-conducting, nociceptive nerve fibers which have little or no myelin (A-delta, C fibers) transmit painful stimuli to the spinal cord where they are then routed to the brain. These smaller diameter fibers can be inhibited by stimulating the large-diameter, fast-conducting, highly myelinated, and proprioceptive sensory nerve fibers (A-beta fibers). Electrical stimulation may decrease the sensation of pain by increasing the activation of the A-beta fibers, "flooding" the pathway to the brain and closing the gate thereby reducing the transmission of pain to the spinal cord (Melzack, 1965; Melzack & Wall, 1968). As the body becomes habituated, more intense stimulation of the A fibers to keep the gate closed to the pain stimulus is required. The gate control system is thought to be located in a segment of the spinal cord known as the substantia gelatinosia in the specialized T-cells (Jessel & Kelly, 1991; Melzack, 1965).

## Endorphin Theory

The second theory attributed to the effects of TENS is known as the endorphin theory or opiate-mediated theory. An extensive amount of research has come out of the field of neuropharmacology in the past 25 years, contributing greatly to understanding pain. Electrical stimulation of areas proximal to the location of pain or to acupuncture or trigger points decreases or modulates the perception of pain (Melzack, Stillwell, & Fox, 1977). Endorphin theory is based on the discovery of natural opiates which are pain suppressors in the body (Bonica, 1990; Kandel, Schwartz, & Jessel, 1991). These endogenous opiates are the body's own natural pain relievers, and are produced by the pituitary gland and in the spinal cord. The pituitary gland produces beta-endorphins and the spinal cord enkephalins. The neurohumeral/neurotransmitter theory suggests that TENS stimulates the body's production of endogenous opiates that interact with receptors and block the perception of pain. These endogenous opiates are effective at decreasing the perception of pain, and mimic the action of narcotic drugs. When administered with a strong, subnoxious intensity at an adequate frequency, TENS can also decrease reliance on pain medication for postoperative pain (Allais et al., 2003; Benedetti, 2007; Bjordal, Johnson, & Ljunggreen, 2003; Goffaux, Redmond, Rainville, & Marchand, 2007; Grond, Meuser, Pietruck, & Sablotzki, 2002; McGaraughty et al., 2005; Washington, Gibson, & Helme, 2000; Zhang et al., 2004).

## Acupuncture Theory

An additional theory postulated to describe the effectiveness of TENS in the management of pain is related to the energy lines or meridians and associated acupuncture points. Some theorists believe that TENS can be used to stimulate the "entry" or acupuncture points along the same meridians used in traditional acupuncture with a resultant decrease in pain perception. Basic acupuncture points are highly innervated and vascularized regions of the body that may overlie the nerves at their superficial aspects. There are basic acupuncture points for a variety of pain syndromes that may lie on or adjacent to the site of pain or are distant from the site of pain. TENS, when applied to these acupuncture points modifies the flow of energy or "chi" through the body—or the meridians—modifying the perception of pain and altering the underlying condition which may have caused the pain. Acupuncture and trigger points are electrically active and exhibit a decreased resistance to the flow of electrical current. It is beyond the scope of this text to review the foundations of acupuncture and the interested reader is urged to research the topic further (Barlas, Ting, Chesterton, Jones, & Sim, 2006; Hong, 2006; Kawakita et al., 2006; Liu, Ouyang, & Yin, 2006; Wu & Yang, 2006). Trigger points are another area that can be stimulated with TENS in order to modulate pain. Trigger points, particularly those in patients with myofascial pain, may cause tissue ischemia. TENS stimulation causes vasodilation to occur, which modifies the ischemic area and decreases pain (Fernandez-de-Las-Penas, Alonso-Blanco, Cuadrado, & Pareja, 2006; Fernandez-de-Las-Penas, Cuadrado, & Pareja, 2006; Gam et al., 1998; Ge, Fernandez-de-las-Penas, & Arendt-Nielsen, 2006; Melzack et al., 1977; Travell, 1976).

## Treatment Parameters of TENS

TENS has been used to manage pain in a variety of musculoskeletal disorders, including low back pain, arthritis, inflammatory disorders of soft tissue, postoperative pain, and other disease processes. There is some controversy and inconclusiveness with regard to the effectiveness of TENS, though inconsistencies in terminology and treatment parameters may account for the discrepancies. There are a variety of claims and protocols offered by the manufacturers that are anecdotal. However, there is wide variability in both the clinical conditions treated using TENS as well as in the treatment parameters and equipment used to treat pain. The clinician needs to respect the uniqueness of each patient and modify the treatment protocols and parameters appropriately. There are no "right or wrong" answers with TENS use, but more of a "trial and error" approach that should be employed. Treatment applications incorporating electrical stimulation for pain control employ pulsed or alternating currents with a variety of combinations of stimulation patterns. TENS equipment provides the clinician with a wide selection of parameters to choose. TENS technologies and equipment are generally characterized by the pulse amplitude, pulse duration or pulse width, and pulse frequency.

There are four primary types of stimulation programs based on the neurological response to the stimulation either reported by the patient or observed in response to the stimulation. The four types of stimulation commonly used are *subsensory level, sensory level, motor level,* and *noxious level.* These various methods of stimulation occur through the manipulation of the electrical current of the TENS units: the pulse rate/frequency, pulse width/duration, and the intensity or amplitude. Modifying these variables and adjusting the parameters may affect the patient's perception of pain, though there is variability in the research (Chesterton et al., 2002; Chesterton, Foster, Wright, Baxter, & Barlas, 2003; Foster, Baxter, Walsh, Baxter, & Allen, 1996).

### TECHNIQUES OF TENS APPLICATION

- *Subsensory level stimulation/CES*: Pain, depression, anxiety
- *Sensory level stimulation*: Acute/chronic pain during occupational tasks and activities
- *Motor level stimulation*: Longer lasting pain relief after TENS treat ment, joint mobilization
- *Noxious level stimulation*: Debridement, painful procedures, passive stretch, joint mobilization

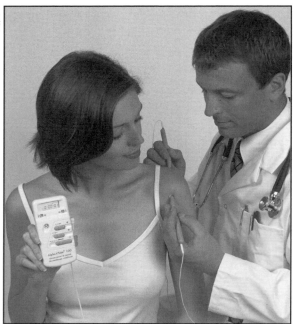

**Figure 10-1.** Microcurrent stimulation. Microcurrent uses a subsensory threshold of electrical current.

## Subsensory Level Stimulation

Subsensory level electrotherapy is also known commercially as microcurrent electrical neuromuscular stimulation (MENS). Subsensory level TENS, may also be referred to as microcurrent electrical therapy (MET) (Figure 10-1). MET uses an electrical current in the microampere range, which is approximately 1,000 times less than that used in conventional TENS applications and below the threshold for sensation. The pulse width or the length of time that the electrical current is being delivered using a microcurrent device is also longer. A microcurrent pulse is approximately 0.5 seconds which is nearly 2,500 times longer than the pulse width in a conventional TENS unit. Subsensory level TENS assumes that microamperage (μA) currents are more effective at enhancing cellular physiology processes. One of the primary premises of microcurrent and its effect on tissue is that "normal" or healthy tissue occurs because of the direct flow of electrical current through the body. When injured, this electrical current flow is disrupted in the affected area with a subsequent cascade of negative events.

Subsensory level stimulation produces currents consisting of the movement of ions in the biological tissues (Hefferman, 1997). These electric currents induced into the tissue are not of sufficient strength or magnitude to produce a recognizable response in the nerve or muscle, and patients do not report any cutaneous sensation or "feeling." Microcurrent helps to realign the flow of electrical current in the body and stimulates the production of ATP, thereby facilitating protein synthesis and tissue healing (Cheng, Van Hoff, & Bockx, 1982).

One of the underlying assumptions of subsensory stimulation is the belief that the body more comfortably and efficiently accepts this low level of electrical energy into its own electrophysiological healing systems. Proponents also contend that the subsensory stimulation closely approximates the naturally occurring bioelectric current found in the body. The low-volt microamperage stimulation is within the range of the body's own physiological currents which enhances comfort and safety (Carley & Wainapel, 1985). Low-level electrical current has also been applied to bone fractures which have been slow to heal and have been found to facilitate bone growth (Spadaro, 1977). Research has been somewhat equivocal with regard to the efficacy of microcurrent in the treatment of pain, as well as TENS (Deyo, Walsh, Martin, Schoenfeld, & Ramamurthy, 1990; Deyo, Walsh, Schoenfeld, & Ramamurthy, 1990; Tan & Thornby, 2000; Tsui & Cheing, 2004; Weber, Servedio, & Woodall, 1994). Additional research on subsensory stimulation using a double blind and placebo-controlled research needs to be completed to further determine the effectiveness of this intervention. (Byl et al., 1994)

Cranial electrotherapy stimulation (CES) is the use of a low-level, pulsed electrical current which is applied to the head primarily for the treatment of both situational and chronic anxiety, depression, insomnia, stress disorders, and drug addiction (Kirsch & Smith, 2000). There is some research that also indicates that it may be useful for treating pain patients, migraine headaches, aggressive behaviors in developmentally disabled individuals, and chronic pain in spinal cord injured individuals (Bronfort et al., 2004; Cameron, Lonergan, & Lee, 2003; Fagade & Obilade, 2003; Gilula & Barach, 2004; Iliukhina et al., 2004; Klawansky, Yeung, Berkey, & Shah, 1994; Lichtbroun, Raicer, & Smith, 2001). CES uses clip electrodes that are attached to the ear lobes. A current of 1 mA or less is used, which is sufficiently strong enough to reach the thalamic area and is sufficient to affect the manufacture and release of neurotransmitters. It should be noted that CES devices use different s than standard mA-current TENS devices. **Standard TENS devices must NEVER be applied transcranially** (Ferdjallah, Bostick, & Barr, 1996). It has been proposed that the effects of CES are primarily mediated through the action on the brain at the limbic system, the hypothalamus, and/or reticular activating system. The reticular activating system regulates electrocortical activity and these are primitive brainstem structures. CES use has been shown to be effective and safe for anxiety and anxiety related disorders. It has also been used for depression and insomnia, muscle tension, decreasing pain in fibromyalgia, reflex sympathetic dystrophy (RSD) or complex regional pain syndrome (CRPS), as well as in treatment of headaches (Alpher & Kirsch, 1998; Smith, 1999; Lichtbroun, Raicer, & Smith, 2001). Further study and research is needed to determine therapeutic parameters and the effect of CES on an individual's occupational performance. Therapists interested in using CES as an adjunct to treatment, should pursue further training and education specific to the use and clinical application of CES (Bronfort, Nilsson, Haas, Evans, Goldsmith, & Assendelft, 2004).

| SUBSENSORY LEVEL PARAMETERS | | |
|---|---|---|
| *Pulse Duration* | *Frequency (pps, bps, Hz)* | *Amplitude* |
| 1 second | < 1 mA | 5 to 20 minute applications, 1 to 3 times daily; subsensory, no noticeable motor or sensory response |

## Sensory Level Stimulation

Sensory level stimulation is also known as "conventional TENS," and consists of stimulation for pain control, which is delivered at pulsed, higher frequencies (50 to 100 pps) with short pulse duration. Conventional TENS is the most commonly used type of TENS and employs amplitudes and durations of stimulation which activate the cutaneous tactile sensory fibers but which are below the motor threshold. Stimulation produces a cutaneous paresthesia (pins and needles) or tingling sensation without muscle contraction if the frequency of stimulation is greater than 10 to 15 pps. Conventional TENS should be considered during the acute stage of injury, but may also be effective for modulating chronic pain. Conventional TENS is based on the gate theory or counter irritation theory, and affects the large afferent (A) fibers, influencing pain transmission. If the frequency of stimulation is less than 7 to 10 pulses per second, patients may experience a "tapping" sensation. The patient's sensory response increases if either the stimulus amplitude or the pulse duration is increased. The most commonly held parameters for sensory level stimulation are in the higher frequencies (50 to 200 pps) with a pulse width of 20 to 100 microseconds (µs). Pulsed or alternating therapeutic currents stimulate the cutaneous sensory primary afferents without a motor response being elicited. Electrode placement should be on or near the location of reported pain. The electrical current is increased to a sensory level perceived by the patient and which is most often a comfortable "tingling" or "buzzing" feeling.

Pain relief is usually of short duration and transient, but can be effective as long as the machine is on and accommodation hasn't occurred. Pain relief is usually noted approximately 5 minutes after initiation of treatment and may last for up to 1 hour when treatment is stopped. The patient should report a reduction or modulation of the pain response with the stimulation, but there is minimal residual analgesia with accommodation frequently occurring (Mannheimer & Lampe, 1984). Because of this, manufacturers of these devices have developed units with current modulators to minimize accommodation during stimulation and which may be left on during the day requiring minimum attention to changing the intensity. Because the unit is on during an extended period of time, these can be used to decrease pain and facilitate performance during occupational tasks. Patients should be instructed to avoid "over-doing it" as their pain threshold may be changed while the stimulation is on, and they may not notice the warning signs of overuse or injury (Figure 10-2).

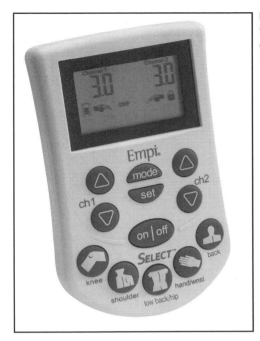

**Figure 10-2.** Select TENS device delivers pain relief through the use of both endorphin release and gate control (Photo courtesy of EMPI Co., Minneapolis, MN).

## SENSORY LEVEL PARAMETERS

| Pulse Duration | Frequency (pps, bps, Hz) | Treatment Time | Amplitude |
|---|---|---|---|
| 50 to 100 µsec | 80 to 100 | 15 to 30 minutes | Tingling, tapping, pins and needles |

**Conditions**: Acute pain, pain associated with positional or dynamic stretch, joint mobilization techniques.

## Motor Level Stimulation

Motor level stimulation occurs when the current becomes strong enough to activate the axons innervating skeletal muscle, causing muscle contractions. Motor level stimulation is often used to treat chronic pain and should produce a noted muscular contraction or fasciculation. Motor level stimulation has also been termed strong low-rate (SLR) or acupuncture like TENS, due to the frequency of stimulation and the concurrent motor level stimulation. Dependent on the frequency stimulation, the tissue response can be one of tremor or twitch-like contractions which occur when the frequency of stimulation is low (<5 pps), or the response can become smooth, isometric, or isotonic tetanic contraction. Increasing the amplitude of the stimulation causes the muscle contractions to become stronger through recruitment of additional motor axons and/or muscle fibers.

Motor level stimulation is characterized by a high amplitude and low frequency, with a frequency below 10 to 20 pps, and typically in the range of 1 to 4 pps. Pulse duration is longer than sensory level stimulation and is most often between a range from 100 to 300 µsec (microseconds). The amplitude should be increased until sufficient to produce strong, visible muscle contraction. Increasing the amplitude to the point of either muscle fasciculation or muscle twitch may be uncomfortable to patients, but should be within their level of tolerance to discomfort. Patients may report a burning or itching feeling during the stimulation. Pain reduction is thought to occur through the gate control theory or more likely due to endorphin release with the duration of analgesia lasting longer than other forms (Low & Reed, 2000). Pain relief may occur approximately 15 to 60 minutes after initiation of treatment with pain relief lasting longer than 1 hour following discontinuation of the treatment. Longer pain relief may be associated with the amount of time it takes the released endorphins to be reabsorbed by the body. Electrodes should be placed over the motor points which correlate with the location of pain or on the segmental nerve roots corresponding with the location of pain and increased until muscle fasciculation is noted (Brosseau et al., 2003; Langley, Sheppeard, Johnson, & Wigley, 1984; Mannheimer & Lampe, 1984).

## MOTOR LEVEL PARAMETERS

| Pulse Duration | Frequency (pps, bps, Hz) | Treatment Time | Amplitude |
|---|---|---|---|
| 150 to 200 μsec | 2 to 10 | 30 to 45 minutes | Muscle twitch, tremor-like, may be smooth, isometric, or isotonic tetantic contraction |

**Conditions**: Used for acute pain conditions and chronic pain conditions.

## Noxious Level (Brief Intense) Stimulation

Noxious level stimulation is known by a number of pseudonyms, including electroacupuncture, hyper-stimulation, or noxious level TENS, and will initially be perceived by the patient as "uncomfortable." These forms of TENS are most often used with chronic pain patients and after other forms of TENS have not been effective in modulating the patient's pain level. Noxious level stimulation can be administered using electrical probe electrodes with a small diameter tip—similar to a pencil in size—or with conventional electrodes. Stimulation can be applied in short applications to acupuncture, motor, or trigger points. In all cases, when the stimulation amplitude is increased to a level which the patient perceives as painful, noxious level stimulation has been reached. Patients will report an uncomfortable or painful stimulus that may be described as burning or needle-like. Noxious stimulation is most often associated with the electrical activation of pain fibers near the site of stimulation and the release of endogenous opiates which modulate the pain perception. The parameters used for noxious level stimulation can produce a motor response, and areas containing superficial motor nerves or motor points should be avoided. Acupuncture meridians which correspond to the painful area can be used as the stimulation points. Brief intense (or noxious) stimulation uses high frequencies of 100 to 200 pps, with pulse duration between 250 to 1000 μsec (Figure 10-3).

Noxious level stimulation is believed to modulate pain through the release of endogenous opiates. Noxious level stimulation produces a surface analgesia of short

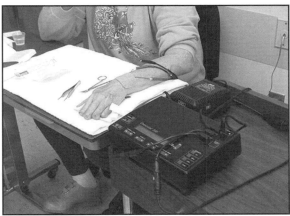

**Figure 10-3.** Noxious level TENS used prior to debridement of digits. Patient is diabetic and underwent amputation to digits following injury caused by "grabbing" her dog's collar.

duration and can be used prior to passive stretch, debridement, or minor surgery. Because noxious level stimulation produces an uncomfortable response, it should be used when other modes of TENS have been unsuccessful. To improve efficacy, patients should also be instructed to remain calm and rested prior to electroacupuncture stimulation parameters (Barlas, Ting, Chesterton, Jones, & Sim, 2006; Fang, Yu, & Li, 1992; He, Lu, Zhuang, Zhang, & Pan, 1985; Liu, 1996).

---

### NOXIOUS LEVEL PARAMETERS

| Pulse Duration | Frequency (pps, bps, Hz) | Treatment Time | Amplitude |
|---|---|---|---|
| 1 ms to 1 sec | 1 to 5 or >100 | 30 seconds per point | Cutaneous paresthesia, noxious may be painful |

**Conditions**: Used for acute or chronic pain syndromes before passive or positional stretching, burn debridement, or minor surgery.

---

## Application and Efficacy

The literature is controversial and unclear on which method of TENS is more effective in the treatment of pain in patients. Rapid development in electrotherapy and increased use of TENS, and the research that followed, occurred in part as an outgrowth of Melzack and Wall's gate theory. Early studies found that TENS use was promising for the reduction of low back pain and overall to modulate pain, but the research lacked consistent terminology and parameter selection and had a variety of methodological and documentation errors and inconsistencies (Farr, Mont, Garland, Caldwell, & Zizic, 2006; Robinson, 1996; Zizic et al., 1995). Ordog (1987) examined the analgesic effect of sensory level TENS on patients with acute traumatic conditions including sprains, lacerations, fractures, and contusions. He concluded that for acute injuries active TENS alone was as effective as Tylenol with codeine in controlling post-traumatic pain. He suggested that active TENS might be the preferred method of pain control in order to avoid the sedative effects of narcotic analgesics.

Other research indicates that TENS inhibits primary hyperalgesia associated with inflammation in a time-dependent manner after inflammation has already developed during both acute and chronic stages (Vance, Radhakrishnan, Skyba, & Sluka, 2007). Denegar (1993) determined that high frequency TENS produced greater reduction in muscle-induced soreness immediately after treatment than low frequency TENS. Denegar and Perrin (1992) also found that TENS and cold produced significantly greater pain relief in delayed onset muscle soreness. Sensory and motor level forms of TENS have been shown to decrease the muscle soreness pain that is often associated with acute inflammatory response. Ainsworth hypothesized that TENS acts through modulating descending influences from supraspinal sites such as rostral ventromedial medulla (RVM) (Ainsworth et al., 2006). Other studies show that the activation of large diameter primary afferents from deep somatic tissues, and not cutaneous afferents, are a factor in causing TENS analgesia (Radhakrishnan & Sluka, 2005). Electroacupuncture TENS has also been shown to decrease pain and improve pain-free hand grip strength in patients with epicondylitis (Tsui & Leung, 2002). Some research is equivocal; MENS, which is subsensory stimulation, does not appear to alter the magnitude of pain in acute inflammatory conditions such as lateral epicondylitis or elbow tendinitis (REFS). However, microcurrent therapy was effective in improving range-of-motion limitations secondary to the late effects of radiation therapy in head-and-neck cancer patients (Lennox, Shafer, Hatcher, Beil, & Funder, 2002). There are no controlled studies demonstrating an analgesic effect of MENS for pain control in acute inflammatory conditions, and further research is needed to optimize microcurrent treatment protocols (Mannheimer & Carlsson, 1979; Robinson, 1996). TENS has also been shown to be effective in the treatment of arthritis, tendinitis, adhesive capsulitis, and for the modulation of pain in aggressive active range of motion programs, multiple sclerosis, and back pain (Al-Smadi et al., 2003; Brosseau et al., 2003; Cannon, 1989; Farr et al., 2006; Mannheimer & Carlsson, 1979; Rizk, Christopher, Pinals, Higgins, & Frix, 1983).

# Interferential Electrical Stimulation

Interferential electrical stimulation (IFS) has also been proposed to be more effective by some clinicians as the current can penetrate deeper due to the interactive effect of the current on the resistance of the skin and superficial tissue. IFS uses two medium frequency electrical currents which are passed through the tissue simultaneously so that their waves cross and intersect causing them to "interfere" with each other. One of the two currents is usually held at 4000 Hz and the other held constant or varied over a range of 4001 to 4100 Hz. High frequency electrical currents are uncomfortable, but because the two electrical currents are delivered out of phase they penetrate through the skin easier and interfere with each other in the deeper tissues where the current crosses (Hansjuergens, 1986; Johnson & Tabasam, 2003a). This amplitude-modulated interference wave has beat frequencies between 1 and 250 Hz, and may induce an analgesic response (Figure 10-4) (Jarit, Mohr, Waller, & Glousman, 2003; Johnson & Tabasam, 2003b).

Interferential currents reportedly can stimulate sensory, motor, and pain fibers. Because of the frequency, the interferential wave meets low impedance when crossing the skin to enter the underlying tissue; therefore, the penetration is deeper. This deep tissue penetration can be adjusted to stimulate parasympathetic nerve fibers for increased blood flow. There are four primary clinical applications for interferential current: *pain relief, muscle stimulation, increased blood flow,* and *edema control.*

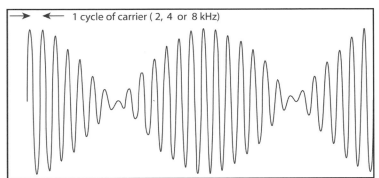

1 cycle of carrier ( 2, 4 or 8 kHz)

**Figure 10-4.** Interferential current waveform.

According to proponents, interferential stimulation differs from TENS because it allows a deeper penetration of the tissue with more comfort which leads to better patient compliance, and increased circulation. This nonlinear effect can lead to more rapid healing. Research, however, has been somewhat equivocal regarding the advantage over more traditional pulsed current or TENS (Cheing & Hui-Chan, 2003; Johnson & Tabasam, 2003b). Parada found that IFS or interferential therapy (IFT), though it has a short-term effect, was effective in decreasing inflammatory pain (Jorge, Parada, Ferreira, & Tambeli, 2006). Further research in the form of well-designed, double-blind studies is required to determine effectiveness of IFC, TENS, and microcurrent devices and to strengthen clinical protocols.

## TENS Electrode Placement

Due to the variability regarding the most effective mode and parameters used for modulating pain in patients, therapists need to be flexible in their selection of TENS technologies and electrode locations. Stimulation sites for electrode placement should be selected based on the problem areas and goals for the patient. Optimal electrode placements should correlate with the initial evaluation which identified the structures and sources of pain. It is important for therapists to consider the degree of skin resistance when selecting electrode sites. An area with greater resistance to the current may require a higher current which is uncomfortable for the patient. There are essentially three identifiable areas that are electrically active and can be used to facilitate current flow into the targeted tissue: *motor points, trigger points*, and *acupuncture points.*

### Motor Points

Peripheral nerves that innervate a painful area and are located superficially can be targeted for direct stimulation. Motor points occur where the peripheral nerve enters the muscle and can also be used as a stimulation point. Less electrical current is necessary to cause a motor response at these areas. Motor points are located in the center of the muscle belly where the motor nerve enters the muscle and a visible contraction is elicited with a minimal amount of stimulation. If a muscle contraction or motor response is desired, electrodes should be placed over the motor point of the selected tissue. The frequency, pulse duration, and intensity should be adjusted to produce the desired clinical response, a muscle twitch, or a tetanic contraction.

### Trigger Points

Areas which are hypersensitive to pressure and electrical stimulation are known as trigger points, and can be located in the skin, fascia, muscle, tendon, ligament, or

**Figure 10-5.** Auricular acupuncture points. These sites can be used with microcurrent (Used with permission of Dr. Daniel Kirsh, Electromedical Products International, Inc. Mineral Wells, Texas).

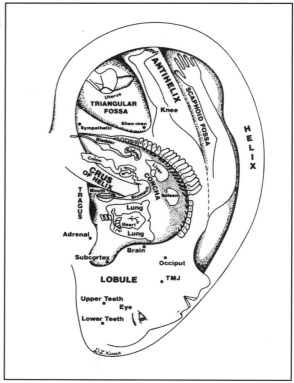

periosteum. Trigger points have a lower resistance to electrical activity and may be painful with compression. Palpation of the trigger point causes referred pain which radiates away from the area and does not always follow a segmental pattern. If the patient displays pain with palpation of the trigger point, the therapist can select the area for electrode placement. Electrodes can be placed over the trigger point or in relation to the zone of referred pain.

## Acupuncture Points

Acupuncture points and the ancient Chinese meridians associated with them can also be used for pain management. Acupuncture points can be targeted along sequential, predefined points, or by treating successive points along the meridian that passes through the painful area. Acupuncture points are located over the entire body and there are a number of charts which have been mapped out to facilitate electrode placement (Barlas, Ting, Chesterton, Jones, & Sim, 2006; Kawakita et al., 2006; Liu et al., 2006).

The acupuncture points and principles are based on thousands of years of Chinese tradition and are identified as meridians. These acupuncture points are highly innervated and vascularized areas that may overlie the nerves at their superficial locations. Electrodes can be placed on a single point or on multiple points concurrently. Stimulation using a predefined sequence of acupuncture points exhibiting a decreased pain threshold along the meridian that passes through the painful area can be also be used (Figure 10-5) (Alimi et al., 2003; Wu & Yang, 2006; Yang, Liu, Kuai, & Gao, 2006).

# Electrodes

The most common adverse reaction to TENS or electrical stimulation is skin irritation. The irritation occurs at the skin-electrode interface and may occur with any of the wide variety of commercially available electrodes. Patients who have sensitivity to adhesive products are the most susceptible. Incidents where patients demonstrate an allergic reaction to an adhesive polymer electrode or who are sensitive and react to the metal snap projection in the center of an electrode should be reported to the manufacturer of the electrodes.

There are a variety of electrode types and sizes that are available, and there is not just one type of electrode that is right for every patient. The primary types of electrodes available include carbon rubber, gel type, or self-adhering. The carbon rubber and gel types of electrodes require the clinician to use a conductive gel and to tape the electrode to the targeted area. Self-adhering electrodes may be single-use or reusable. Patient compliance is usually better when these types of electrodes are used. As a general rule, larger electrodes are used for generalized pain or for multiple electrode setups.

Smaller electrodes are best used for deep localized pain, and smaller self-adhering electrodes may adhere better in certain areas of the body. The density of the current is determined by the size of the electrode with a smaller electrode possessing greater density and producing a greater sensation.

It is vital that the skin is cleaned prior to application of the electrodes. The skin should be washed with water and soap, rinsed, and then blotted dry. Large electrodes should be used on the larger areas of the body, such as the back or leg, and smaller sizes should be used on smaller areas, such as the face and hand. The therapist should use different size electrodes where muscle contractions are easily elicited or hypersensitivity occurs.

Skin burns may occur with excessive stimulation to an area. Burns are more likely to occur with the use of small-area electrodes and care should be used to avoid placing any size electrode too close to another. If there is poor electrical contact between the skin and the electrode, micropunctate burns may occur. Skin irritation and burns may be caused by an improperly applied electrode which does not conform to the contour of the area, or the electrode may lack gel or be too dry. Mechanical stresses caused by the shearing forces between the tape and the skin when the electrodes are removed may also cause an adverse skin reaction. Care should be used when applying tape and the electrodes should be removed from the skin with the movement occurring in the direction that the hair in the region lays. Skin integrity is crucial for effective transmission of the electrical current and should be clean and clear of lesions. Therapists should always carefully inspect the skin for any cuts or disruptions of skin integrity and ensure that the area has normal sensation.

## Electrode Placement

There appears to be a relationship between motor, trigger, and acupuncture points. All are resistant to palpation and can be painful or tender with referred pain. All of these points are electrically active and exhibit a decreased resistance to the flow of electrical energy. This decreased impedance facilitates the flow of electrical current into the tissue and the body. The therapist must be able to identify whether the desired outcome involves a motor response, sensory analgesia, or noxious stimulation for analgesia (Kawakita et al., 2006; Shen, 2001). For initial placement, electrodes can be placed over or contiguous to the site of pain. Stimulation sites also include the tissue overlying the painful area, the superficial points along the peripheral nerves, the specific dermatomes or spinal segmental myotomes, trigger points, motor points, or acupuncture points (Hong, 2006; Johansson, Adolfsson, & Foldevi, 2005; Fernandez-de-Las-Penas, Alonso-Blanco, Cuadrado, & Pareja, 2006). The therapist should monitor the patient's response to the stimulation and move the electrodes to a different site if desired results do not occur (see Appendices A & B).

There are a variety of electrode placements and patterns that can be used with TENS. There are no hard and fast rules regarding electrode arrangements, and therapists should be willing to change their initial electrode placements if the treatment outcomes are less than expected or if the patient experiences pain or discomfort. Electrodes can be placed parallel to the painful site or on either side of a scar or surgical incision; crossed at the site of localized pain; bracketed, which places the electrodes outside the margins of the painful area; or linear, which places the electrodes along the distribution of referred pain, along a peripheral nerve or dermatome. Electrode patterns can be unilateral, bilateral, or contralateral. Electrode patterns that have all electrodes located on the same side of the joint, spine, face, or extremity are referred to as *unilateral*. *Bilateral* electrode placements occur when the electrodes are placed on both sides of a peripheral joint, spine, face, or if the opposite extremity sites are used. *Contralateral* electrode placement is best used when the painful area is irritable or hyperesthetic and inaccessible (see Appendix C).

## Contraindications

Though TENS and electrical stimulation devices provide a safe and effective technology, care should be taken when using electrical stimulation for pain management with some patients, and it is contraindicated for some specific diagnoses and areas (Table 10-1). TENS units should not be used with demand type cardiac pacemakers as it may interfere with their function and performance. Though TENS or electroanalgesia has been used during labor and delivery, the FDA recommends that it not be performed on the trunk or abdomen of pregnant women. Electroanalgesia should also not be applied directly over the eye, in individuals with epilepsy or malignancies, with patients with peripheral vascular disease or infection, or in those with a loss of or decreased sensation.

Electroanalgesia has been used for pain control with patients who have been diagnosed with terminal cancer, but informed consent of the patient should be obtained prior to treatment implementation. TENS is also contraindicated in patients with undiagnosed pain, and electrodes should not be placed over the carotid sinus area or transcerebrally.

Caution should be used when using electroanalgesia on patients with acute pain or immediately postoperatively because the pain serves as a protective function to prevent or to warn of further damage to the tissue or body. TENS use may suppress the sensation of pain which functions as a protective mechanism. As with any medical device or medication, TENS devices should be kept out of the reach of children.

## Table 10-1

### CONTRAINDICATIONS

- Demand-type pacemakers
- Placement over carotid sinus
- Pregnant patients during first trimester
- Anterior neck area
- Cardiac disease (stimulation across the chest)
- Epilepsy (avoid head and neck area)
- Placement over the eyes
- Mucosal surfaces
- Patients with CNS disorders
- Patients with CVAs
- Confused or noncompliant patients
- Children

## CLINICAL CONSIDERATIONS

### Contraindications

- Placement over carotid sinus
- Arterial or venous thrombosis
- Peripheral vascular disease
- Infection
- Decreased sensation
- Pregnancy—over trunk or abdomen
- Never place electrodes transcerebrally
- Undiagnosed pain
- Demand-type cardiac pacemakers
- Over the eyes
- Epilepsy
- Precautions

### Precaution

- Acute pain
- Postoperatively
- Keep out of reach of children
- During occupational tasks or when patients may "over-do" it

# Clinical Reasoning and Application

As with any technology, TENS is used as a part of the overall treatment process. TENS can be a safe and effective adjunct or alternative to traditional pharmacological or surgical interventions when used to modulate pain and facilitate occupational performance. TENS is, however, only one component of the pain modulation continuum. There is a wide variety of equipment, electrode placements, and parameters available, and therapists must be flexible and creative in selecting and applying the technology. As with any intervention, patient compliance and understanding of the treatment and the role TENS may play as a response to the injury or healing process is vital if effective outcomes are to occur.

A thorough evaluation should be completed before the application of TENS to ensure that the intervention is appropriate and indicated for the existing condition. A review of the patient's medical history, pain medications, and a thorough assessment of the patient's presenting condition (including the stage of recovery and level and area of pain) assists in determining treatment alternatives and parameters. The type of pain, length of healing, and psychological reaction and behavior to pain are important characteristics for consideration in the reasoning process. If a patient complains of chronic, generalized pain that is poorly localized and is in response to an injury that occurred months or years ago, the likelihood of positive outcomes for pain modulation using TENS is unlikely. Obtaining a thorough understanding of the individual's occupational performance and the components involved is vital to assist in pain modulation and for preparation for resumption of occupational activities. There are a variety of pain scales available, such as the McGill Pain Questionnaire, and consistent administration of the pain scale assists in determining changes in pain. Before incorporating TENS as part of the treatment protocol, it is important to explain to the patient that TENS itself cannot cure the underlying problem, nor is it the "magic" answer to their pain. Patients who adopt a positive attitude toward the technology and assume responsibility for the intervention will facilitate more positive outcomes.

TENS stimulation is composed of different variables, including pulse rate, pulse width, and intensity. There is no universal agreement as to the optimal TENS mode or electrode placement for a given diagnosis or pathology. Patients, however, do appear to prefer and tolerate low-amplitude conventional TENS, and lower-amplitude formats of other modes such as brief intense, pulse-burst, or modulated. As there are no hard and fast rules governing selection of a specific TENS format, using conventional mode TENS or presetting the duration low and the frequency high are appropriate starting points. Electrodes should be bracketed around the area of pain, or proximal to or on the localized area of pain. When the unit is turned on, the amplitude should be increased until the patient reports a tingling sensation. If there is a good working relationship with the patient and he is accepting of the technology, the patient can adjust the amplitude, self-modulating the sensation and amplitude to the desired sensation. The patient should report a tingling sensation with paresthesia. No muscle response should be noted. Before turning on the TENS, the therapist should preset the pulse duration and frequency. Frequency should be set between 50 to 80 pps, with pulse duration between, 50 to 100 ms. Treatment duration should be a minimum of 20 minutes and a maximum of 60 minutes. Patients should be monitored throughout the course of the treatment with minor adjustments of the stimulation characteristics made as needed. The patient's skin should be examined prior to the implementation of treatment and following the intervention. Stimulation should be discontinued and the electrodes placed in a new location if there is any skin irritation or discomfort.

As with any technology, treatment should be discontinued immediately if the patient is in any distress, or if the patient is unable to tolerate the input. If the patient is able to tolerate the sensation and reports a decrease in pain with an improvement in functional movements, continuation of the stimulation is warranted. If the patient is unable to tolerate the stimulation or is not receiving any decrease in pain, changing the location of the electrodes or readjusting the stimulation parameters may improve the outcome. If the patient continues to complain of discomfort, a different form of TENS should be considered. Other modes of TENS stimulation include acupuncture-like (strong low rate) TENS, brief intense TENS, burst mode (pulse trains) TENS, or hyperstimulation (point stimulation) TENS. Acupuncture-like or strong low rate TENS can be used to provide pain modulation during a chronic phase of pain. Amplitude setting should be strong, yet with a comfortable rhythmic muscle twitch. Frequency is between 1 to 5 pps with pulse duration of 150 to 300 ms. Treatment duration is between 30 to 40 minutes. Brief intense TENS may be used for short-term pain relief and may be most effective prior to painful procedures such as joint mobilization, passive stretch, friction massage, or wound debridement. The amplitude is set to the patient's tolerance, with a frequency between 80 to 150 pps and pulse duration between 50 to 250 ms. Treatment duration is usually short, up to 15 minutes.

The burst mode—or pulse trains TENS—provides characteristics of both high and low rate TENS and may be more tolerable to some patients. The amplitude is set to provide a tingling or paresthesia, with a frequency between 50 to 100 pps, which is cycled in bursts of 1 to 4 pps. The pulse duration is between 50 to 200 ms and the length of the treatment is between, 20 to 30 minutes. Pain relief is usually long lasting with this type of stimulation. Point stimulation or hyperstimulation TENS is used to locate and to stimulate acupuncture or trigger points to a noxious level. As trigger points or acupuncture sites are being targeted, multiple sites may be stimulated depending upon the technique used. The amplitude is strong, and set to the patient's tolerance. Frequency varies from 1 to 5 pps with the pulse duration between 150 to 300 ms. Stimulation continues for 15 to 30 seconds at each point.

Following the treatment, patients should be reevaluated to determine any significant change in their pain level and occupational performance. Use of a pain scale or pain log can assist the patient in tracking changes and assist in determining how long the pain modulation is lasting. Treating acute pain is generally more effective than treating chronic pain and quicker results are seen. Most often, patients will need to use the TENS units at home and they should be receptive and responsible to the use of the equipment. Verbal and written home program instructions should be provided to the patient. Having the patient demonstrate correct use of the equipment in the clinic is necessary. All parameters and controls should be demonstrated to the patient and to any other significant others or family members in order to facilitate patient compliance.

Electrode preparation and placement should be reviewed and anatomical placements highlighted in marker for the patient. Precautions and contraindications should be reviewed and summarized with the patient as well as being documented. A mechanism should be established for patient contact with the department/therapist in case difficulties are encountered, and as with any technology, formative evaluation and specific reevaluation dates should be established prior to the equipment being sent home with the patient.

# Documentation

Documentation for TENS use should include the treatment parameters being utilized, electrode placements, and documentation of any pain scales and drawings. Changes in the patient's condition and subjective reports of sensation during and after the stimulation should be recorded, as well as the type of electrical stimulation, mode of delivery, pulse duration, frequency, intensity, and duration of treatment. Use of a descriptive pain scale or numerical rating scale on a consistent basis aids in reevaluation and adjustments in treatment parameters. Identifying any objective changes in occupational performance and occupational components such as range of motion, improved tolerance or engagement in an activity assist in determining efficacy of the intervention and patient compliance.

# Summary

TENS can be an important adjunct to treatment interventions with patients experiencing pain. Pain is a multifaceted symptom which requires creativity and skill on the part of the therapist to decrease it and facilitate occupational functioning. Because of the variety of equipment, electrode placements, and approaches available to the therapist, patience and persistence in utilizing different TENS modes may be necessary to obtain optimal outcomes for the patient. Careful evaluation and monitoring of the patient's condition is necessary to determine modulation in pain and improvement in occupational performance.

# Case Study

Mrs. M is an active 67-year-old female who was referred for occupational therapy with a diagnosis of status post (s/p) right Colles' fracture, her dominant hand. The injury occurred as a result of a fall from the bottom stair with the patient landing on her flexed wrist. Mrs. M has had the right extremity immobilized in a cast for 6 weeks. The cast was removed 5 days ago. The patient's primary complaints since removal of the cast are "stiffness" and "pain at level 6" on a 1 to 10 pain scale. She has had difficulty "doing anything for myself, even holding onto the fork with my right hand," and the injury and subsequent pain and stiffness have limited her ability to perform basic activities of daily living requiring bilateral movement or stabilization, or any dominant hand activities requiring lifting or prehension. She also complains of her elbow and shoulder "aching" and feeling "stiff and sore." Sensation is intact, though she keeps the extremity in a flexed and guarded position. After evaluating the patient for active movement, AROM and PROM measurements, and circumferential measurements, noting any trophic changes or variations in skin temperature, and examining her x-rays, she is placed on an active treatment program.

Assessment reveals that the impaired function and limitation in occupational performance is due to the fracture and immobilization of the wrist, resulting in pain, swelling, stiffness, and limited motion. Treatment plan includes whirlpool in the initial phase of therapy, ultrasound, gentle joint mobilization, engagement in occupational tasks requiring bilateral hand use, and prehension patterns for the right, and slow, gentle passive stretching. Because the patient reports pain following therapeutic interventions that are stressing the tissue at the end range of motion, and after functional activities, TENS is used as a post-treatment modality with the goal being to decrease the pain. This technology can also be incorporated into the home program to decrease pain, thereby facilitating occupational performance.

## Clinical Reasoning Questions

1. What other clinical condition(s) might have to be ruled out to determine the underlying cause of the patient's pain?

2. What TENS therapeutic parameters might you want to use with this patient?

3. What other physical agents might be effective as part of the treatment process?

4. What precautions might you have to be aware of when using TENS?

5. What electrode placements might you use with this patient and her condition?

# References

Ainsworth, L., Budelier, K., Clinesmith, M., Fiedler, A., Landstrom, R., & Leeper, B. J., et al. (2006). Transcutaneous electrical nerve stimulation (TENS) reduces chronic hyperalgesia induced by muscle inflammation. *Pain, 120*, 182-187.

Alimi, D., Rubino, C., Pichard-Leandri, E., Fermand-Brule, S., Dubreuil-Lemaire, M. L., & Hill, C. (2003). Analgesic effect of auricular acupuncture for cancer pain: A randomized, blinded, controlled trial. *Journal of Clinical Oncology, 21*, 4120-4126.

Allais, G., De Lorenzo, C., Quirico, P. E., Lupi, G., Airola, G., & Mana, O., et al. (2003). Non-pharmacological approaches to chronic headaches: Transcutaneous electrical nerve stimulation, lasertherapy and acupuncture in transformed migraine treatment. *Neurological Sciences, 24*(Suppl 2), S138-42.

Alpher, E., & Kirsch, D. (1998). Traumatic brain injury and full body reflex sympathetic dystrophy patient treated with cranial electrotherapy stimulation. *American Journal of Pain Management, 8,* 124-128.

Al-Smadi, J., Warke, K., Wilson, I., Cramp, A. F., Noble, G., Walsh, D. M., et al. (2003). A pilot investigation of the hypoalgesic effects of transcutaneous electrical nerve stimulation upon low back pain in people with multiple sclerosis. *Clinical Rehabilitation, 17,* 742-749.

Barlas, P., Ting, S. L., Chesterton, L. S., Jones, P. W., & Sim, J. (2006). Effects of intensity of electroacupuncture upon experimental pain in healthy human volunteers: A randomized, double-blind, placebo-controlled study. *Pain, 122,* 81-89.

Benedetti, F. (2007). Placebo and endogenous mechanisms of analgesia. *Handbook of Experimental Pharmacology, 177,* 393-413.

Bjordal, J. M., Johnson, M. I., & Ljunggreen, A. E. (2003). Transcutaneous electrical nerve stimulation (TENS) can reduce postoperative analgesic consumption. A meta-analysis with assessment of optimal treatment parameters for postoperative pain. *European Journal of Pain (London, England), 7,* 181-188.

Bonica, J. (1990). *The managemetn of pain.* Vols I and II. Malvern, PA: Lea & Febiger.

Bronfort, G., Nilsson, N., Haas, M., Evans, R., Goldsmith, C. H., & Assendelft, W. J. et al. (2004). Non-invasive physical treatments for chronic/recurrent headache. *Cochrane Database of Systematic Reviews (Online), 3,* CD001878.

Brosseau, L., Judd, M. G., Marchand, S., Robinson, V. A., Tugwell, P., & Wells, G., et al. (2003). Transcutaneous electrical nerve stimulation (TENS) for the treatment of rheumatoid arthritis in the hand. *Cochrane Database of Systematic Reviews (Online: Update Software), 3,* CD004377.

Byl, N. N., McKenzie, A. L., West, J. M., Whitney, J. D., Hunt, T. K., Hopf, H. W., et al. (1994). Pulsed micro-amperage stimulation: A controlled study of healing of surgically induced wounds in Yucatan pigs. *Physical Therapy, 74,* 201-13; discussion 213-8.

Cameron, M., Lonergan, E., & Lee, H. (2003). Transcutaneous electrical nerve stimulation (TENS) for dementia. *Cochrane Database of Systematic Reviews (Online), 3,* CD004032.

Cannon, N. (1989). Enhancing flexor tendon glide through tenolysis and hand therapy. *Journal of Hand Therapy, 3,* 122-137.

Carley, P. J., & Wainapel, S. F. (1985). Electrotherapy for acceleration of wound healing: Low intensity direct current. *Archives of Physical Medicine and Rehabilitation, 66,* 443-446.

Cheing, G. L., & Hui-Chan, C. W. (2003). Analgesic effects of transcutaneous electrical nerve stimulation and interferential currents on heat pain in healthy subjects. *Journal of Rehabilitation Medicine, 35,* 15-19.

Cheng, N., Van Hoff, H., & Bockx, E. (1982). The effect of electric currents on ATP generation, protein synthesis, and membrane transport in rat skin. *Clinical Orthopedics, 171,* 264-272.

Chesterton, L. S., Barlas, P., Foster, N. E., Lundeberg, T., Wright, C. C., & Baxter, G. D. (2002). Sensory stimulation (TENS): Effects of parameter manipulation on mechanical pain thresholds in healthy human subjects. *Pain, 99,* 253-262.

Chesterton, L. S., Foster, N. E., Wright, C. C., Baxter, G. D., & Barlas, P. (2003). Effects of TENS frequency, intensity and stimulation site parameter manipulation on pressure pain thresholds in healthy human subjects. *Pain, 106,* 73-80.

Childs, A. (2005). Cranial electrotherapy stimulation reduces agression in a violent retarded population: A preliminary report. *Journal of Neuropsychiatry and Clinical Neurosciences, 17,* 548-551.

Denegar, C. (1993). The effects of low-volt microamperage stimulation on delayed onset muscle soreness. *Journal of Sports Rehabilitation, 1,* 95-102.

Deyo, R. A., Walsh, N. E., Martin, D. C., Schoenfeld, L. S., & Ramamurthy, S. (1990). A controlled trial of transcutaneous electrical nerve stimulation (TENS) and exercise for chronic low back pain. *New England Journal of Medicine, 322,* 1627-1634.

Deyo, R. A., Walsh, N. E., Schoenfeld, L. S., & Ramamurthy, S. (1990). Can trials of physical treatments be blinded? the example of transcutaneous electrical nerve stimulation for chronic pain. *American Journal of Physical Medicine & Rehabilitation, 69,* 6-10.

Fagade, O. O., & Obilade, T. O. (2003). Therapeutic effect of TENS on post-IMF trismus and pain. *African Journal of Medicine and Medical Sciences, 32,* 391-394.

Fang, Z., Yu, Q., & Li, Y. (1992). The role of peripheral C afferent fiber in electroacupuncture analgesia. *Acupuncture Research, 17,* 48-53.

Farr, J., Mont, M. A., Garland, D., Caldwell, J. R., & Zizic, T. M. (2006). Pulsed electrical stimulation in patients with osteoarthritis of the knee: Follow up in 288 patients who had failed non-operative therapy. *Surgical Technology International, 15,* 227-233.

Ferdjallah, M., Bostick, F. X.,Jr., & Barr, R. E. (1996). Potential and current density distributions of cranial electrotherapy stimulation (CES) in a four-concentric-spheres model. IEEE *Transactions on Bio-Medical Engineering, 43,* 939-943.

Fernandez-de-Las-Penas, C., Alonso-Blanco, C., Cuadrado, M. L., & Pareja, J. A. (2006). Myofascial trigger points in the suboccipital muscles in episodic tension-type headache. *Manual Therapy, 11,* 225-230.

Fernandez-de-Las-Penas, C., Cuadrado, M. L., & Pareja, J. A. (2006). Myofascial trigger points, neck mobility and forward head posture in unilateral migraine. *Cephalalgia: An International Journal of Headache, 26,* 1061-1070.

Foster, N. E., Baxter, F., Walsh, D. M., Baxter, G. D., & Allen, J. M. (1996). Manipulation of transcutaneous electrical nerve stimulation variables has no effect on two models of experimental pain in humans. *Clinical Journal of Pain, 12,* 301-310.

Fregni, F., Boggio, P. S., Nitsche, M. A., Marcolin, M. A., Rigonatti, S. P., & Pascual-Leone, A. (2006). Treatment of major depression with transcranial direct current stimulation. *Bipolar Disorders, 8,* 203-204.

Gam, A. N., Warming, S., Larsen, L. H., Jensen, B., Hoydalsmo, O., & Allon, I., et al. (1998). Treatment of myofascial trigger-points with ultrasound combined with massage and exercise--a randomised controlled trial. *Pain, 77,* 73-79.

Ge, H. Y., Fernandez-de-las-Penas, C., & Arendt-Nielsen, L. (2006). Sympathetic facilitation of hyperalgesia evoked from myofascial tender and trigger points in patients with unilateral shoulder pain. *Clinical Neurophysiology, 117,* 1545-1550.

Gilula, M. F., & Barach, P. R. (2004). Cranial electrotherapy stimulation: A safe neuromedical treatment for anxiety, depression, or insomnia. *Southern Medical Journal, 97,* 1269-1270.

Goffaux, P., Redmond, W. J., Rainville, P., & Marchand, S. (2007). Descending analgesia - when the spine echoes what the brain expects. *Pain, 130*(1-2), 137-43.

Grond, S., Meuser, T., Pietruck, C., & Sablotzki, A. (2002). Nociceptin and the ORL1 receptor: Pharmacology of a new opioid receptor. *Der Anaesthesist, 51,* 996-1005.

Hansjuergens, A. (1986). Interferential current clarification. *Physical Therapy, 66,* 1002.

He, L. F., Lu, R. L., Zhuang, S. Y., Zhang, X. G., & Pan, X. P. (1985). Possible involvement of opioid peptides of caudate nucleus in acupuncture analgesia. *Pain, 23,* 83-93.

Hong, C. Z. (2006). Treatment of myofascial pain syndrome. *Current Pain and Headache Reports, 10,* 345-349.

Iliukhina, V. A., Kozhushko, N. I., Matveev, I., Ponomareva, E. A., Chernysheva, E. M., & Shaptilei, M. A. (2004). Transcranial micropolarizations in combined treatment of speech and general psychomotor development retardation in children of the senior preschool age. *Zhurnal Nevrologii i Psikhiatrii Imeni S.S., 104, 34*-41.

Jarit, G. J., Mohr, K. J., Waller, R., & Glousman, R. E. (2003). The effects of home interferential therapy on post-operative pain, edema, and range of motion of the knee. *Clinical Journal of Sport, 13,* 16-20.

Jessel, T., & Kelly, D. (1991). Pain and analgesia. In E. Kandel, J. Schwartz & T. Jessel (Eds.), *Principles of neural science.* (3rd ed., pp. 385-399). New York: Elsevier.

Johansson, K. M., Adolfsson, L. E., & Foldevi, M. O. (2005). Effects of acupuncture versus ultrasound in patients with impingement syndrome: Randomized clinical trial. *Physical Therapy, 85,* 490-501.

Johnson, M. I., & Tabasam, G. (2003a). An investigation into the analgesic effects of interferential currents and transcutaneous electrical nerve stimulation on experimentally induced ischemic pain in otherwise pain-free volunteers. *Physical Therapy, 83,* 208-223.

Johnson, M. I., & Tabasam, G. (2003b). A single-blind investigation into the hypoalgesic effects of different swing patterns of interferential currents on cold-induced pain in healthy volunteers. *Archives of Physical Medicine and Rehabilitation, 84,* 350-357.

Jorge, S., Parada, C. A., Ferreira, S. H., & Tambeli, C. H. (2006). Interferential therapy produces antinociception during application in various models of inflammatory pain. *Physical Therapy, 86,* 800-808.

Kandel, E., Schwartz, J., & Jessel, T. (1991). *Principles of neural science.* New York: Elsevier.

Kawakita, K., Shinbara, H., Imai, K., Fukuda, F., Yano, T., & Kuriyama, K. (2006). How do acupuncture and moxibustion act? Focusing on the progress in Japanese acupuncture research. *Journal of Pharmacological Sciences, 100,* 443-459.

Kirsch, D., & Smith, R. (2000). The use of cranial electrotherapy stimulation in the management of chronic pain. A review. *NeuroRehabilitation, 14,* 85-94.

Klawansky, S., Yeung, A., Berkey, C., & Shah, N. (1994). Meta-analysis of randomized controlled trials of cranial electrotherapy stimulation: Efficacy in treating selected psychological and physiological conditions. *Journal of Nervous and Mental Diseases, 183,* 478-485.

Langley, G. B., Sheppeard, H., Johnson, M., & Wigley, R. D. (1984). The analgesic effects of transcutaneous electrical nerve stimulation and placebo in chronic pain patients. A double-blind non-crossover comparison. *Rheumatology International, 4,* 119-123.

Lennox, A. J., Shafer, J. P., Hatcher, M., Beil, J., & Funder, S. J. (2002). Pilot study of impedance-controlled microcurrent therapy for managing radiation-induced fibrosis in head-and-neck cancer patients. *International Journal of Radiation Oncology, Biology, Physics, 54,* 23-34.

Lichtbroun, A. S., Raicer, M. M., & Smith, R. B. (2001). The treatment of fibromyalgia with cranial electrotherapy stimulation. *Journal of Clinical Rheumatology, 7,* 72-78.

Liu, X. (1996). The modulation of cerebral cortex and subcortical nuclei on NRM and their role in acupuncture analgesia. *Acupuncture Research, 21,* 4-11.

Liu, Y. S., Ouyang, Y. Y., & Yin, Y. (2006). Clinical application of electroacupuncture plus chinese medicine in treatment of peripheral facial paralysis. *Chinese Acupuncture & Moxibustion, 26,* 259-260.

Low, R., & Reed, A. (2000). *Electrotherapy explained: Principles and practice.* Oxford, UK: Butterworth-Heinemann.

Mannheimer, J., & Lampe, G. (1984). *Clinical transcutaneous electrical nerve stimulation.* Philadelphia, PA: F.A. Davis.

Mannheimer, C., & Carlsson, C. A. (1979). The analgesic effect of transcutaneous electrical nerve stimulation (TNS) in patients with rheumatoid arthritis. A comparative study of different pulse patterns. *Pain, 6,* 329-334.

McGaraughty, S., Honore, P., Wismer, C. T., Mikusa, J., Zhu, C. Z., & McDonald, H. A., et al. (2005). Endogenous opioid mechanisms partially mediate P2X3/P2X2/3-related antinociception in rat models of inflammatory and chemogenic pain but not neuropathic pain. *British Journal of Pharmacology, 146,* 180-188.

Melzack, R. (1965). Pain mechanisms: A new theory. *Science, 150,* 971-977.

Melzack, R., Stillwell, D. M., & Fox, E. J. (1977). Trigger points and acupuncture points for pain: Correlations and implications. *Pain, 3,* 3-23.

Melzack, R., & Wall, P. (1968). The gate control theory of pain. In A. Soulairac, J. Cahn, & J. Carpentier (Eds.), *Pain: Proceedings of the international symposium on pain.* London: Academic Press.

Ordog, G. (1987). Transcutaneous electrical nerve stimulation versus oral analgesic: A randomized double blind controlled study in acute traumatic pain. *American Journal of Emergency Medicine, 5,* 6-10.

Radhakrishnan, R., & Sluka, K. A. (2005). Deep tissue afferents, but not cutaneous afferents, mediate transcutaneous electrical nerve stimulation-induced antihyperalgesia. *Journal of Pain, 6,* 673-680.

Rizk, T. E., Christopher, R. P., Pinals, R. S., Higgins, A. C., & Frix, R. (1983). Adhesive capsulitis (frozen shoulder): A new approach to its management. *Archives of Physical Medicine and Rehabilitation, 64,* 29-33.

Robinson, A. J. (1996). Transcutaneous electrical nerve stimulation for the control of pain in musculoskeletal disorders. *Journal of Orthopaedic and Sports Physical Therapy, 24,* 208-226.

Rogers, D. R., Eli, S., Rogers, K. R., & Cross, C. L. (2007). Evaluation of a multi-component approach to cognitive-behavioral therapy (CBT) using guided visualizations, cranial electrotherapy stimulation, and vibroacoustic sound. *Complementary Therapies in Clinical Practice, 13,* 95-101.

Shen, J. (2001). Research on the neurophysiological mechanisms of acupuncture: Review of selected studies and methodological issues. *Journal of Alternative and Complementary Medicine, 7*(Suppl 1), S121-7.

Spadaro, J. A. (1977). Electrically stimulated bone growth in animals and man. Review of the literature. *Clinical Orthopaedics and Related Research, 122,* 325-332.

Tan, G., & Thornby, J. (2000). Efficacy of microcurrent electrical stimulation on pain severity, psychological distress and disability. *American Journal Pain Management, 10,* 35-44.

Travell, J. (1976). Myofascial trigger points: Clinical view. In J. J. Bonica, & D. G. Able-Fessard (Eds.), *Advances in pain research and therapy* (2nd ed., pp. 919). New York: Raven Press.

Tsui, M. L., & Cheing, G. L. (2004). The effectiveness of electroacupuncture versus electrical heat acupuncture in the management of chronic low-back pain. *Journal of Alternative and Complementary Medicine, 10,* 803-809.

Tsui, P., & Leung, M. C. (2002). Comparison of the effectiveness between manual acupuncture and Electroacupuncture on patients with tennis elbow. *Acupuncture & Electro-Therapeutics Research, 27,* 107-117.

Vance, C. G., Radhakrishnan, R., Skyba, D. A., & Sluka, K. A. (2007). Transcutaneous electrical nerve stimulation at both high and low frequencies reduces primary hyperalgesia in rats with joint inflammation in a time-dependent manner. *Physical Therapy, 87,* 44-51.

Washington, L. L., Gibson, S. J., & Helme, R. D. (2000). Age-related differences in the endogenous analgesic response to repeated cold water immersion in human volunteers. *Pain, 89,* 89-96.

Weber, M. D., Servedio, F. J., & Woodall, W. R. (1994). The effects of three modalities on delayed onset muscle soreness. *Journal of Orthopaedic and Sports Physical Therapy, 20,* 236-242.

Wu, Z. G., & Yang, Z. G. (2006). On key role of acupoints in elongated needle therapy. *Chinese Acupuncture & Moxibustion, 26,* 685-686.

Yang, H. Y., Liu, T. Y., Kuai, L., & Gao, M. (2006). Electrical acupoint stimulation increases athletes' rapid strength. *Chinese Acupuncture & Moxibustion, 26,* 313-315.

Zhang, R. X., Lao, L., Wang, L., Liu, B., Wang, X., & Ren, K., et al. (2004). Involvement of opioid receptors in electroacupuncture-produced anti-hyperalgesia in rats with peripheral inflammation. *Brain Research, 1020,* 12-17.

Zizic, T. M., Hoffman, K. C., Holt, P. A., Hungerford, D. S., O'Dell, J. R., & Jacobs, M. A. et al. (1995). The treatment of osteoarthritis of the knee with pulsed electrical stimulation. *Journal of Rheumatology, 22,* 1757-1761.

# IONTOPHORESIS

## Learning Objectives

1. Describe the clinical applications for iontophoresis.
2. Discuss the physical concepts and mechanisms related to the transdermal delivery of medication.
3. Describe the physical concepts and terminology of ion movement.
4. Identify common medications used in iontophoresis treatment.
5. Outline clinical decision-making regarding the indications and precautions in the use of iontophoresis as part of the treatment process.

## Terminology

| | |
|---|---|
| Anode | Ion transfer |
| Cathode | Iontophoresis |
| Dermis | Polarity |
| Dosage | Stratum corneum |
| Epidermis | Transdermal |

Iontophoresis is a method of topically delivering medication or ionized drugs into a localized area of tissue by using the force of direct electrical current to create a therapeutic effect. Iontophoresis is a safe and effective way to administer medication because it is essentially painless, nontraumatic, sterile, and relatively noninvasive. Iontophoresis is used by a number of health care professionals in dentistry, dermatology, otorhinolaryngology, and ophthalmology to treat a variety of conditions and has grown in popularity and clinical use by occupational therapists (Banga & Chien, 1998; Glass, Stephen, & Jacobson, 1980).

Occupational therapists frequently utilize iontophoresis to treat inflammatory conditions or to modify scar tissue and manipulate the healing process. It is important for the occupational therapist to have a basic understanding of the mechanism underlying iontophoresis to safely and effectively use it as an adjunct to treatment. Additionally, the occupational therapist should possess a fundamental grounding in the wound healing process and the pathophysiology of the specific diagnoses which are to be treated with iontophoresis. Because we are often using controlled medications and substances in the treatment process there is an inherent responsibility by the occupational therapist to be fully aware of the appropriate indications, dosing, and potential drug interactions. The occupational therapist must also be cognizant of the wide variety of medications and their therapeutic and physiological effects as well as the method of application to ensure a positive clinical outcome.

# History

Iontophoresis is the process of introducing a topically applied medication into the epidermis or mucous membranes of selected tissue (Singh & Maibach, 1993). Literature related to iontophoresis dates as far back as the late 1700s and 1800s. The concept of iontophoresis and ion transfer has been in existence and in use since LeDuc discovered in 1908 that ions could be driven across the skin through the application of an electrical current (LeDuc & MacKenna, 1908). Iontophoresis has grown in popularity with the advent of technological advances of miniaturization and computerization of equipment, as well as the development of effective electrodes to contain the chemicals and facilitate ion transfer. In the past, difficulty with electrodes, lack of electrical safety, and lack of standardization of equipment caused an increased risk of burns and inhibited the widespread use of iontophoresis in the clinic. With greater research and a better understanding of the mechanisms involved in iontophoresis, the risk to the patient has decreased and applications of the treatment technique have grown.

Uses for iontophoresis include administration of local anesthesia, topical application of antibiotics, and, most commonly for occupational therapists, administration of drugs and steroids. A benefit to using iontophoresis is that the medication remains relatively local to the treatment area and is not absorbed in the gastrointestinal tract thereby avoiding some of the complications related to oral medication. In addition, the risk of infection from injections has been eliminated and potential side effects minimized. Iontophoresis can now be performed in a relatively short period of time with positive clinical outcomes and can be an effective alternative to needle injections and oral administration of drugs. When properly applied, medications can be delivered directly to the treatment site without the complications or disadvantages of parenteral delivery. Iontophoresis is also an efficient therapeutic technique because the rate in which drugs are administered can easily be controlled and will remain relatively consistent between treatments (Kanikkannan, 2002; Merino, Kalia, & Guy, 1997). The four basic components of an iontophoretic system include the power source for generating the controlled direct current, the drug containment and dispersive electrodes, the medications, and the skin. However, the skin is considered an unknown variable.

# Biophysiology

Iontophoresis is an active transdermal method in which medications or ionized drugs are topically delivered into localized areas of tissue with direct electrical current Transdermal drug delivery has been widely used in the past to introduce various medications into selected tissue through the skin. Because of certain characteristics of the skin and its permeability, not all medications can be effectively administered this way. The skin effectively acts as a barrier, allowing very few drugs or chemicals to be delivered through the skin. To overcome this barrier and facilitate the movement of the drugs into the tissue, iontophoresis is used. Skin is approximately 3 to 5 mm thick and is composed of three layers: *the epidermis, dermis*, and *hypodermis*.

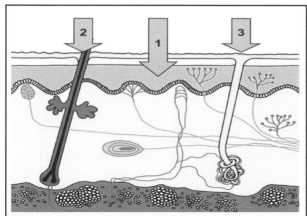

**Figure 11-1.** Hair follicles sweat, and sebaceous glands provide a second entrance into the body for medications. These normal openings in the skin extend deeper through the epidermis, into the dermis, and are more permeable and proximal to the vascular supply (Used with permission from Skin Care Forum, Issue 37, Cognis Deutschland. GmbH & Co. KG, www.scf-online.com).

The primary impediment to the effective penetration of the drug through the skin is the stratum corneum. The stratum corneum is the lipid-rich outermost layer of the epidermis (Christopher, Schebert, & Goos, 1989; Kalia, Naik, Garrison, & Guy, 2004). If the medication is able to penetrate this layer, it then becomes able to passively diffuse into the underlying subcutaneous tissue. There are two primary methods that allow the drug access to the underlying tissue: movement between the intercellular matri, and through the normal openings of the skin.

The skin is relatively permeable to lipophilic or lipid soluble chemicals and acts as a barrier to water-soluble or hydrophilic substances. This lipid layer can be envisioned as the "mortar" between bricks. Small lipophilic molecules are able to pass through this intercellular matrix. The openings found in the normal openings of the skin, such as hair follicles, sweat glands, and sebaceous glands, provide a second entrance into the body for chemicals. Hair follicles, sweat glands, and sebaceous glands extend deeper through the epidermis, into the dermis, and are more permeable and proximal to the vascular supply (Figure 11-1). Applying direct current to the skin assists in moving the chemicals into the subcutaneous tissue (Kalia, Merino, & Guy, 1998; Trommer & Neubert, 2006).

# Basic Principles

The outer layer of the epidermis, the stratum corneum, is composed of cells called *corneocytes,* which are separated by free fatty acids creating a lipid environment. Because of this composition, the stratum corneum becomes an effective barrier to water and other ionic substances, effectively keeping water within the body and preventing foreign material from entering. Iontophoresis delivers ionic drugs across this barrier because the charged drugs help to carry the current to complete an electrical circuit (Riviere & Heit, 1997; Roberts, 1999). Essentially, the direct electrical current moves the ions in a particular direction. The primary physics principle that makes iontophoresis successful is that like charges repel and opposite charges attract. The charged drugs are repulsed by an electrode of the same charge. This can be visualized if you recall taking two magnets and placing the same end together (e.g., positive: positive or negative: negative). When the magnets are placed same end-to-end, the ends of the magnet push the like-charged end of the magnet away.

**Figure 11-2.** Electrical current repels like charged medications into the underlying tissue, crossing the stratum corneum (Used with permission from Skin Care Forum, Issue 37, Cognis Deutschland. GmbH & Co. KG, www.scf-online.com).

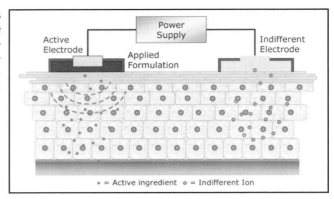

Ions possessing a positive charge can be moved into the epidermis by the positive electrode, and ions which possess a negative charge are propelled by the negative electrode. The negatively charged electrode is known as the cathode, repelling negatively charged ions. The positively charged electrode is known as the anode, repelling positively charged ions. When the electrical current is applied to the electrodes and medication, it repels the negative or positive ions away from the common pole toward the opposite pole facilitating the movement of the ions into the underlying tissue (Riviere & Heit, 1997). When the medication molecules have crossed the outer layer of the skin, the stratum corneum, the drug proceeds to disperse to all local tissues with the highest concentration of the medication being located in the tissues closest to the treatment (electrode) site (Anderson, Morris, Boeh, Panus, & Sembrowich, 2003). Concentrations of the medication are decreased as it moves further away from the electrode (Figure 11-2).

The effectiveness of iontophoresis is dependent on the number of ions transferred, the depth of penetration, the combining of ions chemically with other substances in the skin, and the ability of the individual ion to enter the body (Roberts, 1997; Sanderson, de Riel, & Dixon, 1989). Skin and fat are poor conductors of the electrical current and will resist the flow of the electrical current. Treatment in areas where there are large amounts of adipose tissue or thickened skin may require a higher level of electrical current and care must be taken to monitor the skin condition around the negative electrode due to the chemical changes which occur. Ion penetration extends approximately 1 mm below the electrode surface. The chemical effects from the introduced medication will extend to deeper levels by capillary action and through the biophysical conductance of the current (Kahn, 1995; Trommer & Neubert, 2006; Wang, Thakur, Fan, & Michniak, 2005).

# Application

The typical iontophoresis unit consists of a power source, a "working" or medicated electrode, and an indifferent electrode. Commercially available units, such as Empi's Dupel (St. Paul, MN) and Iomed's Phoresor (Salt Lake City, UT), are small battery powered units which deliver a direct current adjustable by the therapist. The working or active electrode consists of a chamber where the drug is contained (Figure 11-3). The medication or ion which is to be used should be in a charged form and water soluble or in a lipid medium. The indifferent electrode completes the circuit of current. The

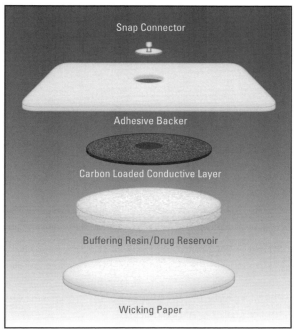

Snap Connector

Adhesive Backer

Carbon Loaded Conductive Layer

Buffering Resin/Drug Reservoir

Wicking Paper

**Figure 11-3.** Dupel's iontophoresis electrode with the drug reservoir. The electrodes come in various sizes and should be selected based on the area of tissue to be treated.

polarity of the active or medicated electrode should consist of the same polarity of the medication desired to deliver to the tissue. Though there is some passive diffusion of the oppositely charged ions, it is not as effective as using the appropriate pole. Like poles repel and unlike poles attract.

The size of the ion also influences the ion delivery. Smaller ions with a lighter molecular weight have a tendency to move quicker and more freely. Larger ions move slower and may be too large to be effectively used with iontophoresis (Glass et al., 1980; Hasson, Wible, Reich, Barnes, & Williams, 1992) The anode (+) produces an acid reaction, with the cathode (-) producing an alkaline reaction. The anode, which is positive, is sclerotic; it hardens tissue and acts as an analgesic. The negatively charged cathode is sclerolytic; it acts as a softening agent and can be used clinically for the management of scars and burns. Most of the commercial electrode pads, such as Empi Corporation, use buffered pads which decrease the acid/alkali buildup at the anode and cathode and could cause chemical burns due to excessive buildup of the chemicals.

The medication being used, should be water soluble and labeled, "…FOR INJECTION, USP" The amount of medication that should be applied to the drug containment reservoir is printed on the electrode packaging. The electrode should be hydrated according to the manufacturer's recommendations so that dry spots will not occur and the electrode will not be overfilled (Figure 11-4). After the medication has dissolved in water or a water-soluble gel, it should be placed on or under the delivery electrode and the delivery electrode should then be positioned on the target area. A dispersive pad should also be placed over a major muscle at least 4 to 6 inches away from the drug electrode.

The ion will penetrate the local subcutaneous tissues and superficial muscles, and enter the systemic circulation when the polarity of the medicated electrode is the same as the ion. After the molecules of the medication have crossed the stratum

**Figure 11-4.** Dosing an iontophoresis medication patch. Each medicated reservoir should be filled according to the manufacturer's recommendation. Avoid overfilling the medicated reservoir.

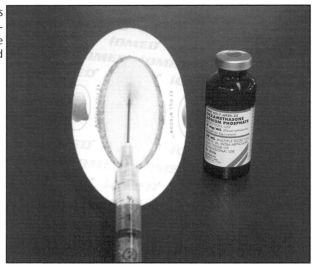

corneum, the drug will disperse to all local tissues and the highest concentration will reside in the tissues that are closest to the treatment (electrode) site.

# Dosage

In iontophoresis, dosage is measured in milliamp-minutes, which is calculated by multiplying the milliamps of the current by the minutes or length of treatment: dosage = milliamps x mins. There are two primary variables affecting the number of ions transported to the tissue, the current amplitude (dosage = mA x mins), and the duration of the current flow (dosage = mA x mins). It is not the volume of the fluid or medication that is being delivered to the underlying tissue, but the ions that are being transported. The volume of the medication being measured into the electrode reservoir does not directly affect the number of ions which are transported, nor does the size of the electrode. Increasing the size of the medicated electrode effectively increases the total treatment area; however, the amount of medication delivered will be the same. The amount of drug delivered to the tissue is determined by the current and the duration of the treatment (current x time).

The volume of medication, assuming it is of the same concentration, will not affect the amount of ions delivered. The significant variables affecting dosage are the current and duration. It is not the total current, but the current density, which determines if a small, safe, and comfortable amount of current is being applied. Most of the commercial units available deliver a maximum current of 4 mA (Anderson et al., 2003). Therapists should use caution in ramping up the maximum current to avoid the possibility of the patient having an allergic reaction to the direct current, known as a galvanic rash. Galvanic rash may occur in those patients with a hypersensitivity to direct current. Ramping up the current too quickly may also be uncomfortable to the patient.

Current density is dependent on the surface area of the electrode and is determined by dividing the current amplitude by the total area of the electrode. To prevent skin irritation or burning, a lower current density, such as $0.5$ mA/cm$^2$, should be used and is effective in transmitting the medication. Many protocols use a current density from

2 mA up to 4 mA, and the clinician should set the parameters based on client tolerance and comfort rather than speed of treatment. There has been some question whether the medication is able to cross the skin barrier and reach a therapeutic level when driven into the tissue quicker than 15 mins (Ting, Vest, & Sontheimer, 2004; Trommer & Neubert, 2006). Further research is necessary to determine the most effective treatment times. A good rule of thumb is to set the current density to patient tolerance, most often making the treatment time between 20 to 30 mins.

There are a number of manufacturers making electrodes and iontophoresis units including Iomed's Phoresor, Empi's Dupel, Life-Tech's Iontophor (Lifetech, Inc., Stafford, TX), and Henley International's Dynaphor (Henley Intl., Sugarland, TX). Most of the current equipment automatically ramp up and ramp down the current, modulate the electrical current, automatically shut off at the end of each treatment, monitor skin resistance, display the treatment status, allow treatment pauses, provide audible and visual alerts, and activate other safety measures through preprogrammed current and time limits. However, the direct current power source, drugs, and electrodes must be used according to the manufacturer's technical guidelines to ensure that the results will be safe, effective, and reproducible. Another treatment option for application of iontophoresis consists of a "patch" with a medicated containment system and a self-contained battery that produces an electric current to carry drug molecules across the skin to underlying tissue (see Figure 11-4). The drug delivery system shuts off automatically when the prescribed dosage of medication has been delivered. These patch delivery systems are single-use and disposable with no external batteries or wires. Because they are self-contained and are worn for approximately 6 to 8 hours before the full dose of drug is delivered, they allow the patient to engage in their daily activities while receiving time-released iontophoresis.

# Indications

Iontophoresis is an effective method of intervention which can be applied to a variety of conditions typically treated by occupational therapists. Most often, iontophoresis is used in the treatment of inflammatory conditions. Equipment manufacturers and researchers have identified a number of other diagnoses and interventions for which iontophoresis is effective, including local anesthesia to decrease joint pain and inflammation and for musculoskeletal inflammatory conditions. Conditions most frequently seen by occupational therapists, and which respond well to the medications and intervention, include carpal tunnel syndrome, epicondylitis, ulnar nerve inflammation, elbow strain/sprain, radiohumeral bursitis, triceps tendinitis, glenohumeral bursitis, hand and wrist tendinitis/tenosynovitis, and DeQuervain's disease (Backstrom, 2002; Banta, 1994; Baskurt, Ozcan, & Algun, 2003; Boskovic, 1999; Cabello Benavente et al., 2005; Riedl, Plas, Engelhardt, Daha, & Pfluger, 2000; Schiffman, Braun, & Lindgren, 1996; Yarrobino, Kalbfleisch, Ferslew, & Panus, 2006). Some manufacturers have developed diagnosis-specific treatment and medication protocols that may be utilized in patient care; however, treatment parameters should always be specific to the patient and the therapist should understand the underlying pathophysiology of the disease and the medications used. It should also be noted that many of the protocols and reports lack the control of structured research, are anecdotal, and should be used with caution.

**Figure 11-5.** Application of iontophoresis for bilateral trigger finger.

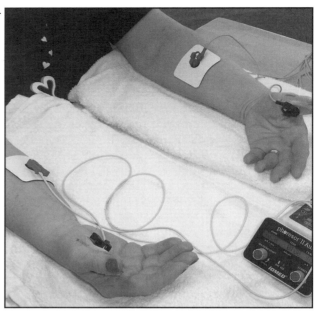

# Medications

There are a large variety of drugs and medications that can be administered using iontophoresis. Therapists should be familiar with the pharmacology, drug interactions, and contraindications of any medications used as part of treatment. A thorough evaluation and patient history should be taken that takes not of current medications the patient may be taking and any known allergies or allergic reactions to medications. Drugs used for iontophoresis must be water-soluble and ionized. Commercially available drugs manufactured by reputable pharmaceutical companies are recommended. Any medications used for iontophoresis should be manufactured to the standards set forth in the U.S. Pharmacopeia (USP) as they will contain the correct stabilizers and preservatives insuring potency and stability until the drug's expiration date. All medication should be discarded by the expiration date on the drug's label. If a sharps needle system is used to transfer the medication from the drug vial to the electrode, it should be appropriately discarded following use. NEVER recap or reuse any needle syringes (see Figure 11-4). Any questions regarding the medications used, their indications, and contraindications should be discussed with the physician or pharmacist before use. Reviewing the electrode manufacturer's recommendations for medication use specific to their electrodes should also be done before using iontophoresis. Medications used must be compatible with the material chosen by the manufacturer for the conductive element. Some combinations of drugs and the elements in the reservoir pad may produce undesirable results and outcomes.

Dexamethasone iontophoresis is perhaps the most widely-applied medication used by therapists due to its anti-inflammatory action. Iontophoresis has been shown to relieve pain and inflammation in tendonitis, osteoarthritis, synovitis, and patellofemoral joint and musculoskeletal problems, and in reducing scar tissue (Aygul, Ulvi, Karatay, Deniz, & Varoglu, 2005; Chandler, 1998; Dakowicz & Latosiewicz, 2005; DuPont, 2004; Gokoglu et al., 2005; Huida, 1998; Schuhfried & Fialka-Moser, 1995; Ting

& Sontheimer, 2001; Williams & Brage, 2004). Use of local anesthetics, such as lidocaine for pain relief, is also a common technique used by the therapist and is based, in part, on anecdotal evidence and research in dentistry and otolaryngology (ears, nose, and throat). Combining the anti-inflammatory benefits of dexamethasone with the anesthetic function of lidocaine is frequently employed. However, there is some controversy as to the effectiveness of this combination due to the negative polarity of the dexamethasone and the positive polarity of the lidocaine (Haga, Shibaji, & Umino, 2005; Pasero, 2006; Russo, Lipman, Comstock, Page, & Stephen, 1980; Sintov & Brandys-Sitton, 2006; Yarrobino, Kalbfleisch, Ferslew, & Panus, 2006). When combining these two drugs, they may "piggy-back" with each other and limit the effectiveness of either or both of the medications. With co-iontophoresis of medications, switching the polarity during the treatment may facilitate more effective penetration of both drugs (Bogner & Banga, 1994; Kassan, Lynch, & Stiller, 1996). A 2% sodium chloride solution has been effective for its sclerotic function on scars and adhesions, while a 2% acetic acid solution has been used for decreasing calcific deposits (Kahn, 1995; Kahn, 1977).

---

## COMMONLY USED DRUGS FOR IONTOPHORESIS

### Clinical Condition—Inflammation

**Glucocorticoids**: Inhibit the synthesis of proinflammatory substances such as prostoglandins and leukotrienes. Inhibit the migration of scavenger WBC's to the site of inflammation.

- *Dexamethasone*: Negative Polarity
- *Decadron*: Negative Polarity

**NSAIDS**

- *Ketaprofen*: Negative Polarity
- *Mecholyl*: Positive Polarity
- *Acetic Acid*: Negative Polarity
- *Voltaren (Diclofenac Sodium)*: Negative Polarity (0.5% to 1%)
- Naprosyn *(Naproxen Sodium)*: Negative Polarity (4% to 8%)

### Clinical Condition—Pain

**Lidocaine** produces an anesthetic effect by blocking the transmission of impulses along the peripheral nerve axons. Sodium channels are bound thus blocked.

**Salicylate** is a potent inhibitor of the enzyme that produces prostaglandins, thereby controlling pain and inflammation.

**Opiods** act on neurons in the CNS to impair the transmission and perception of stimuli.

- *Lidocaine*: Positive Polarity
- *Salicylate*: Negative Polarity
- *Morphine*: Positive Polarity
- *Ketoprofen*: Negative Polarity
- *Magnesium*: Positive Polarity

*continued*

continued from previous page

### Clinical Condition—Scar Tissue and Adhesions

Iodine has a sclerolytic effect though the cellular basis for this action is not clearly defined; has also been shown to increase the extensibility of scar tissue.

- *Iodine*: Negative Polarity
- *Saline*: Negative Polarity (Sodium Chloride)

### Clinical Condition—Soft Tissue Mineralization

The **acetate ion,** which is negatively charged, combines with the insoluble calcium carbonate to form the soluble compound, calcium acetate. This compound is more readily dispersed from the affected tissue by localized blood flow.

- *Acetic Acid*: Negative Polarity (Acetate)

### Clinical Condition—Wounds, Infection

Use of iontophoresis can deliver high doses of antibacterial drugs through the eschar into the underlying avascular tissue. **Zinc** has a bactericidal effect and ability to facilitate tissue growth and repair. It may interfere with metabolic activities in microbial cells, and facilitate tissue healing through zinc's ability to precipitate proteins.

- *Zinc*: Positive Polarity
- *Gentamycin*: Positive Polarity
- *Penicillin*: Negative Polarity

# Indications

As with any therapeutic intervention, the therapist should be well versed in the pathology and physiology of the patient's condition. Understanding what physiological reaction is needed will assist in identifying which medication and ion to use. Therapists should remain current with the changes in medications, precautions and contraindications of the medications selected, and should periodically review product information and new research before applying iontophoresis or any modality. Each patient will bring a unique perspective to the pathology and should be carefully evaluated to determine optimal treatment goals and therapeutic parameters. Selection of the correct ion and the corresponding polarity is vital to obtaining effective outcomes.

Iontophoresis has been shown to be effective for a variety of disorders based in part on the practice emphasis of the researcher or clinician. Dentists have used iontophoresis for treatment of temperomandibular joint disease (TMJ); ENT's have used a 2% copper solution for treating allergic rhinitis; and a 20% zinc oxide ointment has been used to facilitate healing for otitis, dermatitis, ulcerations, and open lesions. The most frequent use of iontophoresis in physical medicine and rehabilitation is for inflammation and for local anesthesia.

# Inflammatory Conditions

Iontophoresis is widely used and indicated in the treatment of localized inflammation. Delivery of water-soluble corticosteroids can be used for many of the inflammatory conditions affecting joints and soft tissue. Corticosteroids are powerful and economical anti-inflammatory agents that will slow the initial movement of both neutrophils and monocytes to an inflammation site and inhibit their rate of activity. Corticosteroids are frequently used to treat acute, inflammatory, and musculoskeletal conditions, as well as well-localized, point-specific injuries. Several corticosteroids are available as $H_2O$ soluble salts that can cause molecules to become negatively charged. Since corticosteroids can inhibit the inflammatory process by decreasing migration into an inflamed area, white blood cell activity is also reduced. Corticosteroids can reduce the "sprouting" that occurs in sensory nerves associated with tissue injury and can minimize systemic side effects such as weight gain, muscle weakness, and behavioral changes. Corticosteroids that are commonly used with iontophoresis include 4 mg/mL dexamethasone sodium phosphate and methyl prednisone sodium succinate.

Iontophoresis can be used for inflammatory conditions of the extremities, spine, or the TMJ. The most commonly-used medication for treating inflammatory conditions using iontophoresis is a 0.4% dexamethasone sodium phosphate with the drug electrode polarity being negative. The dispersive pad polarity should be positive with the recommended dosage for patients with sensitive skin being 2 mA x 12 mins = 24 mA-mins for a small electrode such as the TransQ (IOMED, Salt Lake City, UT) or Dupel Blue (EMPI, St. Paul, MN) which holds 1.5 cc of corticosteroid in the reservoir. For a local anesthetic effect, many therapists use a 4% lidocaine hydrochloride solution. The lidocaine provides a local anesthetic effect for immediate pain relief (Haga et al., 2005; Pasero, 2006; Yarrobino, Kalbfleisch, Ferslew, & Panus, 2006). The amount of medication drawn up and placed into the electrode is dependent on the size of the drug electrode. A small drug electrode holds 1.5 cc of medication with the drug electrode polarity being positive, the dispersive pad polarity being negative. The recommended dosage is 40 mA/mins.

Some therapists will want to combine the two medications for the benefits of both the anesthetic effect and the anti-inflammatory benefits. The medications utilized would be the corticosteroid (0.4% for injection, USP) combined with the local anesthetic of 4.0%. For treatment with both medications, the drug electrode polarity would be negative, with the therapist alternating the polarity of the drug electrode to positive to ensure greatest absorption of both medications. When combining drugs for delivery in iontophoresis, one drug will most often be delivered more effectively than the other and the concentrations of the medications should be adjusted. To achieve an equal dose of a large and small drug, the concentration of the larger, less mobile drug should be increased (Banga & Chien, 1998).

Discussing the medications and their chemical components with the pharmacist helps to ensure the safety, currency, and efficacy of the medication and the treatment.

As most pharmacists dispense IV solutions used for iontophoresis, commercially available products from reputable companies should be used to ensure their purity, concentration, stability, and potential interactions (Batheja, Thakur, & Michniak, 2006; Dixit, Bali, Baboota, Ahuja, & Ali, 2007; Gangarosa, Park, Fong, Scott, & Hill, 1978). Patients should always be questioned as to any known allergies, reactions, or sensitivities to foods or medications. Patients have been known to have a variety of reactions to medications, including anaphylaxis, which can be life threatening. This condition is considered a medical emergency, and should be responded to immediately. Though most often safe and effective, therapists need to recognize that they are introducing potent medications into the patient, and utmost care should and precautions should be taken. **Documented orders from the patient's physician for iontophoresis should always be obtained prior to using iontophoresis**, and any questions or concerns should be directed to the referring physician.

# Precautions and Contraindications

Patients with known sensitivity or allergy to the medications being administered should never have *iontophoresis*. The potential for an *anaphylactic reaction* can be great. Contraindications for the specific medications being used should also be researched by the therapist. Therapists should make sure to discuss with the pharmacist the medications being prescribed by the physician and any related questions. Confirmation of the treatment protocol should be confirmed with the physician. Therapists should refer to the *Physicians Desk Reference*, and should read and keep on file the brochure which comes with each medication.

Care should be used with patients who are pregnant or may be pregnant, as the safety and effectiveness of some medications have not been adequately established. It is better to err on the side of caution! Patients with diabetes who are insulin dependent may notice fluctuations in their blood sugar levels after treatment with corticosteroids. Care should be used when working with diabetic patients who are poorly controlled. Patients should always be asked if they have any known food allergies or sensitivities, particularly those sensitive to sulfites, which are a preservative. Patients with allergies to shellfish may also react to Iodex (GlaxoSmithKline, Philadelphia, PA), which is used for scar management. Iontophoresis should never be placed over skin that is irritated.

---

## CLINICAL CONSIDERATIONS

### Precautions

- Sensitivity to ions
- Abnormal localized reaction of skin
- Drug sensitivities
- Known allergies

### Contraindications

- Known sensitivity or allergies to medication or ions being applied
- Application over skin irritation, bruises, lacerations
- Impaired or absent sensation
- All contraindications identified for electrical stimulation

**Remember: Anaphylaxis is a medical emergency!**

---

# Guide to Application

As with any therapeutic intervention, informing the patient is primary. Properly positioning the patient is important, and the patient should never lie on an electrode, as the area being treated may burn. The therapist should prepare the skin surface by trimming any excess hair with scissors to ensure proper adhesion of the electrodes. Any jewelry should be moved if it could come into contact with the electrodes. Electrode sites should never be shaved due to the possibility of skin irritation. Use of

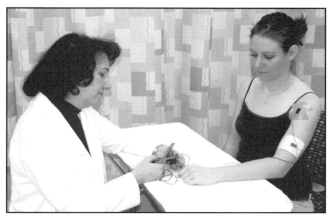

**Figure 11-6.** Iontophoresis application. The medicated electrode is placed over the targeted tissue. Intensity should be set to the patient's tolerance with longer durations providing more comfort.

creams, gels, or other modalities prior to iontophoresis may cause skin irritation and limit drug penetration (Figure 11-6).

1. Hydrate the drug electrode. Use water-soluble 4 mg/mL or 0.4% corticosteroid, frequently labeled "...for injection, USP" It is important that the drug electrode be sufficiently filled to avoid dry spots that may cause some of the units such as the Dupel to shut down or it may cause skin irritation under the electrode.

2. Prepare the electrode sites by cleaning the areas vigorously with alcohol, allowing the skin to dry completely. Do not apply the electrodes if the skin is irritated; apply only on intact skin. Therapists should note the dryness of the skin, excessively oily skin, and the humidity, all of which can influence the resistance of the skin and the effectiveness of the drug delivery.

3. Apply the electrodes. Place the drug electrode on the primary site to be treated. The dispersive electrode should be placed over a major muscle approximately 4 to 6 inches away from the medicated electrode. Binding or compressing the electrodes by using tape or weights should be avoided during treatment.

4. Connect the lead clips to the electrodes. Make sure that the clips are oriented appropriately and keep the clips clean and dry. Avoid pulling on the leads during the treatment and when removing the clips from the electrodes.

5. Begin the treatment. Set the parameters, dependent on the equipment being used. Set the time, set the current, slowly ramping the current up to patient tolerance. Using a lower dosage reduces the chances of skin irritation. Have the patient remain still throughout the session. Most of the equipment available today has dual channels, so the therapist can effectively target two areas for iontophoresis if necessary.

6. After the treatment, a soothing lotion which is nonirritating and has a neutral pH such as aloe-vera gel should be applied to the area. The patient should be well instructed in appropriate skin care, and the therapist should note any erythema or skin breakdown that may occur. If the skin is not intact or lesions develop, iontophoresis should be discontinued or the frequency decreased (Iomed, 1994).

Most protocols recommend administering iontophoresis every other day to minimize the skin irritation from the direct current and to take advantage of the carryover effect or half-life of the dexamethasone from the previous treatment. The patient should notice a decrease in pain or symptomatology after approximately 4 to 6 treat-

**Table 11-1**

| COMMONLY USED IONS FOR INTOPHORESIS | | |
|---|---|---|
| *Medication* | *Therapeutic Indications* | *Polarity* |
| Lidocaine hydrochloride | Analgesia; bursitis, neuritis | + |
| 1% & 2% Sodium salicylate | Analgesia; plantar warts | - |
| Hyaluronidase (Wydase) | Swelling; sprains, strains | + |
| Tap water | Hyperhidrosis of palms/feet | +/- |
| 2% Copper sulfate | Antibacterial, fungicidal; athlete's foot | + |
| 2% Acetic acid solution | Calcium deposits, calcific tendonitis myositis, ossificans; musculoskeletal conditions | - |
| 1 mL 0.4% Decadron dexa-methasone sodium phosphate | Anti-inflammatory, osteoarthritis, bursitis, tendonitis | - |

ments, and the acute inflammation should also subside during that period. If the patient shows continued improvement, the treatment may continue for an additional 9 to 12 sessions if needed. Doubling the amount of medication will have no clinical significance and the treatment should be stopped if the patient is not getting at least 50% relief.

# Summary

Iontophoresis is the application of direct electrical current to enhance drug delivery of ionic drugs from aqueous solutions. Iontophoresis provides a localized concentration of a medication to the tissue while avoiding the difficulties of systemic effects. Iontophoresis can be safely and effectively used with patients who are fearful of the pain associated with intramuscular needle injections. Benefits of iontophoresing medications into specific tissues include the fact that the medication can be delivered to a larger area than for an injection. Using iontophoresis in conjunction with traditional modalities and interventions may provide quicker reduction in patient symptoms, thereby facilitating occupational function. Additionally, the treatment is repeatable, which allows for a longer period of therapeutic exposure to the medication, thereby facilitating therapeutic benefits and outcomes (Backstrom, 2002; Banta, 1994; Gudeman, Eisele, Heidt, Colosimo, & Stroupe, 1997) (Table 11-1).

# Case Study

T. S. is a 41-year-old dental assistant with a diagnosis of right lateral epicondylitis. The patient has been taking nonsteroidal anti-inflammatory drugs (NSAIDs) for the past 6 weeks before being referred to occupational therapy. The patient reports that the medication has provided mild relief, but her symptoms of pain following work or homemaking tasks has continued. The patient reports that she is now having pain and discomfort at rest and when she rolls onto the arm when sleeping. She relates that symptoms are less severe after waking; but that she "hurts more" as the day progresses. She rates her pain during activities at a 7/10, with the pain described as a "constant toothache" in the arm. She does have numbness and tingling in the hand with overuse. She has had increasing difficulty manipulating the equipment at the office. Her occupational tasks at work require her to use both hands to assist the dentist and to manipulate small objects requiring precise movements and static holds. She spends much of the day reaching across the patient or with her arms fully extended, reaching and transferring tools and materials. She has begun to use her nondominant left hand since she is worried that she will drop something while assisting.

Assessment reveals intact skin integrity with the posterior forearm warmer to the touch with a "boggy" feeling. Circumferential measurements reveal a 7-cm increase over the nondominant extremity. This discrepancy may be due to increased muscle bulk of the dominant arm, but wrist and MCP measurements are minimally different. ROM measurements reveal wrist flexion 0 to 55 degrees, wrist extension, 0 to 50 degrees. Pronation is within normal limits (WNL) with supination 0 to 70 degrees. Finger, elbow, and shoulder ROMs are all WNL. Muscle strength is 4/5 with pain on resisted wrist extension. Grip strength on the left is 80#, 45# on the right. There are also noticeable differences in pinch strengths between the dominant and nondominant hand. She exhibits increased pain, with palpation along the lateral epicondyle and the radiohumeral joint. Joint distraction and anterior-posterior glides are restricted.

The patient's signs and symptoms are consistent with lateral epicondylitis, with point tenderness over the extensor tendon origin, pain with wrist loading in extension, and limited wrist movement. The patient is educated in work modification and joint protection techniques, including a HEP requiring icing of the elbow as needed after her patients. She is provided with a soft wrist splint for the right and instructed to wear during the day when manipulating objects or when in a static position. Treatment plans include ice massage and iontophoresis using 0.4% dexamethasone sodium phosphate with the drug delivery electrode placed over the area of point tenderness. TS noted marked improvement following the third treatment using iontophoresis. She remarked that she was, "finally able to sleep without pain waking me up." Because of her improvement, a full course of nine applications of iontophoresis was continued.

Iontophoresis was used to decrease the inflammation and was used as a component of the treatment protocol including stretching exercises and joint mobilization. When the inflammation was decreased and the symptoms abated, involvement in occupational activities simulating the work related movements were implemented to strengthen the weakened muscles and to problem solve possible ergonomic adaptations and movements.

## Clinical Reasoning Questions

1. What was the underlying cause of the injury?
2. What phase of healing was the injured tissue in and how was this determined?
3. What other physical agents might be appropriate to use with this patient?
4. What signs and symptoms did the patient display to confirm the diagnosis?
5. What adaptations might be provided to this patient to prevent further reinjury and following successful resolution of her condition?

# References

Anderson, C. R., Morris, R. L., Boeh, S. D., Panus, P. C., & Sembrowich, W. L. (2003). Effects of iontophoresis current magnitude and duration on dexamethasone deposition and localized drug retention. *Physical Therapy, 83*, 161-170.

Aygul, R., Ulvi, H., Karatay, S., Deniz, O., & Varoglu, A. O. (2005). Determination of sensitive electrophysiologic parameters at follow-up of different steroid treatments of carpal tunnel syndrome. *Journal of Clinical Neurophysiology: Official Publication of the American Electroencephalographic Society, 22*, 222-230.

Backstrom, K. M. (2002). Mobilization with movement as an adjunct intervention in a patient with complicated de quervain's tenosynovitis: A case report. *Journal of Orthopaedic and Sports Physical Therapy, 32*, 86-94; discussion 94-7.

Banga, A., & Chien, Y. (1998). Iontophoretic delivery of drugs: Fundamentals, developments and biomedical applications. *Journal of Controlled Release, 1.*

Banta, C. A. (1994). A prospective, nonrandomized study of iontophoresis, wrist splinting, and antiinflammatory medication in the treatment of early-mild carpal tunnel syndrome. *Journal of Occupational Medicine, 36*, 166-168.

Baskurt, F., Ozcan, A., & Algun, C. (2003). Comparison of effects of phonophoresis and iontophoresis of naproxen in the treatment of lateral epicondylitis. *Clinical Rehabilitation, 17*, 96-100.

Batheja, P., Thakur, R., & Michniak, B. (2006). Transdermal iontophoresis. *Expert Opinion on Drug Delivery, 3*, 127-138.

Bogner, R., & Banga, A. (1994). Iontophoresis and phonophoresis. *U. S. Pharmacist, 8*, 14.

Boskovic, K. (1999). Physical therapy of subjective symptoms of the cervical syndrome. *Medicinski Pregled, 52*, 495-500.

Cabello Benavente, R., Moncada Iribarren, I., de Palacio Espana, A., Hernandez Villaverde, A., Monzo, J. I., & Hernandez Fernandez, C. (2005). Transdermal iontophoresis with dexamethasone and verapamil for peyronie's disease. *Actas Urologicas Espanolas, 29*, 955-960.

Chandler, T. J. (1998). Iontophoresis of 0.4% dexamethasone for plantar fasciitis. *Clinical Journal of Sport Medicine, 8*, 68.

Christopher, E., Schebert, C., & Goos, M. (1989). The epidermis. In M. Greaves, & S. Schester (Eds.), *Pharmacology of the skin* (1st ed.). Berlin: Springer-Verlag.

Dakowicz, A., & Latosiewicz, R. (2005). The value of iontophoresis combined with ultrasound in patients with the carpal tunnel syndrome. *Roczniki Akademii Medycznej w Bialymstoku (1995), 50 Suppl 1*, 196-198.

Dixit, N., Bali, V., Baboota, S., Ahuja, A., & Ali, J. (2007). Iontophoresis - an approach for controlled drug delivery: A review. *Current Drug Delivery, 4*, 1-10.

DuPont, J. S., Jr. (2004). Clinical use of iontophoresis to treat facial pain. *Cranio: The Journal of Craniomandibular Practice, 22*, 297-303.

Gangarosa, L. P., Park, N. H., Fong, B. C., Scott, D. F., & Hill, J. M. (1978). Conductivity of drugs used for iontophoresis. *Journal of Pharmaceutical Sciences, 67*, 1439-1443.

Glass, J. M., Stephen, R. L., & Jacobson, S. C. (1980). The quantity and distribution of radiolabeled dexamethasone delivered to tissue by iontophoresis. *International Journal of Dermatology, 19*, 519-525.

Gokoglu, F., Fndkoglu, G., Yorgancoglu, Z. R., Okumus, M., Ceceli, E., & Kocaoglu, S. (2005). Evaluation of iontophoresis and local corticosteroid injection in the treatment of carpal tunnel syndrome. *American Journal of Physical Medicine & Rehabilitation, 84*, 92-96.

Gudeman, S. D., Eisele, S. A., Heidt, R. S. Jr, Colosimo, A. J., & Stroupe, A. L. (1997). Treatment of plantar fasciitis by iontophoresis of 0.4% dexamethasone. A randomized, double-blind, placebo-controlled study. *American Journal of Sports Medicine, 25*, 312-316.

Haga, H., Shibaji, T., & Umino, M. (2005). Lidocaine transport through living rat skin using alternating current. *Medical & Biological Engineering & Computing, 43*, 622-629.

Hasson, S. M., Wible, C. L., Reich, M., Barnes, W. S., & Williams, J. H. (1992). Dexamethasone iontophoresis: Effect on delayed muscle soreness and muscle function. *Canadian Journal of Sport Sciences, 17*, 8-13.

Huida, P. P. (1998). Current approaches to the treatment of patients with systemic scleroderma. *Likars'Ka Sprava/Ministerstvo Okhorony Zdorov'Ia Ukrainy, (1)*, 122-126.

Iomed, Inc. (1994). *Phoresor application guide.* Salt Lake City, UT: Iomed.

Kahn, J. (1995). *Principles and practice of electrotherapy.* London: Churchill Livingstone.

Kahn, J. (1977). Acetic acid iontophoresis for calcium deposits. *Physical Therapy, 57*, 658-659.

Kalia, Y. N., Merino, V., & Guy, R. H. (1998). Transdermal drug delivery. clinical aspects. *Dermatologic Clinics, 16*, 289-299.

Kalia, Y. N., Naik, A., Garrison, J., & Guy, R. H. (2004). Iontophoretic drug delivery. *Advanced Drug Delivery Reviews, 56*, 619-658.

Kanikkannan, N. (2002). Iontophoresis-based transdermal delivery systems. *BioDrugs, 16*, 339-347.

Kassan, D. G., Lynch, A. M., & Stiller, M. J. (1996). Physical enhancement of dermatologic drug delivery: Iontophoresis and phonophoresis. *Journal of the American Academy of Dermatology, 34*, 657-666.

LeDuc, S., & MacKenna R. (1908). *Electric ions and their use in medicine*. London: Rebman Ltd.

Merino, V., Kalia, Y. N., & Guy, R. H. (1997). Transdermal therapy and diagnosis by iontophoresis. *Trends in Biotechnology, 15*, 288-290.

Pasero, C. (2006). Lidocaine iontophoresis for dermal procedure analgesia. *Journal of Perianesthesia Nursing, 21*, 48-52.

Riedl, C. R., Plas, E., Engelhardt, P., Daha, K., & Pfluger, H. (2000). Iontophoresis for treatment of Peyronie's disease. *Journal of Urology, 163*, 95-99.

Riviere, J. E., & Heit, M. C. (1997). Electrically-assisted transdermal drug delivery. *Pharmaceutical Research, 14*, 687-697.

Roberts, D. (1999). Transdermal drug delivery using iontophoresis and phonophoresis. *Orthopaedic Nursing, 18*, 50-54.

Roberts, M. S. (1997). Targeted drug delivery to the skin and deeper tissues: Role of physiology, solute structure and disease. *Clinical and Experimental Pharmacology & Physiology, 24*, 874-879.

Russo, J., Jr., Lipman, A. G., Comstock, T. J., Page, B. C., & Stephen, R. L. (1980). Lidocaine anesthesia: Comparison of iontophoresis, injection, and swabbing. *American Journal of Hospital Pharmacy, 37*, 843-847.

Sanderson, J. E., de Riel, S., & Dixon, R. (1989). Iontophoretic delivery of nonpeptide drugs: Formulation optimization for maximum skin permeability. *Journal of Pharmaceutical Sciences, 78*, 361-364.

Schiffman, E. L., Braun, B. L., & Lindgren, B. R. (1996). Temporomandibular joint iontophoresis: A double-blind randomized clinical trial. *Journal of Orofacial Pain, 10*, 157-165.

Schuhfried, O., & Fialka-Moser, V. (1995). Iontophoresis in the treatment of pain. *Wiener Medizinische Wochenschrift (1946), 145*, 4-8.

Singh, J., & Maibach, H. I. (1993). Topical iontophoretic drug delivery in vivo: Historical development, devices and future perspectives. *Dermatology (Basel, Switzerland), 187*, 235-238.

Sintov, A. C., & Brandys-Sitton, R. (2006). Facilitated skin penetration of lidocaine: Combination of a short-term iontophoresis and microemulsion formulation. *International Journal of Pharmaceutics, 316*, 58-67.

Ting, W. W., & Sontheimer, R. D. (2001). Local therapy for cutaneous and systemic lupus erythematosus: Practical and theoretical considerations. *Lupus, 10*, 171-184.

Ting, W. W., Vest, C. D., & Sontheimer, R. D. (2004). Review of traditional and novel modalities that enhance the permeability of local therapeutics across the stratum corneum. *International Journal of Dermatology, 43*, 538-547.

Trommer, H., & Neubert, R. H. (2006). Overcoming the stratum corneum: The modulation of skin penetration. A review. *Skin Pharmacology and Physiology, 19*, 106-121.

Wang, Y., Thakur, R., Fan, Q., & Michniak, B. (2005). Transdermal iontophoresis: Combination strategies to improve transdermal iontophoretic drug delivery. *European Journal of Pharmaceutics and Biopharmaceutics, 60*, 179-191.

Williams, S. K., & Brage, M. (2004). Heel pain-plantar fasciitis and achilles enthesopathy. *Clinics in Sports Medicine, 23*, 123-144.

Yarrobino, T. E., Kalbfleisch, J. H., Ferslew, K. E., & Panus, P. C. (2006). Lidocaine iontophoresis mediates analgesia in lateral epicondylalgia treatment. *Physiotherapy Research International, 11*, 152-160.

# Chapter 12

# Low Level Laser and Light Therapy

## Learning Objectives

1. Define low level laser therapy (LLLT).
2. Describe the difference between LED, SLD, and LLT devices.
3. Describe the physical properties of the electromagnetic spectrum.
4. Discuss the different types of electromagnetic radiation used clinically.
5. Discuss the physiological effect of electromagnetic radiation.
6. Identify the precautions and contraindications for electromagnetic radiation.
7. Describe the clinical indications for the use of diathermy.

## Terminology

| | |
|---|---|
| Collimation | Monochromatic |
| Electromagnetic radiation | Nonometers |
| Light emitting diode (LED) | Photobiomodulation |
| Low-level laser therapy (LLLT) | Wavelength |

## Laser Theory

There has been a great deal of research, interest, and use in laser and light therapy in rehabilitation, with a plethora of manufacturers developing new equipment for a variety of clinical applications. Lasers have been used in Europe for many years and are gaining more widespread acceptance in the United States with the advent of a number of US Food and Drug Administration (FDA) approved devices. Because of science fiction movies, the general public and many therapists may have misconceptions of how lasers work in rehabilitation and what they can do. A common misconception is that the laser is "hot." The common image of a laser is from a science fiction movie of somebody getting "vaporized" by a laser beam, so there is a natural hesitancy to explore low-level laser therapy as an additional tool in the occupational therapy toolbox. There are some lasers used in medicine and surgery which have a thermal effect and which are used to cauterize or ablate tissue or for other purposes.

In rehabilitation, low-level laser therapy (LLLT) or "cold" lasers as they are sometimes called, are the forms of laser and energy that are used for a variety of therapeutic reasons and clinical conditions. Other common terms used for phototherapy or laser therapy, include photobiomodulation, soft lasers, low energy or low intensity lasers, or just laser therapy. Some of the confusion in use arises due to the equipment manufacturer's terms and by their claims. The energy produced through the visible spectrum can be produced by either light emitting diodes (LEDs), super luminous diodes (SLDs), or from low-level laser diodes. Most of these phototherapy devices use light which is within the visible red and infrared spectrum between 600 and 1000 nanometers (nm). Visible red light has been used for centuries in the treatment of various conditions and the healthy benefit of sunshine was documented by the Greeks and Romans. We are all aware of the effect the sun has on skin if we fail to use the correct sun screen (sunburn), and the effect of sunlight and the specific color spectrum of light on mood and personality, the "winter blues," (seasonal affective disorder). LEDs, SLDs, and LLLT use the light energy spectrum to facilitate biochemical changes in the treated tissue with a cascade of physiochemical effects occurring following exposure to the wavelengths.

# History

Lasers fall within the category of electromagnetic radiation and produce energy in the form of visible and invisible light. Electromagnetic radiation consists of both electric and magnetic fields and can transmit energy without the need for a medium. Electromagnetic radiation is also able to be transmitted through the vacuum of space. Electromagnetic radiation is classifed into a "spectrum" according to wavelength, frequency, and quantum energy. The spectrum of electromagnetic radiation includes electrical energy, radio, microwave, infrared, the visible spectrums which we can see visually as "light", ultraviolet, x-rays, and gamma rays. We perceive this form of "light" radiation as colors, which range from red, ~700 nm, to violet which has a shorter wavelength of ~400 nm. At the higher end of the electromagnetic spectrum, the particles are moving at very high velocities and create high-energy radiation like X-rays and gamma-rays.

Laser is an anacronym for light amplification by stimulated emission of radiation. The underlying principles for lasers were first described by Albert Einstein in 1917's work, *On the Quantum Theory of Radiation*. Research into lasers and their applications grew in significance during the 1960's facilitated by the arms race and search for weapons grade lasers for military applications. Building on earlier research and theory, Theodore Maiman developed the first LASER device, which produced a mechanism capable of amplifying a monochromatic light (red) at a specific wavelength. This research led to the development of "hot" or high power lasers which have been refined to their current use in surgery and medicine. Building on this initial work, Endre Mester began experimenting with a laser in an attempt to destroy tumor cells. Though he believed that he was using a "high" power laser (>500 mW) in an attempt to destroy them, he was in fact, using a "low" level, "red" light laser, which appeared to facilitate the healing process of the surgical implant site. Further experiments using the laser demonstrated that other forms of wounds, ulcers, and bedsores also healed more quickly using the intervention (Mester, Ludany, & Seller, 1968; Mester, Spry, Sender, & Tita, 1971; Mester, Mester, & Mester, 1985). Mester concluded that rather than having a destructive effect, the low levels of light facilitated tissue healing.

Conceptually, as small amounts of sunlight can be beneficial, large amounts can be destructive, causing sun burns. The ultraviolet rays of the sun can be powerful influences on the body in small, controlled amounts. Sun exposure is perhaps the most important source of vitamin D because exposure to sunlight provides most humans with their vitamin D requirement (Holick, 1994). Ultraviolet rays from the sun trigger vitamin D synthesis in skin through the action of the ultraviolet B waves that convert ergosterol in the skin into vitamin D. Ergosterol belongs to the steroid family (Holick, 1994; Holick, 2002). Ten minutes of daily exposure to sunlight supply us with all the vitamin D that is required by the body. Exposure to sunlight also stimulates the pineal gland, which produces tryptamines (one form of which is melatonin), which keeps our internal "clock" aware of night and day and the changing seasons. Conversely, unprotected exposure to the suns rays for as little as 30 minutes can cause sunburn, and potential skin damage, which can lead to skin cancer due to the ultraviolet radiation. Skin cancer makes up half of all new cases of cancer in the United States and is a growing concern. Additionally, melanomas developing at different body sites are associated with distinct patterns and amounts of sun exposure (Whiteman, Stickley, Hughes, Davis, & Green, 2006). All of these biophysiological effects are due to exposure to the specific wavelengths of the light. Similarly to the effect of the suns rays on the body and tissue, high intensity lasers can possess either a thermal or heat effect on physiological tissue; while cold or LLLT, the form used for rehabilitation can also impact the healing process and physiological response of treated tissue.

Lasers can be either high level energy or intensity (hot), or low-level energy or intensity (cold). The use of lasers in medicine has been gaining in popularity and use, though low-level laser therapy has not been as readily used or accepted in physical medicine in the United States as it has in Europe, Asia, and other parts of the world. Part of this may be due to the time consuming process of receiving FDA approval for new equipment. There was some initial hesitancy on the part of the FDA to approve LLLT, and it has only been since 2002 that the FDA cleared laser devices and LED equipment for the treatment of a variety of conditions including carpal tunnel syndrome, cervical neck pain, low back pain, joint pain, generalized muscle pain, and to facilitate the healing process. Laser equipment that does not receive FDA approval is considered experimental and therapists should be aware of potential limitations or concerns in using the equipment clinically. Equipment which has been approved by the FDA is most often stated as such by the manufacturer. Prior to using LLLT, clinicians should review state regulatory laws related to physical agents to ensure that there are no limitations in effect which might limit or prohibit laser therapy by occupational therapists. Currently, only Nebraska's licensing law prohibits occupational therapists from using LLLT.

## Mechanism of Action

Light is a form of energy that we can "see" and consists of a stream of particles known as photons. Light energy is transmitted in "waves" and "streams" of photons which possess unique characteristics and movements and exhibit both electrical and magnetic properties, the electromagnetic spectrum. Photons vibrate at different rates and also vary in terms of their energy. The electromagnetic spectrum includes radio waves, infrared radiation, ultraviolet rays, x-rays, cosmic radiation, and the visible light that we see. Each of these various waves consists of photons that vary in vibration rates and energy as well as possess different wavelengths. The differing energy levels account for the variations in tissue changes and effects, with gamma or x-rays tending to ionize matter and destroy tissue, while radio waves, which have a lower energy and longer wave, have minimal if any effect on tissue.

Unlike the ambient light produced by a light bulb that contains many differing wavelengths dispersed throughout the room, laser light is considered *monochromatic, coherent*, and *collimated*. Laser light is monochromatic, which means that it is light consisting of a single, defined wavelength, and if in the visible spectrum, seen in only one color (red). The laser beam is also collimated, which means that there is little divergence of the photons away from the central core or column; with the photons moving parallel to each other in one direction. The laser beam is more focused, and allows for deeper penetration into the underlying tissue than a non-collimated or non-focused light which is more dispersive. The laser beam is also coherent with the photons emitted being of the same wave length and the waves being in phase with one another. Laser light occurs when photons are amplified and stimulated, causing them to collide with other excited electrons, thereby releasing more photons.

Other forms of light therapy have been found to be effective in treatment (Ross, 2006). There are other technologies and equipment available which are often marketed or misunderstood as being a "laser," but which are not true lasers. They may vary in energy density and intensity, and are biologically independent from each other (Sommer, Pinheiro, Mester, Franke, & Whelan, 2001). LEDs and SLDs use monochromatic light with a narrow spectrum and may have many of the same therapeutic effects or benefits of true lasers. SLDs are "super luminious," meaning they are brighter in intensity than LEDs and are an additional option in treatment. Primary differences between these forms of light therapy (LEDs and SLDs to LLLT) occur in wavelength, duration, and depth of penetration. The critical factor among competing light forms is in the dose and wavelength; with a therapeutic dose to facilitate tissue healing or modulate pain being between 600 to 1,000 nm. LEDs and SLDs may have the same physiochemical effect, but may take longer to reach the therapeutic threshold in the treated tissue (Figure 12-1).

# Biophysiological Effects

Like other physical agent modalities, there are some basic components necessary to produce lasers. The primary components of a laser system consist of a power supply, a lasing medium, which is a material that generates the laser light and can be a gas, liquid, or solid; a pumping device, which is used to elevate the electrons to an "excited" energy level; and a cavity or containment device, which holds the reflecting surfaces and directs the beam propagation. There are a variety of laser devices on the market that are used in medicine and dentistry (Figure 12-2). According to the type of their active medium, lasers can be classified as solid, gas, semiconductor, and liquid. There are two primary forms of lasers used in the United States: the helium neon (HeNe) or gallium arsenide (GaAs) laser. The HeNe laser creates a laser in the red light spectrum with a wavelength of 633 nm while the GaAs lasers produce a wavelength of 904 nm. The HeNe laser will penetrate less deeply and produces a laser light with a shorter wavelength and higher frequency. The GaAs laser will penetrate deeper and will produce a lower frequency and longer wavelength. As the laser energy and beam penetrate the underlying tissue, the energy is also absorbed, reflected, refracted and transmitted, similar to ultrasound energy. Most of the laser light between 300 to 1000 nm will be absorbed in the superficial layer of tissue within the first 3 to 4 mm of tissue (Goldman & Rockwell, 1971).

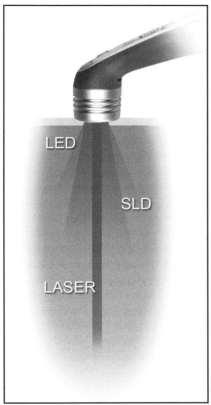

**Figure 12-1.** Depth of laser light penetration—LED, SLD, and LASER.

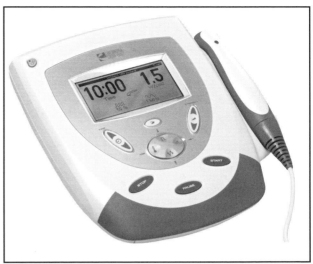

**Figure 12-2.** Vectra Genisys Laser system (Photo courtesy of Chattanooga Group).

The exact mechanism of action of LLLT is still not completely understood. The basic feature of LLLT is to modulate cell behavior without causing a significant temperature increase. During irradiation of a tissue with a laser beam, an interaction between cells and photons takes place, a photochemical reaction. After a cell absorbs the photon, the photon stops existing, and its energy is incorporated into the molecule which has absorbed it. Once this energy is transferred to different biomolecules, it can be transferred to other molecules as well. The energy transferred to the molecule can increase its kinetic energy, and activate or deactivate enzymes or alter the physical or chemical properties of main macromolecules (Matic, Lazetic, Poljacki, Duran, & Ivkov-Simic, 2003).

The characteristics of the light delivery systems can be determined by looking at beam properties, transmission, and thermal properties. The delivery of continuous wave or pulsed laser energy—contact or noncontact—will determine the contribution of optical, thermal, and mechanical effects to the tissue (Verdaasdonk & van Swol, 1997). Also similar to ultrasound, the output of the lasers can be continuous or pulsed to decrease the average power output. For most applications, the energy produced in the laser is administered using a handheld applicator which, in some cases, looks similar to an ultrasound head or transducer. As the laser beam leaves the applicator, the laser beam will eventually diverge and spread out over the area being treated

**Figure 12-3.** Laser applicators (Photo courtesy of Chattanooga Group).

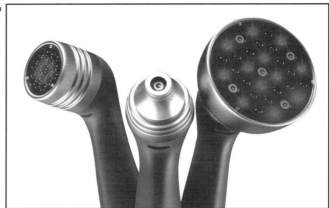

resulting in a decrease in intensity the further away from the source. The overall depth of penetration depends on the tissue which is being treated and the frequency of the laser. Laser light with a wavelength of 600 to 1300 nm will penetrate to a depth of 1 to 4 mm with lower wavelengths limiting the depth of penetration. A laser utilizing a wavelength of 632 nm will penetrate to a depth of approximately 1 to 2 mm, while an 830 nm wavelength may penetrate to a depth of 4 mm or more (Figure 12-3).

The output or amount of energy that is administered to the underlying tissue is measured in terms of joules (J), which is equivalent to 1 watt (W)/second. The output of the laser can be continuous or pulsed, which effectively reduces the average power and affects the treatment time, increasing it if a specific amount of energy is required for a specific condition. The dosage of the laser is documented as Joules per square centimeter ($J/cm^2$). The energy of the laser—the dose being administered to the tissue is related to three factors: the output of the laser in mW (milliwatt), the length of time the tissue is being exposed to the light (measured in seconds), and the overall emitting surface area of the laser beam in $cm^2$. Unlike ultrasound, treatment times are dramatically decreased when using LLLT due to the amount of energy being delivered to the tissue. As a general rule of thumb, some research has indicated that chronic conditions respond better to higher dosages of up to 4.0 $J/cm^2$, while acute conditions respond to lower-energy applications in the range between 0.05 and 1 $J/cm^2$ (Oshiro & Calderhead, 1988).

Though the depth of penetration may appear to be limited, all frequencies will impact the physiological processes at a deeper level due to the stimulating effect on the metabolic processes at the deeper cellular levels. LLLT has an anti-inflammatory effect. Energy densities or parameters that produced an anti-inflammatory effect have varied between 1 and 2.5 $J/cm^2$ and also decreased edema. Research suggests that low power laser irradiation possibly exerts its anti-inflammatory effects by stimulating the release of adrenal corticosteroid hormones (Albertini et al., 2004). LLLT has been used in the management of tendinopathy and arthritis. Results from in vitro and in vivo studies have suggested that inflammatory modulation is one of several possible biological mechanisms of LLLT action. LLLT at a dose of 5.4 J per point can reduce inflammation and pain in activated Achilles tendonitis and may therefore have potential in the management of diseases with an inflammatory component (Bjordal, Lopes-Martins, & Iversen, 2006). An energy density of 1.2 and 2.4 $J/cm^2$ facilitated the healing of third-degree burns in rats, and also acted as an anti-infective agent, inducing the destruction of *staphylococcus aureus* and *Pseudomonas aeruginosa* in the healing tissue (Bayat, Vasheghani, & Razavi, 2006). Other research has shown that phototherapy increases cell growth and impairs protein secretion of fibroblasts. Fujihara found that phototherapy acts as a proliferative stimulus on osteoblast-like cells and could be used as a coadjuvant in bone clinical manipulation in order to accelerate bone regeneration (Fujihara, Hiraki, & Marques, 2006).

Clinically and anecdotally, other commonly noted parameters are between 3 $J/cm^2$ to 5 $J/cm^2$ with treatment applications two to three times per week. Patients may note improvement in their condition within three to five treatments with the course of treatment ranging from eight to ten total visits. Research, however, has been somewhat equivocal with parameters and settings and the manufacturers also espouse a variety of potential treatment parameters or recommendations. Some studies have found settings using 8 J effective for carpal tunnel, while doses between 0.4 to 19 J with power densities of 5 to 21 $mW/cm^2$ effective for treating joint capsules, while using short duration, high dosage applications being more effective than low doses with longer duration. A dose of 5 $J/cm^2$ stimulated mitochrondrial activity on fibroblasts and cell proliferation and viability, while higher doses in the range of 10 and 16 $J/cm^2$ had the opposite effect (Bjordal, Couppe, Chow, Tuner, & Ljunggren, 2003; Hawkins & Abrahamse, 2006; Kymplova, Navratil, & Knizek, 2003; Padua, Padua, Aprile, & Tonali, 1998; Weintraub, 1997). The clinician should continue to evaluate the research and clinical studies to further determine the effectiveness and treatment parameters of LLLT for wound healing and musculoskeletal conditions (Brosseau et al., 2000; Brosseau et al., 2005).

LLLT and phototherapy use light to penetrate the skin and underlying tissue to facilitate the healing process through stimulation and activation of enzymatic activity at the cellular level creating a cascading of effects. There is some research that indicates that LLLT in specific wavelengths stimulates activity in the mitochondria and is used to synthesize adenosine triphosphate (ATP). The ATP is used to stimulate and drive a variety of metabolic processes, including the synthesis of DNA, RNA, proteins, and enzymes that is necessary and responsible for cell regeneration and tissue repair. Phototherapy and LLLT also have been found to impact tissue repair and pain control by altering nerve conduction velocity and somatosensory evoked potentials as well as modulating prostaglandins and hyperemia of underlying tissues. The net effect and outcome of these physiochemical changes are pain modulation and facilitation of tissue repair The research on lasers, though positive, has also been equivocal. A primary difficulty in the research and the inconclusivity of the research is due in part to variability in the design and methodology, as well as in the parameters used. Further research is warranted to better establish therapeutic parameters for clinical applications (Enwemeka et al., 2004; Herascu, Velciu, Calin, Savastru, & Talianu, 2005; Khadra, Ronold, Lyngstadaas, Ellingsen, & Haanaes, 2004; Khadra, 2005; Pourzarandian, Watanabe, Ruwanpura, Aoki, & Ishikawa, 2005; Reddy, 2004; Reddy, Gill, & Rochon, 2006; Sun & Tuner, 2004; Woodruff et al., 2004).

## Applications and Indications

The primary uses for LLLT have been in the areas of dentistry, wound or fracture healing, in the treatment of musculoskeletal conditions, and in modulating pain. Laser use in wound healing has been purported to stimulate phagocytosis, fibroplasia, and increase circulation. Surgical wounds, chronic wounds, and animal studies including fractures have been researched. A meta-analysis of 24 animal experiments and human clinical studies concluded that LLLT had a significant positive effect on the healing process in the areas of accelerating the inflammatory process, strengthening collagen synthesis as well as improving overall tensile strength of the wound, and decreasing both the healing time and overall size of the wound (Enwemeka et al., 2004; Woodruff et al., 2004). Musculoskeletal conditions and pain including trigger points, back, neck, and elbow pain may also benefit from LLT. Rheumatoid arthritic patients also noticed decreases in pain, swelling, stiffness, and medication use following laser therapy. A meta-analysis investigating LLLT therapy in the treatment of tissue repair and pain control also found a positive effect for laser phototherapy on tissue repair in the areas of collagen formation, rate of healing, tensile strength, overall time for wound closure, number and rate of degranulation of mast cells, and flap survival. The most effective wavelength of laser light for tissue repair was 632.8 nm, with 780 nm least effective. There was also a concurrent positive treatment effect for pain control (Enwemeka, 1989; Enwemeka et al., 2004). Myofascial neck pain was also found to be effectively treated using LLLT, which not only modulated the pain, but also improved functional ability and quality of life. LLLT was also found to be effective in the treatment of myofascial pain and fibromyalgia (Gur et al., 2002; Gur, Sarac, Cevik, Altindag, & Sarac, 2004; Hakguder, Birtane, Gurcan, Kokino, & Turan, 2003).

Though in relative infancy in the United States, LLLT and phototherapy hold great promise as an adjunctive, preparatory tool for the occupational therapist in treating a variety of clinical conditions. As laser therapy gains greater acceptance and use, further research will help to clarify the parameters and conditions most amenable to this intervention. Clinicians are encouraged to continue to monitor the research related to laser and phototherapy to stay current with applications and therapeutic parameters.

## CLINICAL APPLICATIONS

- **Pain management:** Neck pain, back pain
- **Musculoskeletal conditions:** Carpal tunnel syndrome, rheumatoid arthritis, osteoarthritis, fibromyalgia, temporomandibular joint dysfunction
- **Inflammatory conditions:** Bursitis, tendonitis, soft tissue conditions
- **Wound healing:** Diabetic ulcers, venous ulcers, bedsores, mouth ulcers, fractures, tendon ruptures, ligament tears, improving tensile strength
- **Lymphedema**

# Precautions and Contraindications

As with any physical agent modality, care must be used during treatment application and the patient's condition and response to treatment carefully monitored. Laser therapy, if applied in the correct doses, can be a safe and effective intervention. Because lasers use collimated light, damage to the eyes can occur if the beam is directed toward the eyes or when viewing the beam or its specular reflections off of a smooth surface area. The laser beam should never be directed at the eyes, and the patient should be instructed to not look directly at the laser beam. Obviously, any other patients, family members or staff should also follow the same precautions and protect their vision if in the vicinity of the treatment.

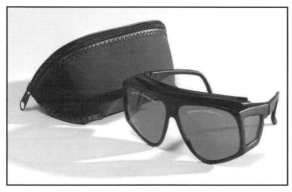

**Figure 12-4.** Protective goggles should always be warn by patient and therapist during laser application.

The patient and clinician should both wear goggles or eye protection that provides the appropriate optical density for the wavelength or laser which is being used (Figure 12-4). Failure to protect the eyes is precautionary though the laser energy can be of sufficient intensity to cause partial or complete loss of vision and blindness. Direct application to the eyes is contraindicated.

Lasers should not be applied to the vagus nerve or over the carotid sinus, or in patients with decreased sensation, infected tissue, or an active hemorrhage. Application over the gonads and sexual organs and the epiphyseal plates of children should be avoided. Lasers should not be applied over tumors or cancerous lesions, or over the endocrine glands.

## CLINICAL CONSIDERATIONS

### Precautions

- Fever
- Over gonads
- Epiphyseal plates in children
- Decreased sensation or mentation/orientation
- Infections
- Carotid sinus
- Epilepsy

### Contraindications

- Irradiation over the fetus or uterus during pregnancy
- Irradiation over the endocrine glands
- Patients with sensitivity to light or idiopathic photophobia
- Hemorrhages
- Irradiation to the eyes
- Cancer or tumors

# Documentation

As with all physical agent modalities, subjective comments from the patient and consistent monitoring of the patient are required to safely administer laser therapy. When documenting on the laser protocol, attention should be paid to the location and area that is being treated and any distinguishing features such as skin irritation, lacerations, etc. The dosage of the laser should be written in "$J/cm^2$" for each application. Additionally, the laser power in W, the treatment time for each area, the frequency and type of laser being used, as well as if the application mode (i.e., continuous or pulsed) should be charted daily. Any subjective and objective comments or observations as well as the patient's response to the intervention should be specified.

# Diathermy

Diathermy is most often used for its deep heating capabilities through the application of high radiofrequency currents to the underlying tissue. Deep heating is caused by the conversion of energy into heat as it passes through the tissue. Heating of deeper structures can be obtained through the application of high frequency electrical currents, (short wave diathermy), or through the application of electromagnetic waves (microwave radiation). Short wave diathermy and microwave diathermy devices can be modulated in either a continuous or pulsed mode generating heat in the underlying tissue when the intensity is increased to a sufficient level (Goats, 1989a).

## Mechanism of Action

Short wave diathermy devices (SWD) most commonly use a radiofrequency electromagnetic field of 27.12 MHz. There are different frequency ranges depending on the equipment which will affect specific tissue types at different depths. The output of the SWD can be modified to be delivered in either a continuous or pulsed mode. The application of the high-frequency electromagnetic energy (SWD) generates heat in the underlying tissue due to the resistance of the tissue to the passage of the energy. The physiological effects of continuous SWD are thermal with deeper tissues being heated to a depth of 2 to 5 cm. As with all thermal agents, temperature rise is dependent on the specific properties of the tissue being treated, thermal conductivity of the tissue, and the duration of application. An advantage to using SWD is that the overall area that can be heated will be larger than those covered by a hot pack or ultrasound. The physiological effects of diathermy are consistent with the application of heat and include increased tissue temperature, increased blood flow, increased membrane permeability, increased enzymatic reactions, increased metabolic rate, tissue extensibility, decreased joint stiffness, increased pain threshold, and facilitation of tissue healing (Balogun & Okonofua, 1988; Berna, Sanchez, Madrigal, Rodenas, & Berna, 2002; Conradi & Pages, 1989; Draper, Castro, Feland, Schulthies, & Eggett, 2004; Dziedzic, Hill, Lewis, Sim, Daniels, & Hay, 2005; Garrett, Draper, & Knight, 2000; Guler-Uysal & Kozanoglu, 2004; Hill, Lewis, Mills, & Kielty, 2002; Jan, Chai, Wang, Lin, & Tsai, 2006; Robertson, Ward, & Jung, 2005; Xu, Feng, Zeng, & Xu, 1999). Shortwave diathermy can be administered through capacitance or induction techniques. Capacitor electrodes create a strong electrical field impacting the tissue through the movement of small electrical fields or eddy currents. These units use two capacitance electrodes which are spaced apart with the underlying tissue becoming part of the circuit. Induction methods use either a cable which is wrapped over the extremity or treatment area, or drum, both which use alternating electric current flowing through the wires. The drum is placed over the treatment area and with the flow of electrical current in the coil produces a magnetic field and eddy current in the tissue. Capacitive electrodes in general, produce a more superficial heating effect as compared to inductive methods (Bansal, Sobti, & Roy, 1990; Lehmann, McDougall, Guy, Warren, & Esselman, 1983; Oosterveld, Rasker, Jacobs, & Overmars, 1992). Microwave diathermy units consist of a power supply which provides energy to a magnetron which produces a high frequency alternating current. The alternating current produces an electromagnetic field over the treated tissue, focusing the energy into a smaller area. Microwave radiation provides a more superficial effect in the tissue and is more prone to the potential for burning of the skin or fat tissue due to the development of standing waves and reflection (Conradi & Pages, 1989; Fadilah, Pinkas, Weinberger, & Lev, 1987).

The primary factor whether the tissue temperature will increase is the overall amount of energy which is absorbed by the tissue. This is determined by the intensity of the electromagnetic field and the type of tissue which is being treated. Tissue that offers the greatest resistance to current flow develops higher levels of heat. Subcutaneous fat and tissue that has a high fat content insulates and resists the flow of electrons and have a tendency to overheat. Pulsing the signal allows the tissue to cool as the heat dissipates during the off cycle of the pulse (Conradi & Pages, 1989; Draper, Knight, Fujiwara, & Castel, 1999; Pasila, Visuri, & Sundholm, 1978). Pulsed diathermy is achieved by the electronics of the instrument interrupting the output at different intervals. An advantage to diathermy is that it can heat larger areas than therapeutic ultrasound or hotpacks and does not cause periosteal burning. Reflection of the waves, however, can lead to hot spots in other areas due to reflection and must be taken into account. The patient's electrical impedance or resistance of the tissue to the energy flow, becomes part of the patients own circuit during treatment. The shortwave diathermy unit will generate a high-frequency electrical current producing both an electrical and magnetic field within the treatment tissue. Newer, pulsed short wave diathermy units use a drum electrode producing a magnetic field which creates eddy currents in the underlying tissue. The patient should only feel a comfortable level of heat during the treatment. Treatment times vary between 15 to 20 minutes or up to a maximum of 30 minutes long to achieve desired physiological effects.

## Indications

In general, the clinical application of continuous shortwave diathermy would be a consideration for the desired effect of a thermal response in the treatment tissue. Pulsed shortwave diathermy, and microwave diathermy also have nonthermal effects which may be desired for a variety of musculoskeletal conditions. Clinical application may be warranted for selectively heating joint structures, for decreasing stiffness, increasing tissue extensibility and improving blood flow to an area, and decreasing pain (Balogun & Okonofua, 1988; Bansil & Joshi, 1975; Berna et al., 2002; Draper, et al., Goats, 1989; McCann & Sherar, 2006). Pulsed short wave diathermy has been shown to facilitate tissue healing, decrease edema and inflammation, reabsorb hematomas, and decrease pain (Balogun & Okonofua, 1988b; Brucker, Knight, Rubley, & Draper, 2005; Callaghan, Whittaker, Grimes, & Smith, 2005; Draper, Castro, Feland, Schulthies, & Eggett, 2004; Dziedzic, et al., 2005; Jan, et al., 2006; Jiang, Zhu, Luo, Wang, & Jiang, 2004; Laufer, Zilberman, Porat, & Nahir, 2005; Pasila et al., 1978; Seiger & Draper, 2006).

## Precautions

Care should always be taken when using diathermy as the equipment produces diffuse radiation during use. Consistent with any thermal modality, consideration of all contraindications and precautions identified in earlier chapters should be of significance. Because the units produce radiation, the therapist should not stand close to the machine. Some research has found an increase in the risk of miscarriage of pregnant therapists who were frequently exposed to microwave diathermy. Exposure to shortwave diathermy during pregnancy, however, did not increase the risk of miscarriage in the study (Hocking & Joyner, 1995; Ouellet-Hellstrom & Stewart, 1993). Some studies, however, have noted an increase in spontaneous abortion and abnormal fetal development, specifically, low birth rate in therapists exposed or using SWD, though another study did not find statistic significance (Larsen, Olsen, & Svane, 1991; Lerman, Jacubovich, & Green, 2001; Taskinen, Kyyronen, & Hemminki, 1990). Because of the current research findings related to diathermy and pregnancy, it is better to err on the side of caution and it is recommended that therapists should avoid using SWD and microwave diathermy during pregnancy.

## Contraindications

Diathermy will cause an increase in tissue temperature and may therefore, be contraindicated in any clinical condition where increased temperature may produce negative effects. Traumatic, acute inflammatory conditions, ischemia, or application over areas of decreased sensitivity should be avoided. Contraindications include patients with metal implants, pacemakers, implanted or transcutaneous neural stimulators. Watches, jewelry should also be removed before application and the patient should not be positioned on metal furniture during the application. Diathermy units should also be kept away from other types of medical devices or equipment such as TENS units. Diathermy should never be applied to the eyes, testes or over the epiphyseal plates of children or over areas of malignancy (Frey, 2004; Jiang et al., 2004; Jones, 1976; Macca et al., 2007; Ruggera, Witters, von Maltzahn, & Bassen, 2003; Shields, O'Hare, Boyle, & Gormley, 2003; Shields, O'Hare, & Gormley, 2004).

# Case Study

A 37-year-old female who has been performing piece work in an area shop, is referred for therapy with a diagnosis of bilateral carpal tunnel syndrome. The patient is an active individual who "enjoys" her work and job. She relates that her symptoms have been getting progressively worse. She states that initially, following her work, she noticed burning, tingling, and "numbness" in the palm of her hand which then "moved" up into her fingers. Symptoms are most noticeable in her thumb, index finger, and middle finger. She has attempted to "self-treat" and has been wearing a soft wrist splint at night and soaking her hands in the evening. Her employer will not allow her to wear the splint while at work due to "safety concerns." Upon evaluation, you note that the patient frequently "shakes" her hands and wrist in an attempt to alleviate her symptoms. Sensation is impaired in the palmar aspect of both hands, thumb, index finger, and middle finger, with paresthesia worse on the right hand. Grip and pinch strength are slightly decreased, but the patient is more concerned with the "tingling and numbness" and denies any difficulty manipulating objects. Patient tests positive for Phalen's test.

➤ *Impression*: Signs and symptoms consistent with bilateral carpal tunnel syndrome.

➤ *Intervention*: Due to its therapeutic effect on inflammation and carpal tunnel, you decide to implement intervention using LLLT as an adjunct to the patient's treatment. Treatment parameters are between 1 to 3 J/cm$^2$ and are applied over the median nerve and palmar trigger point.

## Clinical Reasoning Questions

1. What other therapeutic interventions will be necessary to treat this patient?
2. Will the patient require any adaptive equipment or modifications to her home or work routines?
3. What other physical agent modalities could be used adjunctively rather than LLLT?
4. What signs and symptoms indicated that the patient had carpal tunnel?
5. Are there any precautions or contraindications you should explore prior to using LLLT?

# References

Albertini, R., Aimbire, F. S., Correa, F. I., Ribeiro, W., Cogo, J. C., & Antunes, E., et al. (2004). Effects of different protocol doses of low power gallium-aluminum-arsenate (ga-al-as) laser radiation (650 nm) on carrageenan induced rat paw ooedema. *Journal of Photochemistry and Photobiology, 74*, 101-107.

Balogun, J. A., & Okonofua, F. E. (1988). Management of chronic pelvic inflammatory disease with shortwave diathermy. A case report. *Physical Therapy, 68*, 1541-1545.

Bansal, P. S., Sobti, V. K., & Roy, K. S. (1990). Histomorphochemical effects of shortwave diathermy on healing of experimental muscular injury in dogs. *Indian Journal of Experimental Biology, 28,* 766-770.

Bansil, C. K., & Joshi, J. B. (1975). Effectiveness of shortwave diathermy and ultrasound in the treatment of osteo-arthritis of the knee joint. *Medical Journal of Zambia, 9,* 138-139.

Bayat, M., Vasheghani, M. M., & Razavi, N. (2006). Effect of low-level helium-neon laser therapy on the healing of third-degree burns in rats. *Journal of Photochemistry and Photobiology, 83*, 87-93.

Berna, J. D., Sanchez, J., Madrigal, M., Rodenas, J., & Berna, J. D.,Jr. (2002). An alternative approach to the treatment of mammary duct fistulas: A combination of microwave and ultrasound. *American Surgeon, 68*, 897-899.

Bjordal, J. M., Couppe, C., Chow, R. T., Tuner, J., & Ljunggren, E. A. (2003). A systematic review of low-level laser therapy with location-specific doses for pain from chronic joint disorders. *Australian Journal of Physiotherapy, 49*, 107-116.

Bjordal, J. M., Lopes-Martins, R. A., & Iversen, V. V. (2006). A randomised, placebo controlled trial of low-level laser therapy for activated achilles tendinitis with microdialysis measurement of peritendinous prostaglandin E2 concentrations. *British Journal of Sports Medicine, 40*, 76-80; discussion 76-80.

Brosseau, L., Robinson, V., Wells, G., Debie, R., Gam, A., & Harman, K., et al. (2005). Low level laser therapy (classes I, II and III) for treating rheumatoid arthritis. *Cochrane Database of Systematic Reviews (Online), 4*, CD002049.

Brosseau, L., Welch, V., Wells, G., deBie, R., Gam, A., & Harman, K., et al. (2000). Low level laser therapy (classes I, II and III) in the treatment of rheumatoid arthritis. *Cochrane Database of Systematic Reviews (Online), 2*, CD002049.

Brucker, J. B., Knight, K. L., Rubley, M. D., & Draper, D. O. (2005). An 18-day stretching regimen, with or without pulsed, shortwave diathermy, and ankle dorsiflexion after 3 weeks. *Journal of Athletic Training, 40*, 276-280.

Callaghan, M. J., Whittaker, P. E., Grimes, S., & Smith, L. (2005). An evaluation of pulsed shortwave on knee osteoarthritis using radioleucoscintigraphy: A randomised, double blind, controlled trial. *Joint, Bone, Spine : Revue Du Rhumatisme, 72*, 150-155.

Conradi, E., & Pages, I. H. (1989). Effects of continuous and pulsed microwave irradiation on distribution of heat in the gluteal region of minipigs. A comparative study. *Scandinavian Journal of Rehabilitation Medicine, 21*, 59-62.

Draper, D. O., Castro, J. L., Feland, B., Schulthies, S., & Eggett, D. (2004). Shortwave diathermy and prolonged stretching increase hamstring flexibility more than prolonged stretching alone. *Journal of Orthopaedic and Sports Physical Therapy, 34*, 13-20.

Draper, D. O., Knight, K., Fujiwara, T., & Castel, J. C. (1999). Temperature change in human muscle during and after pulsed short-wave diathermy. *Journal of Orthopaedic and Sports Physical Therapy, 29*, 13-8; discussion 19-22.

Dziedzic, K., Hill, J., Lewis, M., Sim, J., Daniels, J., & Hay, E. M. (2005). Effectiveness of manual therapy or pulsed shortwave diathermy in addition to advice and exercise for neck disorders: A pragmatic randomized controlled trial in physical therapy clinics. *Arthritis and Rheumatism, 53*, 214-222.

Einstein, A. (1917). On the quantum theory of radiation. *Phys Zeitschrift, 18*, 121.

Enwemeka, C. S. (1989). The effects of therapeutic ultrasound on tendon healing. A biomechanical study. *American Journal of Physical Medicine & Rehabilitation, 68*, 283-287.

Enwemeka, C. S., Parker, J. C., Dowdy, D. S., Harkness, E. E., Sanford, L. E., & Woodruff, L. D. (2004). The efficacy of low-power lasers in tissue repair and pain control: A meta-analysis study. *Photomedicine and Laser Surgery, 22*, 323-329.

Fadilah, R., Pinkas, J., Weinberger, A., & Lev, A. (1987). Heating rabbit joint by microwave applicator. *Archives of Physical Medicine and Rehabilitation, 68*, 710-712.

Frey, F. J. (2004). Microwave-induced heating injury. *Therapeutische Umschau. Revue Therapeutique, 61*, 703-706.

Fujihara, N. A., Hiraki, K. R., & Marques, M. M. (2006). Irradiation at 780 nm increases proliferation rate of osteoblasts independently of dexamethasone presence. *Lasers in Surgery and Medicine, 38*, 332-336.

Garrett, C. L., Draper, D. O., & Knight, K. L. (2000). Heat distribution in the lower leg from pulsed short-wave diathermy and ultrasound treatments. *Journal of Athletic Training, 35*, 50-55.

Goats, G. C. (1989). Continuous short-wave (radio-frequency) diathermy. *British Journal of Sports Medicine, 23*, 123-127.

Goldman, L., & Rockwell, J. (1971). *Lasers in medicine.* New York: Gordon & Breach.

Guler-Uysal, F., & Kozanoglu, E. (2004). Comparison of the early response to two methods of rehabilitation in adhesive capsulitis. *Swiss Medical Weekly, 134*, 353-358.

Gur, A., Karakoc, M., Nas, K., Cevik, R., Sarac, J., & Demir, E. (2002). Efficacy of low power laser therapy in fibromyalgia: A single-blind, placebo-controlled trial. *Lasers in Medical Science, 17*, 57-61.

Gur, A., Sarac, A. J., Cevik, R., Altindag, O., & Sarac, S. (2004). Efficacy of 904 nm gallium arsenide low-level laser therapy in the management of chronic myofascial pain in the neck: A double-blind and randomize-controlled trial. *Lasers in Surgery and Medicine, 35*, 229-235.

Hakguder, A., Birtane, M., Gurcan, S., Kokino, S., & Turan, F. N. (2003). Efficacy of low-level laser therapy in myofascial pain syndrome: An algometric and thermographic evaluation. *Lasers in Surgery and Medicine, 33*, 339-343.

Hawkins, D. H., & Abrahamse, H. (2006). The role of laser fluence in cell viability, proliferation, and membrane integrity of wounded human skin fibroblasts following helium-neon laser irradiation. *Lasers in Surgery and Medicine, 38*, 74-83.

Herascu, N., Velciu, B., Calin, M., Savastru, D., & Talianu, C. (2005). Low-level laser therapy (LLLT) efficacy in post-operative wounds. *Photomedicine and Laser Surgery, 23*, 70-73.

Hill, J., Lewis, M., Mills, P., & Kielty, C. (2002). Pulsed short-wave diathermy effects on human fibroblast proliferation. *Archives of Physical Medicine and Rehabilitation, 83*, 832-836.

Holick, M. (2002). Vitamin D: The underappreciated D-lightful hormone that is important for skeletal and cellular health. *Current Opinion in Endocrinology and Diabetes, 9*, 87-98.

Holick, M. (1994). McCollum award lecture, 1994: Vitamin D: New horizons for the 21st century. *American Journal of Clinical Nutrition, 60*, 619-630.

Hocking, B., & Joyner, K. (1995). Re: "miscarriages among female physical therapists who report using radio- and microwave-frequency electromagnetic radiation." *American Journal of Epidemiology, 141*, 273-274.

Jan, M. H., Chai, H. M., Wang, C. L., Lin, Y. F., & Tsai, L. Y. (2006). Effects of repetitive shortwave diathermy for reducing synovitis in patients with knee osteoarthritis: An ultrasonographic study. *Physical Therapy, 86*, 236-244.

Jiang, J., Zhu, F. Q., Luo, J., Wang, L. F., & Jiang, Q. (2004). Severe burn of penis caused by excessive short-wave diathermy. *Asian Journal of Andrology, 6*, 377-378.

Jones, S. L. (1976). Electromagnetic field interference and cardiac pacemakers. *Physical Therapy, 56*, 1013-1018.

Khadra, M. (2005). The effect of low-level laser irradiation on implant-tissue interaction. in vivo and in vitro studies. *Swedish Dental Journal Supplement, 172*, 1-63.

Khadra, M., Ronold, H. J., Lyngstadaas, S. P., Ellingsen, J. E., & Haanaes, H. R. (2004). Low-level laser therapy stimulates bone-implant interaction: An experimental study in rabbits. *Clinical Oral Implants Research, 15*, 325-332.

Kymplova, J., Navratil, L., & Knizek, J. (2003). Contribution of phototherapy to the treatment of episiotomies. *Journal of Clinical Laser Medicine & Surgery, 21*, 35-39.

Larsen, A. I., Olsen, J., & Svane, O. (1991). Gender-specific reproductive outcome and exposure to high-frequency electromagnetic radiation among physiotherapists. *Scandinavian Journal of Work, Environment & Health, 17*, 324-329.

Laufer, Y., Zilberman, R., Porat, R., & Nahir, A. M. (2005). Effect of pulsed short-wave diathermy on pain and function of subjects with osteoarthritis of the knee: A placebo-controlled double-blind clinical trial. *Clinical Rehabilitation, 19*, 255-263.

Lehmann, J. F., McDougall, J. A., Guy, A. W., Warren, C. G., & Esselman, P. C. (1983). Heating patterns produced by shortwave diathermy applicators in tissue substitute models. *Archives of Physical Medicine and Rehabilitation, 64*, 575-577.

Lerman, Y., Jacubovich, R., & Green, M. S. (2001). Pregnancy outcome following exposure to shortwaves among female physiotherapists in israel. *American Journal of Industrial Medicine, 39*, 499-504.

Macca, I., Scapellato, M. L., Carrieri, M., di Bisceglie, A. P., Saia, B., & Bartolucci, G. B. (2007). Occupational exposure to electromagnetic fields in physiotherapy departments. *Radiation Protection Dosimetry*, (in press).

Matic, M., Lazetic, B., Poljacki, M., Duran, V., & Ivkov-Simic, M. (2003). Low level laser irradiation and its effect on repair processes in the skin. *Medicinski Pregled, 56*, 137-141.

McCann, C., & Sherar, M. D. (2006). The use of a dispersive ground electrode with a loosely wound helical coil for interstitial radiofrequency thermal therapy. *Physics in Medicine and Biology, 51*, 3851-3863.

Mester, E., Ludany, M., & Seller, M. (1968). The simulating effect of low power laser ray on biological systems. *Laser Review, 1*, 3.

Mester, E., Mester, A. F., & Mester, A. (1985). The biomedical effects of laser application. *Lasers in Surgery and Medicine, 5*, 31-39.

Mester, E., Spry, T., Sender, N., & Tita, J. (1971). Effect of laser ray on wound healing. amer J surg. *American Journal of Surgery, 122*, 523-535.

Oosterveld, F. G., Rasker, J. J., Jacobs, J. W., & Overmars, H. J. (1992). The effect of local heat and cold therapy on the intraarticular and skin surface temperature of the knee. *Arthritis and Rheumatism, 35*, 146-151.

Ouellet-Hellstrom, R., & Stewart, W. F. (1993). Miscarriages among female physical therapists who report using radio- and microwave-frequency electromagnetic radiation. *American Journal of Epidemiology, 138*, 775-786.

Oshiro, T., & Calderhead, R. (1988). *Low level laser therapy: A practical introduction.* Chichester, United Kingdom: Wiley.

Padua, L., Padua, R., Aprile, I., & Tonali, P. (1998). Noninvasive laser neurolysis in carpal tunnel syndrome. *Muscle & Nerve, 21*, 1232-1233.

Pasila, M., Visuri, T., & Sundholm, A. (1978). Pulsating shortwave diathermy: Value in treatment of recent ankle and foot sprains. *Archives of Physical Medicine and Rehabilitation, 59*, 383-386.

Pourzarandian, A., Watanabe, H., Ruwanpura, S. M., Aoki, A., & Ishikawa, I. (2005). Effect of low-level er:YAG laser irradiation on cultured human gingival fibroblasts. *Journal of Periodontology, 76*, 187-193.

Reddy, G. K. (2004). Photobiological basis and clinical role of low-intensity lasers in biology and medicine. *Journal of Clinical Laser Medicine & Surgery, 22*, 141-150.

Reddy, M., Gill, S. S., & Rochon, P. A. (2006). Preventing pressure ulcers: A systematic review. *Journal of the American Medical Association, 296*, 974-984.

Robertson, V. J., Ward, A. R., & Jung, P. (2005). The effect of heat on tissue extensibility: A comparison of deep and superficial heating. *Archives of Physical Medicine and Rehabilitation, 86*, 819-825.

Ross, E. V. (2006). Laser versus intense pulsed light: Competing technologies in dermatology. *Lasers in Surgery and Medicine, 38*, 261-272.

Ruggera, P. S., Witters, D. M., von Maltzahn, G., & Bassen, H. I. (2003). In vitro assessment of tissue heating near metallic medical implants by exposure to pulsed radio frequency diathermy. *Physics in Medicine and Biology, 48*, 2919-2928.

Seiger, C., & Draper, D. O. (2006). Use of pulsed shortwave diathermy and joint mobilization to increase ankle range of motion in the presence of surgical implanted metal: A case series. *Journal of Orthopaedic and Sports Physical Therapy, 36*, 669-677.

Shields, N., O'Hare, N., Boyle, G., & Gormley, J. (2003). Development and application of a quality control procedure for short-wave diathermy units. *Medical & Biological Engineering & Computing, 41*, 62-68.

Shields, N., O'Hare, N., & Gormley, J. (2004). An evaluation of safety guidelines to restrict exposure to stray radiofrequency radiation from short-wave diathermy units. *Physics in Medicine and Biology, 49*, 2999-3015.

Sommer, A. P., Pinheiro, A. L., Mester, A. R., Franke, R. P., & Whelan, H. T. (2001). Biostimulatory windows in low-intensity laser activation: Lasers, scanners, and NASA's light-emitting diode array system. *Journal of Clinical Laser Medicine & Surgery, 19*, 29-33.

Sun, G., & Tuner, J. (2004). Low-level laser therapy in dentistry. *Dental Clinics of North America, 48*, 1061-76, viii.

Taskinen, H., Kyyronen, P., & Hemminki, K. (1990). Effects of ultrasound, shortwaves, and physical exertion on pregnancy outcome in physiotherapists. *Journal of Epidemiology and Community Health, 44*, 196-201.

Verdaasdonk, R. M., & van Swol, C. F. (1997). Laser light delivery systems for medical applications. *Physics in Medicine and Biology, 42*, 869-894.

Weintraub, M. I. (1997). Noninvasive laser neurolysis in carpal tunnel syndrome. *Muscle & Nerve, 20*, 1029-1031.

Whiteman, D., Stickley, M., Hughes, M., Davis, M., & Green, A. (2006). The biomedical effects of laser application. *Journal of Clinical Oncology, 24*, 3172-3177.

Woodruff, L. D., Bounkeo, J. M., Brannon, W. M., Dawes, K. S., Barham, C. D., & Waddell, D. L., et al. (2004). The efficacy of laser therapy in wound repair: A meta-analysis of the literature. *Photomedicine and Laser Surgery, 22*, 241-247.

Xu, H., Feng, L., Zeng, Z., & Xu, S. (1999). Experimental study on ultrashort wave therapy on the healing of fracture. *Bulletin of Hunan Medical University, 24*, 125-127.

# NMES Hand Rehabilitation Guide

Utilizing Neuromuscular Electrical Stimulation (NMES) for the treatment of hand and finger dysfunction is a widely accepted adjunctive rehabilitation tool. When used correctly, it can assist in a patient's functional recovery from either an orthopedic or neurologic injury. Proper application of an NMES program will depend first upon a complete clinical evaluation and the establishment of the treatment plan and goals. The next steps in a successful application of NMES include:

1. Device selection

2. Parameter selection

3. Electrode placement

4. Patient education

## Finger Flexion

➤ **Electrodes**: (–) the smaller electrode is over the motor point of the muscle mass most likely to produce finger flexion without activating wrist flexors (the area for finger stimulation is closer to the ulnar border of the forearm). (+) on the distal aspect of the flexor digitorum muscle belly.

➤ **Waveform**: Asymmetrical

➤ **Rate**: 35 pps. May use higher rate if needed for patient comfort.

➤ **Mode**: Not applicable (single channel use)

➤ **On-/off-ratio**: 1:3 most programs, 1:3 to 1:1 endurance, 1:5 power

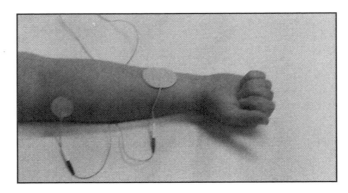

# Finger Extension

➤ **Electrodes**: (–) the smaller electrode is over the motor point of the muscle mass most likely to produce finger extension without activating wrist extensors (the optimal area to stimulate finger extension is distal to that for wrist extension). (+) on the distal aspect of the extensor muscle belly.

➤ **Waveform**: Asymmetrical.

➤ **Rate**: 35 pps. May use higher rate if needed for patient comfort.

➤ **Mode**: Not applicable (single channel use).

➤ **On-/off-ratio**: See finger flexion

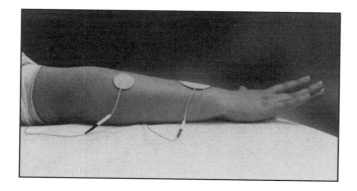

# Thumb Opposition

➤ **Electrodes**: (–) lateral border of the thenar eminence. (+) placed on either the dorsal or volar forearm.

➤ **Waveform**: Asymmetrical.

➤ **Rate**: 35 pps. May use higher rate if needed for patient comfort.

➤ **Mode**: Not applicable (single channel use).

➤ **On-/off-ratio**: 1:3 most programs, 1:3 to 1:1 endurance, 1:5 power.

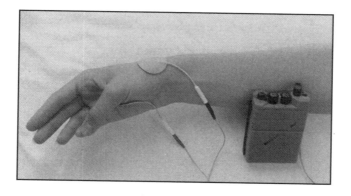

# Lumbrical Grip

➤ **Electrodes**: (–) proximal to the pisiform bone. (+) volar surface of the forearm (this placement stimulates the 3rd and 4th lumbricals and all of the dorsal and palmar interossei).

➤ **Waveform**: Asymmetrical.

➤ **Rate**: 35 pps. May use higher rate if needed for patient comfort.

➤ **Mode**: Not applicable (single channel use).

➤ **On-/off-ratio**: 1:3 most programs, 1:3 to 1:1 endurance, 1:5 power.

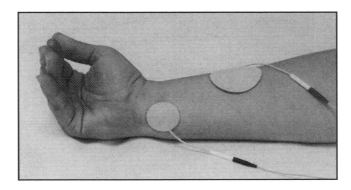

# Power Grasp—Dual Channel

➤ **Electrodes**: *Channel one*: (–) optimal finger flexion placement; (+) over the flexor tendon. *Channel two*: (–) optimal intrinsic activation; (+) over the flexor tendon (stimulation of both the extrinsic and intrinsic finger flexors can produce a powerful grip).

➤ **Waveform**: Asymmetrical.

➤ **Rate**: 35 pps. May use higher rate if needed for patient comfort.

➤ **Mode**: Synchronous (S).

➤ **On-/off-ratio**: 1:3 most programs, 1:3 to 1:1 endurance, 1:5 power.

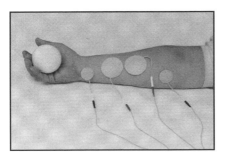 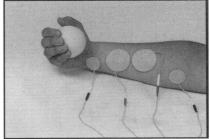

# Clinical Tips

1. Use of a larger electrode on the positive lead will improve patient comfort.

2. A smaller electrode on the motor point may help in specific muscle recruitment but will increase current density and may decrease patient comfort.

3. Do not cut through the electrode connector wire if trimming an electrode.

4. A denervated condition will require direct current because the peripheral nerve is not intact.

5. Treatment duration should be based upon rate of fatigue. Fatigue may occur rapidly during hand applications due to the small size of the muscle(s) being stimulated. Note: the higher the rate (pps), the more rapidly fatigue will occur.

# Bibliography

American Physical Therapy Association. (2001). Guide to physical therapist practice. Second edition. *Physical Therapy, 81*(1).

Baker, L. L, Wederich, C. L., McNeal, D. R., Newsam, C., & Waters, R. L. (2002). *Neuromuscular electrical stimulation: A practical guide* (4th ed.). Downey, CA: Los Amigos Research and Education Institute, Inc.

Baker, L. L., Yeh, C., Wilson, D., & Waters, R. L. (1979). Electrical stimulation of wrist and fingers for hemiplegic patients. *Physical Therapy, 59*(12), 1495-1499.

Bertoti, D. (2000). Electrical stimulation: A reflection on current clinical practice. *Assitive Technology, 12*, 21-32.

Chae, J., Bethoux, F., Bohinc, T., Dobos, L., Davis, T., & Friedl, A. (1998). Neuromuscular stimulation for upper extremity motor and functional recovery in acute hemiplegia. *Stroke, 29,* 975-979.

Chae, J., & Yu, D. (2000). A critical review of neuromuscular electrical stimulation for treatment of motor dysfunction in hemiplegia. *Assistive Technology, 12,* 33-49.

Kraft, G. H., Fitts, S. S., & Hammond, M. C. (1992). Techniques to improve function of the arm and hand in chronic hemiplegia. *Archives of Physical Medicine and Rehabilitation, 72*, 220-227.

Powers, W. S. (2001). Use of electrical stimulation in the recover of upper extremity function after proximal radial nerve injury from anterior shoulder dislocation. *Physical Therapy Case Reports, 4*(3), 122-129.

Reprinted with permission from EMPI, Inc., Minneapolis, MN.

# NMES PARAMETER OVERVIEW

Neuromuscular Electrical Stimulation (NMES) is the use of electricity to stimulate the nerves that correspond to a targeted muscle or muscle group and cause it to contract. It requires an intact peripheral nerve and healthy muscle tissue.

## Clinical Indications for NMES

➤ Retard or prevent disuse atrophy

➤ Muscle re-education

➤ Maintain or increase joint mobility

➤ Increase local blood circulation

➤ Relax muscle spasm

➤ Prevent venous thrombosis in calf muscles immediately following surgery

Treatment decisions should be based on a full patient evaluation and individualized for each patient. Consult your device manual for specific instructions for use, indications, contraindications, precautions and warnings.

The following parameter options should be considered to ensure the successful use of NMES.

## Pulse Duration

➤ Pulse durations between 200 to 400 microseconds (ms) are typically used.

## Amplitude (Intensity)

➤ Affects the magnitude of muscular response. Higher amplitudes will generate an increase in the number of motor units activated.

## On-/Off-Time (Duty Cycle)

➤ Affects the fatigue rate. Initial treatments with NMES may require longer off-times to delay onset of fatigue.

➤ Typical on/off ratios: ??

➤ Muscle re-education: Minimum 1:3.

➤ Muscle spasm: 1:1.

# Channel Selection

➤ Use of 1 channel vs 2 channel.

➤ *Synchronous*: Channel 1 and channel 2 will deliver stimulation simultaneously.

➤ *Asynchronous* (Reciprocal): Stimulation will alternate between channel 1 and channel 2.

➤ Channel 2 delay: After a short delay, stimulation from channel 2 occurs following the onset of channel 1. Length of delay may be selected. (Useful when treating muscle groups with specific firing patterns.)

# Waveform Selection

➤ Symmetrical: Large muscles.

➤ Asymmetrical: Small muscles.

# Electrode Size

➤ Use the largest electrode that provides the desired response, without causing overflow to the other muscles.

# Electrode Placement

➤ Symmetrical waveform: Both electrodes active; use negative over the motor point.

➤ Asymmetrical waveform: Negative electrode is more active; place over the motor point.

➤ *Note*: Distance between electrodes will determine depth of current: greater distance = deeper current flow.

# Rate Selection

➤ Affects the quality of a muscle contraction and fatigue.

➤ Rates in range of tetany: 25 to 50 pps; higher rates to elicit muscle fatigue (80pps).

➤ Using the minimum rate that produces a good, tetanized contraction will help to control onset of fatigue.

# Ramp Up/Down Time

➤ Aids comfort of treatment and can be used to mimic normal recruitment.

➤ 0 to 3 seconds is typical; longer ramp time may be beneficial in minimizing stretch reflex when spasticity is a factor.

# Bibliography

Baker, L. L., Parker, K., & Sanderson, D. (1983). Neuromuscular electrical stimulation for the head injured patient. *Physical Therapy, 63,* 1967-1974.

Currier, D. P., & Mann, R. (1983). Muscular strength development by electrical stimulation in healthy individuals. *Physical Therapy, 63*, 915-921.

Delitto, A., Rose, S. J., McKowen, J. M., et al. (1988). Electrical stimulation versus voluntary exercise in strengthening thigh musculature after anterior cruciate ligament surgery. *Physical Therapy, 68,* 660-663.

Gould, N., Donnermeyer, D., et al. (1983). Transcutaneous muscle stimulation as a method of retard disuse. *Clinical Orthopaedics & Related Research, 178,* 190-197.

Halback, J. W., & Straus, D. (1980). Comparison of electro-myo stimulation to isokinetic training in increasing power of the knee extensor mechanism. *Journal of Orthopaedic & Sports Physical Therapy, 2,* 20-24.

Liberson, W. T., Holmquist, H. J.,  Scot, D., & Dow, M. (1961). Functional electrotherapy: Stimulation of the peroneal nerve synchronized with the swing phase of the gait of hemiplegic patients. *Archives of Physical Medicine & Rehabilitation, 42,* 101-105.

Munsat, T. L., McNeal, D. R., & Waters, R. L. (1976). Preliminary observations on prolonged stimulation of peripheral nerve in men. *Archives of Neurology, 33,* 608-617.

Peckham, P. H., Mortimer, J. T., & VanDer Meulen, J. P. (1973). Physiologic and metabolic changes in white muscle of cat following induced exercise. *Brain Research, 50,* 424-429.

Romeo, J. A., Sanderd, T. L., Schreoeder, R. V., & Fahey, T. D. (1982). The effects of electrical stimulation of normal quadriceps on strength and girth. *Medicine & Science in Sports & Exercise, 14,* 194-197.

Selkowitz, D. M. (1985). Improvement in isometric strength of the quadriceps femoris muscle after training with electrical stimulation. *Physical Therapy, 65,* 186-196.

Soo, C. L., Currier, D. P., & Threlkeld, A. J. (1988). Augmenting voluntary torque of healthy muscle by optimization of electrical stimulation. *Physical Therapy, 68,* 333-337.

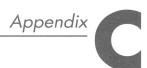

# MET AND CES TREATMENT PROTOCOLS

## Modified Auriculotherapy for MET

Use Alpha-Stim (EPI, Mineral Wells, TX) ear clip electrodes over the area of the ear corresponding to neuromusculoskeletal disorders for 30 seconds to 1 minute per area. Place both ear clips on the same ear unless a full cranial electrotherapy stimulation (CES) treatment is provided immediately following the modified auriculotherapy treatment.

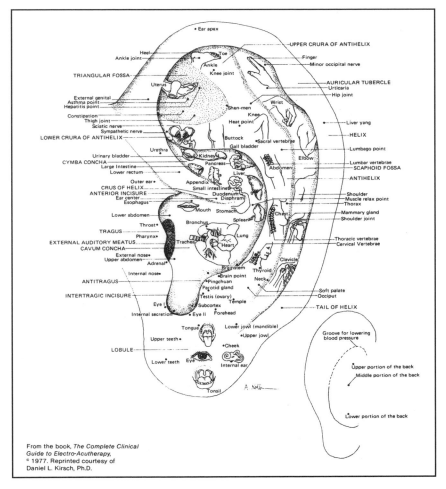

From the book, *The Complete Clinical Guide to Electro-Acutherapy,* © 1977. Reprinted courtesy of Daniel L. Kirsch, Ph.D.

# Alpha-Stim Probe and
# Electrode Treatment Protocol Guidelines

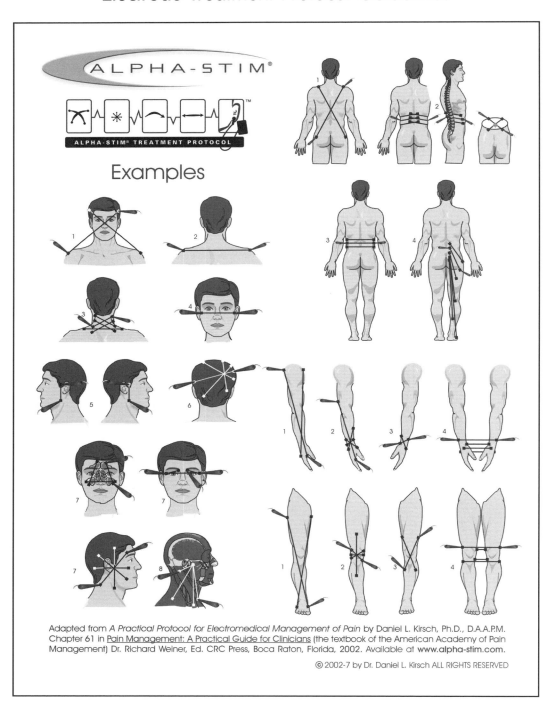

Adapted from *A Practical Protocol for Electromedical Management of Pain* by Daniel L. Kirsch, Ph.D., D.A.A.P.M. Chapter 61 in <u>Pain Management: A Practical Guide for Clinicians</u> (the textbook of the American Academy of Pain Management) Dr. Richard Weiner, Ed. CRC Press, Boca Raton, Florida, 2002. Available at **www.alpha-stim.com.**

Use Alpha-Stim probes for 10 to 30 seconds per point. Distances are based on the average adult male. Two cm = width of the thumb at base of the thumbnail. Six cm = width of 4 digits (minus thumb). Use two probes or one probe and one self adhesive electrode with the electrode placed away from the point being treated on the midline of the body.

# INDEX

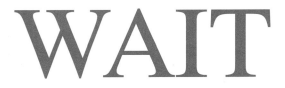

# WAIT ...*There's More!*

*SLACK Incorporated's Health Care Books and Journals offers a wide selection of products in the field of Occupational Therapy. We are dedicated to providing important works that educate, inform and improve the knowledge of our customers. Don't miss out on our other informative titles that will enhance your collection.*

**Low Vision Rehabilitation: A Practical Guide for Occupational Therapists**
*Mitchell Scheiman, OD, FCOVD, FAAO; Maxine Scheiman, MEd, OTR/L, CLVT; Stephen G. Whittaker, OTR, PhD, CLVT*
360 pp., Hard Cover, 2007, ISBN 10: 1-55642-734-4,
ISBN 13: 978-1-55642-734-3, Order# 37344, **$49.95**

**Understanding and Managing Vision Deficits: A Guide for Occupational Therapists, Second Edition**
*Mitchell Scheiman, OD*
400 pp., Soft Cover, 2002, ISBN 10: 1-55642-528-7,
ISBN 13: 978-1-55642-528-8, Order# 35287, **$44.95**

**Physical Agent Modalities: Theory and Application for the Occupational Therapist, Second Edition**
*Alfred Bracciano, EdD, OTR*
328 pp., Soft Cover, 2008, ISBN 10: 1-55642-649-6,
ISBN 13: 978-1-55642-649-0, Order# 36496, **$54.95**

Please visit
# www.slackbooks.com
### to order any of these titles!
### 24 Hours a Day...7 Days a Week!

**Attention Industry Partners!**
Whether you are interested in buying multiple copies of a book, chapter reprints, or looking for something new and different — we are able to accommodate your needs.

**Multiple Copies**
At attractive discounts starting for purchases as low as 25 copies for a single title, SLACK Incorporated will be able to meet all of your needs.

**Chapter Reprints**
SLACK Incorporated is able to offer the chapters you want in a format that will lead to success. Bound with an attractive cover, use the chapters that are a fit specifically for your company. Available for quantities of 100 or more.

**Customize**
SLACK Incorporated is able to create a specialized custom version of any of our products specifically for your company.

*Please contact the Marketing Communications Director of the Health Care Books and Journals for further details on multiple copy purchases, chapter reprints or custom printing at 1-800-257-8290 or 1-856-848-1000.*

*\*Please note all conditions are subject to change.*

**CODE: 328**

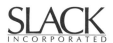

SLACK Incorporated • Health Care Books and Journals
6900 Grove Road • Thorofare, NJ 08086
**1-800-257-8290** or 1-856-848-1000
Fax: 1-856-848-6091 • E-mail: orders@slackinc.com • Visit: www.slackbooks.com